The Detox Miracle Sourcebook

RAW FOODS AND HERBS FOR
COMPLETE CELLULAR REGENERATION

Robert Morse, N.D.

KALINDI PRESS
Chino Valley, Arizona

Cover design: Kim Johansen
Layout design: Bookworks, Inc.
Layout: Kadak Graphics

ISBN: 978-1-935826-19-4

KALINDI PRESS
P.O. Box 4410
Chino Valley, AZ 86323
800-381-2700
www.kalindipress.com

This book was printed in the U.S.A. on acid-free paper using soy ink.

An earlier version of this book was published by the author, as: *True Healing: The Science and Practice of Detoxification*. Previous ISBN: 0-9701253-9-9

This book is dedicated first to God, which is all I live for and try to express in every moment. God is the greatest healing power of all. I acknowledge also the hierarchy of God, including all the living and ascended masters, saints, saviors and angels who help keep God's creation in balance. Finally, it is dedicated to my personal staff members who have labored for hundreds of hours through the years to bring this book to light.

Unless we put medical freedom in the constitution, the time will come when medicine will organize itself into an undercover dictatorship to restrict the art of healing to one class of men and deny equal privileges to others which will constitute the Bastille of medical science.
        —Dr. Benjamin Rush, a signer of the Declaration of Independence

No one can overcome a health problem using the same mind-set that created the problem.
        —Thomas Edison

In health there is no disease.
You do not find cancer in healthy tissue.
        —Robert Morse, N.D.

Contents

Chapter 5   The Nature of Disease — 138

Chapter 6   Eliminating Disease Through Cleansing and Rebuilding Tissue — 182

Chapter 7   Eating For Vitality — 213

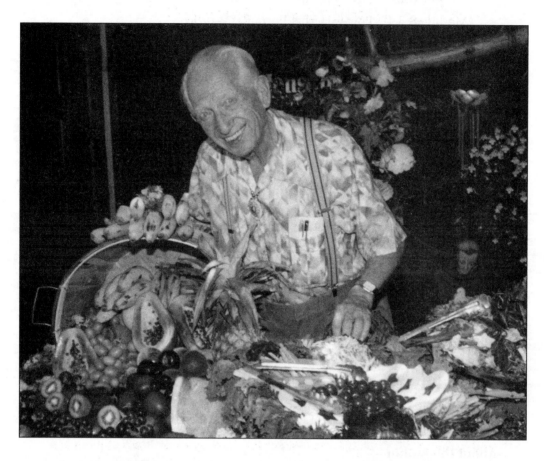

Dr. Bernard Jensen enjoying Nature's bounty of raw foods.

Acknowledgements

A special recognition to my good friend Dr. Bernard Jensen who spent the last sixty years of his life fighting human ignorance in the field of true nutrition and vitality. His pioneering work in Iridology, "The Master Science," is known throughout the world. We have spent many hours talking about vitality and longevity.

A special recognition to my friend Dr. Rudy Splavic, N.M.D., who could feel a hair under seven sheets of paper. He was one of Dr. Stone's personal students in the art of polarity and manipulation work. His tremendous knowledge is deeply acknowledged and will be greatly missed.

I acknowledge the following individuals and their pioneering efforts in health and other related fields. They are truly God-men and God-women in their own right: Professor Arnold Ehret (mucus and detoxification awareness); Professor Hilton Hotema (George Clements) (fruitarian advocate); Bernard McFadden (fasting and energy healing); Ann Wigmore (wheat grass juice); Herbert M. Shelton (fasting and raw food); John Tilden, M.D. (toxemia); Stanley Burroughs (lemon juice fasting); Dr. John Christopher (master herbalist pioneer); Ladean Griffin (health pioneer); Norman W. Walker (raw juice therapy); Bruce Copen, Ph.D. (naturopathy); Paul Bragg (fasting and raw foods); John Hoxey (herbal and health pioneer); C.L. Kervran (biological transmutations); Benedict Lust (founder of naturopathy); Dr. Rife, M.D. (cancer and virus pioneer); Hereward Carrington (fruitarian pioneer); "Nature's First Law" Group (renewing the consciousness of raw food eating); Tompkins and Bird (energetics of foods); Sebastian Kneipp (hydrotherapy); John W. Keim (Amish healer); J.H. Rausse (hydrotherapy and nutrition); Jethro Kloss (herbal healer); Paul Twitchell (mapping the heavens); Darwin Gross (a true master); Dr. Harvey Kellogg (detoxification), and T.C. McDaniel, D.O. (chemistry).

Special thanks to Brenda, Tony, Kathie, Theresa and Jennifer for all their help and valuable assistance in putting this information together in a cohesive form and for helping to keep our organization a true God company.

There are so many great healers and scientists that I couldn't possibly mention them all. I send my humblest apologies to those whom I did not mention. A great healer or scientist is not swayed by humanity's conditioning or monetary systems. Rather, he or she forges ahead seeking truth so all can benefit.

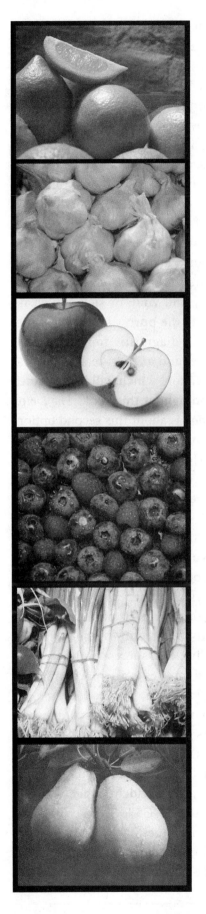

Introduction

Welcome to a fantastic journey into vitality. Health is one of our greatest assets, and many refer to the body as a temple, or a vehicle that carries around the true Self while we're on this planet. However, we often treat our cars better than we treat our bodies.

The information contained in this book was not taken from double-blind studies, from misconstrued facts and figures of treatment agencies, or from "bought-and-paid-for" scientific research. I wrote this book based on thirty years of self-experience, and from clinical observation of thousands of patients who used my programs to overcome their toxic conditions and diseases.

Basically, we have two choices to make when we develop a condition or disease: **Treatment** or **Detoxification**. If we choose treatment, we have two additional choices. The first choice is *allopathic* **(pharmaceutical) medicine**, which is the status-quo medical or chemical approach. The second choice is *natural* **(traditional) medicine**, which uses products made from natural sources or herbs to treat the symptoms. If we choose the allopathic approach to "fight" our disease, it is important to understand that allopathic medicine offers only three types of treatment for any condition: **chemical medicines, radiation or surgery**.

Pharmaceutical companies spend a lot of money developing drugs and training medical (allopathic) doctors in how to use these chemical medicines in the presence of disease. But, "curing" the disease (in the sense of removing its cause, not just its symptoms) is not a part of this type of thinking. Diseases are incurable in the allopathic approach—which is a totally a "treatment"-based modality. Chemical medicines are used for everything from simple headaches and fevers to degenerative conditions, like Parkinson's disease or cancer.

The second form of treatment in allopathic medical procedures is some type of burning or radiation. This is used in most diagnostic procedures (X-rays, for example) and some treatment procedures, especially but not limited to cancer.

The third procedure that the allopathic medical profession can use to treat a problem or condition is surgery. Surgery is simply the removal of "bad" tissue that is causing the problem. If the disease is cancer of the breast, simply remove the breast and the patient is "cured."

Natural medicine, or what I will refer to as "traditional medicine," differs from the allopathic approach. Natural medicine simply treats disease with natural products (those made from animal, plant or mineral substances) or herbs, which are found in nature. The science of natural medicine has been around for hundreds of thousands of years, at one level or another.

Most of the substances used in natural medicine have no damaging side effects, while most chemical medicines have some degree of harmful side effects. However, it is fair to say that some natural products used without proper wisdom can still create harm. Supplementing calcium in the presence of a parathyroid weakness, for example, results in stone formation or excessive free calcium. In general, the diagnostic procedures used in natural medicine including iridology, kinesiology, pulsing, hair or tissue analysis, and many others are non-invasive and not harmful to the patient whatsoever.

Most health care systems today, including allopathic, naturopathic and homeopathic medicine, are treatment-based modalities. Treating symptoms *never* cures the "causes." Until a genuine cure has been effected, we will always be suffering in some form. The alternative to treatment is *True Naturopathy (detoxification)* a little known science of nature that has been used for hundreds of years, by hundreds of thousands of people and animals worldwide. It has restored health and vitality to their physical, emotional and mental bodies. Detoxification encompasses the sciences of chemistry, biochemistry, botanical science and physics, and has always been at the heart of true healing. For that reason, detoxification should be at the heart of natural medicine today, but has been forgotten in our modern world of "treatment."

Detoxification is not a system of treatment or a way to remove symptoms; it is a system of curing by addressing the cause of the disease. It involves the understanding that the body is the healer, and that energy is at the core of healing. It also sheds light on the true cause of disease— the destruction of energy. Energy or the destruction of energy results from what we eat, drink, breathe, put on our skin, and from what we think and feel. These are the six ways we either make ourselves healthy and vital, or sick and weak.

Naturopathy is the purest form of healing. Its procedures and diagnostic tools are all totally non-invasive, and at its core are alkalization and detoxification, which will be explained in great depth throughout this book. *The Detox Miracle Sourcebook* is about this second option, true healing through detoxification and its related sciences. However, the approach taken here never puts science above the power of God and nature, as science is only the study of what *already is*.

My success with true detoxification in chronic and degenerative issues has been recognized worldwide. Out of 100 people who come to us with various types of cancer, approximately 70 percent cure themselves, 20 percent can't do the program and 10 percent are too advanced or don't want to live. Our success with regeneration in spinal cord injuries is also phenomenal: a thirty-two-year-old female, who had severed her upper cervical spine (a C3-C4 spinal cord severation) twelve years previously, came to our clinic. In eleven months she had complete feeling and movement throughout her body. A young Amish man who had a tractor accident, which left him a quadriplegic at the C4-C5 level, in six months had total feeling in his toes.

One of the hardest parts of this program is working with the mind. Like a computer, you get out what you put in. This book will supply you with the most up-to-date and thorough information you need to feed your mind and thus educate yourself about the miraculous healing system of your body. It will cover some physiology, chemistry, physics and nutrition all in a way that you can understand and immediately use. It will also encourage you to "change your mind" from one of toxic thinking to one of natural and pure thinking.

Most people live to eat; I would like you to start thinking about *eating to live,* and this book will show you how to do that. What you eat has a direct effect upon your health, and I have proven this year-in and year-out on hundreds of clients. I have seen cancer, time and time again, cleaned out by the body. Also, diabetes, coronary artery disease and arthritis all eliminated. I have seen spinal cord injuries reconnect and nerve damage from strokes, multiple sclerosis and the like, heal.

There is no magic or mystery to health or disease. Disease is a natural process! When we understand how the body works, and what causes the tissues in the body to fail, we will then understand what causes disease symptoms, and how to reverse it.

This book will take you on a journey with many important stops along the way. You will learn about the species your physical body comes from; how your body works; the nature of disease. And finally, what health is. One of the premises of this book is that health is really very simple, yet we spend a large part of our time and money trying to achieve it. *The Detox Miracle Sourcebook* will help you to understand your species, and encourage you toward eating in harmony with your anatomical, physiological and biochemical processes. This will give you vitality and a disease-free life.

Allow yourself the time and discipline to *become alive again through detoxification!* Put your heart, self-discipline and soul into it. Detoxification will be one of the greatest things you do for yourself in your lifetime.

NOTE: As this book was written for the health-care practitioner and lay person alike, some chapters are more scientifically based than others. For myself, I say: "Keep it simple!" Pass over those chapters that might confuse you at first. Come back later and read them to better understand your body and how it works. Your body is a very complex machine, but keeping it healthy is very simple.

A Personal Journey

I was raised in a small town in Indiana. The typical diet in this part of the country consisted of lots of dairy products, refined sugars, grains and, of course, meat three times a day. Dairy products and refined sugars are very mucus forming, consequently I became addicted to nose drops, as my sinus cavities were always blocked. I also developed severe constipation, which led to bleeding hemorrhoids. Along with all this came migraine headaches, about every three days. When I was taken to one specialist after another, the stories I would hear, hypothesizing over the cause of these severe headaches, after a while became a

joke. Obesity was another side effect of this type of diet. If I were not connected consciously to God in these early years, depression would have overcome my life. My love for God and life has always dominated my life, giving me an inward joy.

In the late 1960s I became a raw-food eater. I was reading books by Ehret, Jensen, Hotema, McFaddin, Tilden (see Bibliography), and a dozen other great healers, about the common sense concepts of not destroying the foods you eat before you eat them. I read about breatharianism and the ability to live off of oxygen, hydrogen,

Nature's Way

1. Natural (nature's) health is not alternative medicine. Natural health is traditional medicine.

2. Nature's way is hundreds of thousands of years old. Chemical medicine is only 125 years old.

3. Since the advent of chemical medicine, disease has skyrocketed.

4. Medicine should only consist of natural remedies that alkalize, clean and regenerate the body.

carbon, nitrogen, etc. Since all elements are made up of these higher atoms in the first place, it made sense to me that if our consciousness was in the right place we could survive at this level. Souls that survive at this level are known as "God eaters." Since I wanted to know God more than anything else, this fit perfectly for me. I decided I would live in remote areas and attempt this level of consciousness. Becoming a hermit, I started the process of eliminating the heavy or low-vibrational foods, including meats and grains. I also wanted to stop eating vegetables, which left me with a diet of only fruits and nuts. Finally, I decided to get away from all acid-forming foods as well, so I stopped eating the nuts. With those choices I had become what is called a "fruitarian." I lived exclusively on fresh, raw fruits.

My goal was still to attempt to live on pure air only. I had read about a Catholic nun who lived high in the mountains of Tibet and only ate snow, and about several others who had reportedly obtained this same refined level of survival. To move in this direction, my next step was to limit my fruit eating to one type only. According to my plan, after several months on one type of fruit I could then stop all intake of food as we know it and I would have obtained my goal. Of course this was a very radical approach to experiencing God, but I had set my mind on it and had strong self-discipline. I read a lot of Professor Hotema's work on the power of organic oranges as a complete food so I decided that these would be my only food.

I was a fruitarian for approximately four years, out of which I lived six months exclusively on oranges. I had discovered a special organic orange garden created by a person I considered to be a very high soul. Nature must have been looking out for me during those times because this orange garden had a bumper crop, and the grower was able to supply me with navel oranges for the entire year.

During this period as a fruitarian I began to experience the truth of Arnold Ehret's work about the tremendous rejuvenational powers of the body. I could cut myself and feel no pain. There was no bleeding, and the wound would be healed in the next day or two. Remember that my goal was to stop eating the oranges and live exclusively on air! But the problem was that my energy levels became so high that I couldn't stay in my body. I was traveling "out of body" into some of the most magnificent worlds of God that exist beyond the normal human experience. I felt like I merged with God, leaving "me" behind. I became unlimited. I had no point of reference, as I wanted or desired nothing. I was totally fulfilled. My love for God and all life intensified beyond words. The difficulty was that I was young, physically, and I was immature with this level of God realization. As I could not communicate in this world anymore, especially with humans, I decided, for survival's sake, that I needed to "ground" myself and go on to teach others about the tremendous healing power of raw foods and the unlimited awareness that we each possess. So, after several years of living in remote areas I moved back to "civilization." I knew then that I wanted to dedicate my life to helping others rejuvenate themselves and to teaching the beauty of God to a world that starves for both.

Since that point I have opened several health food stores and became degreed as a biochemist, naturopath, master herbalist and iridologist. I have been teaching about God and vitality ever since, and traveling throughout the world sharing with others the magic and secrets of health. I had a small clinic in Portugal for a number of years and I represented the United States several times in worldwide symposiums.

Twenty-five years ago I opened a health clinic that I still manage. Based on my experiences I can tell you that there are no incurable diseases, only incurable people. I have also spent many years working in emergency medicine, which used to be one of my hobbies, and I have seen both allopathic medicine and traditional (herbal) medicine in action. While emergency medicine is *fantastic,* allopathic medicine, in general, kills hundreds of thousands of people per year, while traditional medicine (or botanical medicine) saves hundreds

of thousands of lives per year. I invite you to join me in learning and using God's natural laws to heal and rejuvenate yourself.

My work has been both inspired and supported by the work of Dr. Bernard Jensen, a world-renowned healer and author of many outstanding books (see Bibliography). Years ago, Dr. Jensen consulted me about his wife's health and we became instant friends. We immediately recognized a spiritual bond, as we shared a similar passion for and commitment to a mission of love and healing. *The Detox Miracle Sourcebook* reflects our experiences and viewpoints on true healing.

Always seek truth. Open your heart totally to God. If you desire anything, desire God. All else will come to you. Always be and give love. Become alive again (in all your bodies) physically, emotionally, mentally and spiritually.

NOTE: Check Glossary for unfamiliar terms.

Getting Started
10 Ways To Be Successful

As you prepare to use the information presented in this book, here is an overview. This is what it takes to be successful. These ten principles or recommendations will help you tremendously in achieving success and the health and vitality you want from your detoxification and regeneration process. These points will be covered in depth as you continue to work with this book.

1. The diet is your number one key to success. What you eat, drink, breathe and what you put on your skin is how you bring the outside world in. Study and learn the concepts in this book about a raw food diet. The greater percentage of raw fruits and vegetables (salads) you eat, the greater your success will be. If you have cancer, a spinal

cord injury, multiple sclerosis, Parkinson's or any other chronic or degenerative condition, you will want to consume a 100 percent raw, "live" food diet of fruits and vegetables (salads) only.

2. Invite the help of a healthcare professional who has experience in the use of raw foods and other natural detoxification procedures, like fasting. Especially with illnesses like cancer and other chronic, degenerative conditions, it is beneficial to have guidance and support throughout your healing process. Ultimately you are responsible for yourself, but there are many valuable resources to assist you in making this journey into vibrant health.

3. Find someone who is adept at "reading" the iris of the eye (a science known as iridology).

This is one of nature's greatest and, at present, only types of soft tissue analysis. It will give you a road map of your strengths and weaknesses. It will also indicate your congestive (lymphatic) and chemical accumulations. This is invaluable in helping you to address your glandular or organ weaknesses. For this I recommend an herbal (formula) program. Use herbs to address your cellular weaknesses and to move and clean your lymphatic system, GI tract, and lungs. (See Resource Guide for herbal companies that supply such formulas.)

Almost 100 percent of homo sapiens have glandular weaknesses. Begin this process by taking the "What Is Your Body Telling You" Self-Assessment Questionnaire found in Chapter 5 to determine yours.

Use the Basal Temperature Study Test (found in Appendix A) for thyroid function to determine your level of thyroid function. This is extremely important when considering calcium utilization and metabolism.

If you have high or especially low blood pressure, you know you have adrenal gland weakness. Again, check your Self-Assessment Questionnaire to determine other side effects of adrenal gland weaknesses.

4. Always "move" your lymph system. Everyone has a stagnant lymph system to one degree or another. All your cells need to eat and excrete, and your lymph system is your sewer system. Your lymph nodes are your septic tanks. Keep them cleaned out! Use an herbal formula for your kidneys and eat lots of fruits. Clean and enhance your GI tract with raw foods and a restorative intestinal herbal formula. Avoid laxatives or purgatives, acidophilus, bifidophilus, or any other intestinal flora. Your intestinal flora will restore itself. Exercise (like walking or swimming) is extremely important in moving your lymph system, especially in your lower extremities.

Let yourself sweat! Your skin is your largest eliminative organ. Keep it clean and stimulated with skin brushing, regular showers, hot and cold showers, and by sweating.

5. You will want to spend a month on an herbal parasite formula (see Resource Guide at the back of this book to find excellent herbal companies that carry these). This will help get rid of the larger worms, flukes, etc. It will also help reduce your microorganisms (candida, bacterias, etc.) that affect your desire for foods.

6. Clean your liver and enhance your pancreas for about a month or so before starting on your detoxification program. *See Chapter 8* for suggestions about supporting and cleansing these organs with herbs and herbal formulas. If you have diabetes or you're excessively thin you will probably need three months or so.

7. If you're on chemical medications, don't worry. There are very few possible interactions with this program and these herbal formulas. If you're on high blood pressure medication, simply watch your blood pressure. This program can bring down your blood pressure fast. Use common sense. If your blood pressure is low, lowering it further with chemical meds might not be too smart.

SCIENTIFIC FACTS

Most chemicals weaken and destroy cells. Chemotherapy causes high acidosis and destroys cells causing future cancer or the spreading (metastasis) of cancer.

Radiation inflames, burns and destroys cells (tissues), and can cause cancer to metastasize.

If your blood pressure is low, you must work to get it normalized by enhancing and regenerating your adrenal glands. Diabetes (Type II) is very easy to overcome in most cases. If you're on insulin, watch your blood sugars. The same principle applies as with high blood pressure.

9. As you detoxify and regenerate, your body will go through symptoms of a "healing crisis." This is normal, natural and positive. As you understand about the healing crisis you'll understand what "diseases" truly are. See Chapter 5. Remember, disease symptoms manifest from two sources—congestion and cellular weakness.

10. Finally: Attitude, attitude, attitude! Enjoy what you're doing. Always remember why you're getting your body (or physical vehicle) healthy. Your body is your mobility in this physical world. Many of your weaknesses are genetically passed to you. Your toxicity may have developed in utero, so give it time to be released. Vibrant health in this world does not occur overnight. Sometimes it's hard work—but well worth it. It connects you with life, love and God.

May the blessings be!

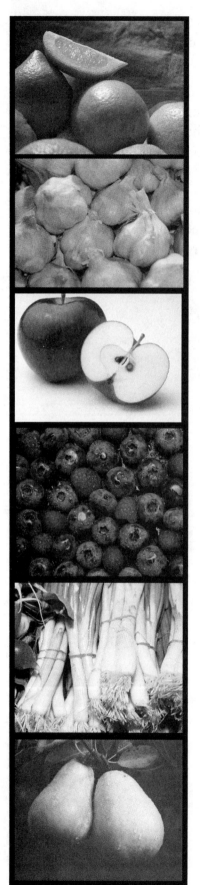

CHAPTER ONE

Understanding Our Species

I am constantly being asked what my secrets are for regenerating and making the physical body vital again. There have been hundreds of books written about health and nutrition, most of which are variations on other people's hypotheses or old ideas, which never seem to change. Some are plainly foolish. On the shelves of your local bookstore you will find books on blood types, mega-dosing with vitamins and minerals, high protein diets, and the like. Some of these programs are highly toxic to the body, in my experience, and actually kill many people each year.

I think health is much less complex than these books indicate. My approach is simply: **Eat the foods that are biologically suited for your species.** This might seem to be oversimplified or plain confusing, but let's take a moment to explore and determine just what type of species we are.

Imagine yourself standing somewhere in the plains or jungles of Africa. Look out over a vast landscape and see elephants, giraffes, deer, hippos, silverback apes, chimpanzees, snakes, birds of all kinds, lions, cheetahs, and many other animals. Now if I ask you one simple question: "Which of these animals do we 'homosapiens' look like?" which one would you pick? The primates, of course. These are frugivores, as we are. Now some might say that this is far too simplistic a comparison on which to build our case. Okay, then let's kill (I would never) one animal from each species and bring them back to the lab. Let's dissect each animal and look at its anatomy and physiology to determine which one we humans most resemble, internally.

The list that follows designates the four classes of vertebrates (carnivores, omnivores, herbivores and frugivores), highlighting the differences among them.

NOTE: Remember to check the Glossary for unfamiliar terms.

☼ Anatomical and Physiological Differences of Vertebrates

CARNIVORES

Includes:
Cats, cheetahs, lions, etc.

Diet:
Mainly meats, some vegetables, grass
and herbs

Digestive system:
Tongue—very rough (for pulling and tearing)
Salivary glands—none
Stomach—simple structure; small round sacks;
strong gastric juices
Small intestine—smooth and short
Liver—50 percent larger than that of humans;
very complex with five distinct chambers;
heavy bile flow for heavy gastric juices

Eliminative system:
Colon—smooth, non-sacculated, minimal
ability for absorption
GI tract—three times the length of the spine

Extremities (limbs):
Hands (upper front)—claw type
Feet (lower back)—claw type
Quadrupeds—walks on all four

Integumentary system:
Skin—100 percent covered with hair
Sweat glands—uses tongue, and has sweat
glands in foot pads only

Skeletal system:
Teeth—incisor teeth in front, molars behind
with large canine teeth for ripping
Jaws—unidirectional, up-and-down only
Tail—yes

Urinary system:
Kidneys—(urine) acid

OMNIVORES

Includes:
Birds (including chickens, turkeys, etc.),
hogs and dogs

Diet:
Some meat, vegetables, fruits, roots
and some barks

Digestive system:
Tongue—moderate to rough
Salivary glands—underactive
Stomach—moderate gastric acids (HCL and
pepsin)
Small intestines—somewhat sacculated, which
accounts for their ability to eat vegetables
Liver—complex and larger proportionally than
that of humans

Eliminative system:
Colon—shorter than human colon, with
minimal absorption
GI tract—ten times the length of the spine

Extremities (limbs):
Hands—hoofs, claws, and paws
Feet—hoofs, claws, and paws
Quadrupeds—walks on all four extremities;
except for birds, which have and walk
on two legs only

Integumentary system:
Skin—smooth, oily, hair or feathers
Sweat glands—very minimal; only around
snout (hogs) and foot pads (dogs) and
none on birds

Skeletal system:
Teeth—tusk-like canine teeth or beaks
Jaws—multi-directional
Tail—yes

Urinary system:
Kidneys—(urine) acid

HERBIVORES

Includes:
Horses, cows, sheep, elephants, deer, giraffes

Diet:
Vegetables, herbs and some roots and barks

Digestive system:
Tongue—moderately rough
Salivary glands—alkaline digestion starts here
Stomach—oblong, ringed, and the most complex (as a rule, has four or more pouches or stomachs); weak stomach acids
Small intestines—long and sacculated for extensive absorption
Liver—similar to human (slightly larger in capacity)

Eliminative system:
Colon—long and sacculated (ringed) for extensive absorption
GI tract—thirty times the length of the spine

Extremities (limbs):
Hands (upper)—hoofs
Feet (lower)—hoofs
Quadrupeds—walks on all four extremities

Integumentary system:
Skin—pores with extensive hair covering entire body
Sweat glands—includes millions of perspiration ducts

Skeletal system:
Teeth—twenty-four molars, five on each side of each jaw and eight incisors (cutting teeth) in the front part of the jaws
Jaws—multi-directional, up-and-down, side-to-side, forward and backward creating a grinding effect
Tail—yes

Urinary system:
Kidneys—(urine) alkaline

FRUGIVORES

Includes:
Humans and primates (apes, chimpanzees, monkeys)

Diet:
Mainly fruits, nuts, seeds, sweet vegetables and herbs

Digestive system:
Tongue—smooth, used mainly as a shovel
Salivary glands—alkaline digestive energies start here
Stomach—oblong with two compartments
Small intestines—sacculated for extensive absorption
Liver—simple and average size, not large and complex, like carnivores

Eliminative system:
Colon—sacculated for extensive absorption
GI tract—twelve times the length of the spine

Extremities (limbs):
Hands (upper)—fingers for picking, peeling and tearing
Feet (lower)—toes
Walks upright on two extremities

Integumentary system:
Skin—pores, with minimal hair
Sweat glands—includes millions of perspiration ducts

Skeletal system:
Teeth—thirty-two teeth: four incisors (cutting), two cuspids (pointed), four small molars (bi-cuspids), and six molars (no long canine or tusk-type teeth)
Jaws—multi-motional, dimensional, up-and-down, backward and forward, side-to-side, etc.
Tail—some

Urinary system:
Kidneys—(urine) alkaline

After dissecting and observing different species' anatomical structures and physiological processes we come to the same conclusion: Humans are frugivores, like it or not.

The human is the only species that is confused about what to eat. As children we are instinctual in what we want to eat. I can fill a large table with every type of food that humans eat, and put a small child in front of the table. Guess which foods they will always go to? Fruits and flowers—the high energy, colorful foods. That is because we are frugivores, not omnivores. If a human were truly a carnivore, he or she would enjoy catching a live animal, ripping it apart, and eating it as it is . . . and I don't know of too many people who enjoy this.

It is not difficult to understand that we need to start eating as our biological makeup demands. On top of this, we need to realize that no animal cooks its food before eating it. Zookeepers learned years ago never to feed cooked foods to any animal, as this will cause them to sicken and die. I don't know of any veterinarian who encourages people to feed their house pets from the table. Why? Simple. Our pets will get the same diseases we have. Cooking your food destroys it. It changes the chemistry and severely reduces its electrical energy.

God intended food for life, not death. God is about life, energy, love and happiness. Of course, we can have the other too: depression, anger, hate and ego. It is always our choice. A healthy vital physical body can also make our emotional and mental bodies healthy. Health breeds awareness and joy for living, which most people have lost.

All of humankind is biologically the same. Our physiological processes and our anatomical makeup are virtually the same, whether we are from China, India or America. However, the consciousness (awareness), the activity level, and the parts of the body used all make a difference in the types of foods we generally eat or crave. Don't make getting healthy complicated. Keep it simple. Foods can bind you to this world or set you free. If you have never experienced this, then start the journey now into a new world of vitality. Seek to be free from the chains of food addictions that undermine your health and create bondage to the lower aspects of God.

I invite you to become vital again and enjoy the rewards of life. Recondition your mind and retrain your emotions to enjoy the simplicity of eating raw fruits, vegetables, nuts and seeds. Understand your species and eat the foods that will make your body healthy.

"The ancient Greeks, before the time of Lycurgus, ate nothing but fruit," (Plutarch) and *"each generation reached the age of 200 years."*
— Onomacritus of Athens

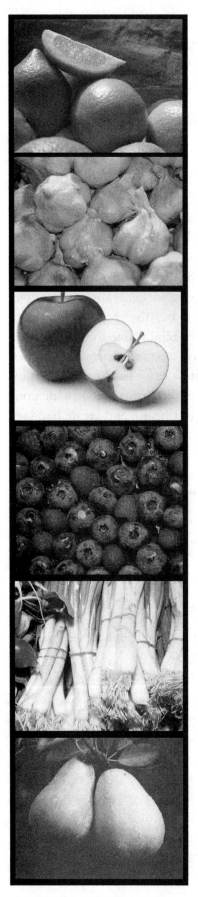

CHAPTER TWO

How the Body Works

A ny soul that has a physical body should understand the basics of the body's operation. "Why do we eat and what happens to the food we eat?" is the question to ask. When we understand the answer, we will begin to appreciate the nature of health and disease.

Food consumption is vital—most life forms on this planet need to consume some sort of "food" to exist and maintain expression, and most people will die if they stop eating, although there have been a few exceptions to this rule. A handful of individuals have consumed only air, which consists of carbon, oxygen, hydrogen and nitrogen (these elements are the sugars, fats and proteins at higher frequencies). This scenario, however, is extremely rare and one must be very spiritually connected to achieve this. Personally, I have never met anyone who could do this, although I've met some extremely aware spiritual masters and teachers.

We eat for additional energy. We know that our cells are cities within themselves and are conscious entities; each cell knows its specific duties. We know that spirit—the life force, consciousness, or whatever you wish to call it—is the inner force that holds and molds life into forms and gives it awareness. Nevertheless, cells need an external source of energy to sustain themselves in activity.

Most people chew and swallow their food without thought of how or why it is utilized within the body. *We assume that if it's edible, it's useable by the body.* This just simply isn't so. This chapter will explore the ways that the body breaks down and uses the foods we eat, and how it eliminates the by-products of these foods.

Eating, digesting, absorbing, utilization, and elimination are ongoing and consistent processes. When one or more of these processes is impaired, the body as a whole begins to suffer. It may take many years for a major symptom to appear, but appear it will. There are always signs along the way, however, including fatigue, obesity, excessive thinness, bags under the eyes, rashes, constipation and/or diarrhea, to name just a few.

☼ The Four Basic Processes

DIGESTION

First, when we consume any food it must go through a "digestive" process, or a process whereby the body breaks down the structures of the food into building materials and fuels. The body requires these raw materials for energy to function and also to build and repair itself.

The breakdown of food is accomplished through enzyme action, which starts in the mouth, where carbohydrates, sugars and fats begin their alkaline digestion. The stomach also produces a digestive enzyme called pepsin; an acidic enzyme released by HCL (hydrochloric acid) for initial protein digestion. The rest of digestion takes place in the small bowel, which is alkaline in nature. When our foods are not properly broken down, either from a weak pancreas, stomach and intestinal tract, or from bad food combinations, one will experience gas formation from fermentation and/or putrefaction. The greater the gas problems, the greater the weakness and/or bad diet choices.

The body breaks down the foods you eat into the following: **Proteins** are broken down into amino acids for building and repair material. **Carbohydrates** (starches and complex sugars) are broken down into simple sugars for fuel. **Fats** are broken down into fatty acids and glycerol, for building, repair and emergency needs.

It is important to remember that we have alkaline digestive enzymes in the mouth for carbohydrate and fat digestion. We have acid (pepsin) digestive enzymes in the lower stomach for initial protein digestion. Then we have alkaline digestive enzymes in the pancreas and throughout the first part of the small intestinal tract to finish up the job for proteins, starches, sugars and fats. It is also important to understand that most of our processes are **alkaline** in nature.

Digestion is the first process that must take place in a healthy body and many people fail right here. If you are very thin or lack adequate muscle tissue, it is a strong probability that your body has not been digesting (breaking down) your foods adequately.

ABSORPTION

Once foods are broken down, we must now absorb these building materials, fuels and other components, which include: tissue salts, vitamins, tannins, alkaloids, flavins, and the like. These components are now carried by the bloodstream to the cells for energy, stimulation, building and repairing, or stored for future use. Absorption is accomplished through the villi (fingerlike projections on the surface of certain membranes) and small pores all along the mucous membranes of the small and large intestines. This absorption should be simple, but most people's intestines become impacted with a thick rubber-like substance called "**mucoid plaque.**" This thick plaque, which develops in the GI tract, is made of gluten, mucus, foreign protein, and other food by-products that act more like glue than nutrition! Refined sugars, grains, meats, and dairy products are the foods that are most responsible for the formation of this plaque. This "mucoid plaque" blocks the nutritional components of our foods from being adequately absorbed into the body. (I have seen patients who have eliminated buckets of this "black" plaque from their intestines.)

Most of us fail in the second stage of food utilization to some extent because of this congestive mucoid plaque. Again, if you are thin, malnourished or lack adequate muscle tissue, a malabsorption issue must be considered.

UTILIZATION

We must get nutrition to and into our cells. The blood system and its highways (the vascular system) are the transport system. Most of the absorbed nutrition must first pass inspection by the liver, which can create further chemical changes, store nutrients, or pass them on unchanged to the rest of the body for utilization. The number of processes the liver can carry out is miraculous. It can create its own amino acids, change sugars to fats, and vice versa. It can create or destroy.

Now a little secret. This is where the importance of acid and alkaline comes in. If our body (including our blood) becomes more acidic, our nutrition becomes anionic (coagulating). In other words, our building materials (fats, fuels, minerals, and other compounds) start sticking or clumping together. Most of the foods commonly eaten by humans are acid forming. Acidity, which is heat-producing, causes inflammation in the walls of the vascular highway and throughout the body. Lipids (fats) begin sticking to the walls of the vessels in hopes of buffering this inflammation. But lipid bonding also causes lipid stones, such as gallbladder and liver stones. Cholesterol is the most common anti-inflammatory lipid that the body uses to fight this inflammation. When the tissues become acidic and thus inflamed, the liver will produce more cholesterol to fight it. But that means that blood cholesterol levels begin to elevate. Minerals too start bonding and form "rock-type" stones, which show up as kidney stones, bone spurs, and the like.

Cell membrane walls have tiny portholes that will not allow this "clumped" nutrition to be absorbed. When red blood cells start clumping together, blocking proper oxygen transport, or utilization, this creates cellular starvation, which causes hypo-active conditions of glands and organs, loss of systemic energy, loss of muscle tissue, and finally death.

Many glands supply hormones, steroids, and the like, to assist utilization. As these glands become hypo- or underactive as described above, the utilization of calcium and other constituents is affected, creating many disease symptoms. For example, one of the jobs of calcium is to help transport nutrients across cell membrane walls. When the thyroid gland becomes hypoactive this slows or stops calcium utilization, which has a domino effect, causing cellular starvation. This, of course, makes tissue even weaker and the cycle just gets worse and worse until death. Most people fail in the utilization of their nutrition to some degree.

ELIMINATION

What goes in must, for the most part, come out. If it comes out looking the same way it went in, that's a problem. (You should not see undigested foods, except corn, in your stools.) When the elements in food are broken down into their simplest forms for utilization by the cells, there are many by-products from this process—including gases, acids, cellular wastes, undigested proteins, and unused material like vitamins and minerals —that need to leave the body.

The body is always trying to eliminate in ways that we often do not understand. An example would be cold and flu-like symptoms, where sneezing, coughing, sweating, aching, fevers, and diarrhea are experienced. These symptoms are elimination processes used by the body to purge itself of mucus, parasites, toxins, and the like.

If we do not eliminate our wastes, we build congestion *interstitially* (around cells) and *intracellularly* (inside cells), causing further cellular decay and death. Good elimination means moving our bowels three times a day, urinating adequately, sweating, and breathing properly. All of us fail in this category to some extent or another. By correcting digestion, absorption, utilization, and elimination we can regain our energy, build vitality and vibrancy, and live a disease-free life.

☼ The Body's Systems

Structures and Functions

Your physical body is comprised of many systems, which in a combined effort keep it alive and well. These systems make up the organs, glands, blood supply, lymph tissue, muscles, bones, etc. Each system has its own unique job to do to support the whole. As previously stated, these systems depend upon each other for the running, maintenance and repair of the body as a whole entity.

The infrastructure of the human body is like a society: The glandular system is the government. The nervous (electrical) system is the information highway, without which communication throughout the cities (cells, organs and glands) is crippled. The police department consists of small immune cells called lymphocytes (white blood cells), neutrophils, basophils, and macrophages. For added protection we have the military, which are the NK (natural killer) cells the large T and B cells. Of course there are factories, like the liver, bone marrow, glands and some organs. And trash pick-up and waste disposal are done by the lymphatic system, colon, kidneys, lungs and skin. However, without general laborers a society would have all chiefs and nothing would get done. The majority of the cells in the body act as laborers. These cells comprise all the systems, including the skeletal system (bones), muscular system, and connective tissue.

Most of this society's food is supplied externally by what we feed the body. However, many nutrients are grown by "farmers" called bacteria. It is through their actions and transmutation techniques that many co-enzymes (vitamins or helpers) are produced.

Stepping down into a smaller world we find the cells themselves. Each cell is a city unto itself—a microcosm of the larger society of the whole body. God's worlds are merely a reflection of each other, as all life forms and structures require other life forms and structures to exist. Consciousness, or the awareness behind all things, is the driving force.

In the following pages of this section I have detailed the various systems and their structures and functions that comprise the physical body.

CIRCULATORY SYSTEM

STRUCTURES — Heart, vascular system (arteries, capillaries and veins), and the blood (also part of the digestive system).

FUNCTIONS — The circulatory system is comprised of the pathways within the body, through which the physical life force of the body flows. It distributes nutrients, building materials and fuels for cellular life and activity; works with the lymphatic system in removing metabolic and other wastes from the body; helps keep the body alkaline; is used to help regulate body temperature; and carries oxygen for oxidation purposes (antioxidant and biological transmutation responses).

DIGESTIVE SYSTEM

STRUCTURES — Mouth and salivary glands, stomach, small intestines (duodenum, jejunum and ileum), pancreas, liver, gallbladder.

FUNCTIONS — The digestive system employs mechanical (teeth) and chemical (enzymatic) action for the breakdown of coarse foods and compounds into simple structures for absorption and utilization purposes. It allows for biological and biochemical transmutation of elements and complexes into more usable or storable compounds or substances.

ELIMINATIVE SYSTEMS

STRUCTURES — Colon, lymphatic system, urinary system, immune system and the integumentary system (skin).

FUNCTIONS — The elimination of wastes and by-products from metabolism and digestion. Elimination of pathogens and mucus from the lymphatic system. Excess water elimination.

The eliminative system encompasses several other systems, which are complete systems within themselves. They are the **intestinal system, lymphatic system, urinary system, integumentary system** and **immune system.**

Intestinal System (Colon)

STRUCTURES — There are five sections to the colon. The first section, which is valved and connected to the jejenum (small bowel), is called the cecum. Then there is the ascending portion, which trails upward against gravity toward the right lower lung and liver area. The transverse portion travels across your abdomen toward the left side. Next it curves downward, becoming the descending portion. It then curves again, and becomes the sigmoid portion. Finally, it curves one last time, ending with the rectal portion. The average human colon is five to six feet long.

FUNCTIONS — Wastes and by-products from digestion are eliminated through the large intestine (called the colon). The lymph system also eliminates one-third or more of its wastes through the colon. Wastes from metabolism that enter the blood and lymph system are carried to the kidneys, skin, and colon, to then be eliminated. The colon is truly the "sewer system" and must be in a state of good health in order for the whole body to be in a good state of health.

Lymphatic System

STRUCTURES — Spleen, thymus, appendix, tonsils, lymph nodes, lymph vessels and lymph fluid.

FUNCTIONS — The lymphatic system is one of the most vital systems in the body. Its job includes removing cellular wastes, removing excessive fat-soluble compounds from the gastrointestinal tract, and serving as the "house" of the immune system. It creates white blood cells and antibodies, and is truly the battlefield of "the good vs. the bad," where immune cells battle pathogens, including bacteria, yeasts, viruses and other unwanted intruders. The lymph system is also a carrier of nutrients to various parts of the body. It serves as both the police force and part of the body's septic system. It becomes heavily congested with excessive mucus and lymph from dairy products and refined and complex sugars. This causes a type of congestion that most people are unaware of except when their sinus cavities or lung tissues let them know it.

Urinary System

STRUCTURES — Kidneys, bladder, ureters and urethra.

FUNCTIONS — The filtration and elimination of excess H_2O, nutrients and metabolic wastes and by-products from the body is the job of the urinary system. It helps regulate the sodium/potassium balance, and works with the acid-alkaline balance. Urine is about 95 percent waste and 5 percent dissolved substances.

Integumentary System

STRUCTURES — Skin, nails, hair, oil and sweat glands.

FUNCTIONS — This system provides protective and outer covering for the physical body. The skin is the body's largest eliminative organ and aids in the elimination of wastes and by-products from metabolism. The integumentary system maintains body temperature.

Immune System

STRUCTURES — Lymphatic system, which includes the thymus and spleen, bone marrow, immune cells (lymphocytes, monocytes, basophils, macrophages, T-lymphocytes, B-cells, helper T and B cells, etc.), the liver and parasites (toxin eaters).

FUNCTIONS — To protect the body from pathogens (foreign enemies), antigens (foreign proteins), parasites and the like, that could harm or destroy it. The immune system is truly the police force of the body.

GLANDULAR SYSTEM (ENDOCRINE)

STRUCTURES — The pituitary gland, pineal gland, thyroid and parathyroid glands, thymus, adrenal glands, pancreas (including the islets of Langerhans), glands within the intestinal mucosa, ovaries and testes.

FUNCTIONS — The regulation of all the activities of the body from breathing, nerve response, and temperature changes, to elimination. This is all accomplished through hormones, neurotransmitters, steroids, and the like. The glandular system is tied into our emotional and mental bodies as well.

MUSCULAR SYSTEM

STRUCTURES — Muscles, tendons and connective tissue.

FUNCTIONS — Movement, strength and skeletal support. Transportation of heat.

NERVOUS SYSTEM

STRUCTURES — The brain, spinal cord (Central Nervous System), the autonomic nervous system, sensory organs (eyes, ears, nose, olfactory nerves, etc.).

FUNCTIONS — The nervous system is truly the information highway of the body. It is divided into two main systems: the autonomic (ANS)

nervous system, and the central nervous system (CNS). The autonomic system is further divided into two branches, the sympathetic and parasympathetic systems.

REPRODUCTIVE SYSTEM

STRUCTURES — Testes, ovaries, sperm, ova, mammary glands, and prostate gland. The reproductive system works in conjunction with the glandular system.

FUNCTIONS — Reproduction via conception, the continuation and improvement (supposedly) of a species.

RESPIRATORY SYSTEM

STRUCTURES — Lungs, trachea, bronchi, bronchial tubes, and alveoli.

FUNCTIONS — Ingestion of the body's main source of energy—"oxygen." Oxygen allows for oxidation to take place within the body. The respiratory system removes carbon dioxide; helps regulate the acid-base balance of the body; and brings hydrogen, carbon, nitrogen, etc., into the body. These elements are life's most basic foods.

SKELETAL SYSTEM

STRUCTURES — All the bones and cartilage that comprise the physical body. There are 206 bones in the human body: Head—twenty-nine bones. Upper extremities—sixty-four bones. Trunk—fifty-one bones. Lower extremities—sixty-two bones.

FUNCTIONS — The skeletal system gives form and structure to the physical body. It also allows for various movements of the limbs. Our bones are oftentimes a source of calcium when they shouldn't be.

☀ The Cell

In Modules 2.1 and 2.2 we have already laid out the basics, presenting the overall systems of the body. Modules 2.5 and 2.13 will detail each of these various systems (circulatory system, immune system, glandular system, etc.), the organs and glands that comprise them, as well as their related functions.

Before we discuss the systems, organs and glands, however, let's start at the beginning: with the cell. As all of creation is made up of atoms, so your body—bones, tissues, organs and glands—is made up of cells.

The body has over 75 trillion cells, each as individual as you are. They each perform a specific function, while all working together in harmony to form a social (body) consciousness. In other words, all your cells depend upon each other and work together for the life and functioning of the body.

As the microcosm is a reflection of the macrocosm, a body is a reflection of each of its cells, each being a society unto itself. Each cell is actually like a completely self-sustaining city, taking care of all its own functions, with two exceptions. All cells need an **external source of energy** (or connection) to this world, and they all need to **eliminate their wastes**. Let's examine the "city" or "universe" of the cell.

There are many different systems or structures within a city (like the highway department, for instance) that perform specific functions aimed at the survival and productivity of that city. The same is true within each cell. It has a courthouse (**nucleus**) where all the records (genetic information) are kept. Within the courthouse (nucleus) you have government employees (**nucleoli**) who carry out the daily activities and needs that are required for the "men in the field" (**ribosomes**). All of the above determine the individuality of the cells and their functions.

The atmosphere and the living substance of a cell is called **cytoplasm**. The city (or cell) is surrounded and protected by a wall and gate system called the **plasma membrane** or **cell wall membrane**. This "cellular wall" has gatekeepers that allow or disallow substances into the cell.

The courthouse (nucleus) is also surrounded by a protective and functional wall called the **nuclear envelope**. There are workers that carry information (substances) from the courthouse (nucleus) to the city and from the city (body or cytoplasm) to the nucleus. These workers are called the **endoplasmic reticulum** (ER for short).

Extra-cellular substances = substances outside the cells

Intra-cellular substances = substances inside the cells

The **Golgi apparatus** is named for Camillo Golgi (individuals who discover things like to put their names on them). Golgi was an Italian histologist who uncovered the function of these curved stacks of membrane-bound sacs within cells, which act as factories. They collect, modify, package and distribute the proteins and lipids that are manufactured by the ER. These proteins are present in large amounts in the pancreas, salivary glands, liver, and other organs.

In our cities we have transporters and storage facilities. These are called **vesicles** within cells. **Secretory vesicles** break off from the Golgi apparatus with the materials manufactured by the ER, and carry these to the outer cell membrane wall, where this material is then dumped or carried out into the world of the body. Some vesicles act as holding tanks until the "created" or "manufactured" product is needed. An example of this is the hormone **insulin**, which is held in vesicles in the beta cells of the pancreas. When the body's blood glucose levels rise, these vesicles then release their stored insulin into the blood to assist cellular utilization of glucose.

As in any city, we need protection from invaders. Many cells act as protectors of the body. These are called **immune cells**. Within each cell, the **lysosomes** are vesicles that contain a variety of **enzymes** that are used for intracellular sanitation and elimination (digestive) functions. **Macrophages** (the white blood cells, or WBCs, for example) ingest bacteria (antigens or pathogens). The lysosomes within your cells "eat" or "digest" (break apart) and destroy the invader.

Now what's a city without power? The powerhouse for a cell is its **mitochondria**. These are bean- or rod-shaped **organelles** (specialized organs or structures) that produce, store and release **adenosine triphosphate (ATP)**. This is the energy source for most chemical reactions within the cell. Mitochondria use oxygen (oxidative metabolism) which allows ATP to be produced.

The skeletal portions of the cells (or the "structures" of the city) are called **cytoskeleton**, which is made up of proteins (chained and bound amino acids). Within the cytoskeleton there are several structures, all of which play a role in its flexibility, shape and size. These are called microtubules, microfilaments and intermediate filaments.

It is noteworthy to mention that some cells have **cilia**, which are hair-like extensions from the outer membrane wall. They can vary in number from one to thousands. Their coordinated job is to move mucus. You can especially see this in the respiratory tract where mucus is secreted by the lymphatic mucosa of the lining of the lungs and bronchi. The action of the cilia allows the body to keep its lungs clear of dust

or other particles that could damage (or affect) its functions.

Some cells have what are called **microvilli**, which are projections of the outer cell membrane wall. This is especially true of kidneys and intestinal wall cells where additional absorption of nutrients is necessary.

Now you can see how a cell "acts like" and is "created like" a city. All the worlds (creations) of God are just a mirror reflection of each other, from the **macrocosm** (the largest "world") to the **microcosm** (the smallest).

To understand the nature of your cells, it's also important to understand the different ways that nutrients or elements can enter through the cell membrane wall. Basically, there are two conditions **diffusion** or **osmosis** that allow this process to happen.

How Nutrients Enter the Cells

DIFFUSION
Molecules or substances move from a higher or greater concentration of particles into a lesser concentration in a solution. A common example of this is how a concentrated sugar cube disperses in a glass of water.

OSMOSIS
This is a type of diffusion in which molecules or substances move from a less concentrated solution to a higher or more concentrated solution or fluid. Osmosis and the rate of osmosis depend upon several factors that facilitate this action. First and primarily, the osmotic pressures on each side of the cell membrane wall. Secondly, the permeability of the membrane. Thirdly, the electrical potential across the membrane wall and its pores.

A great percentage of osmosis and "facilitated" diffusion requires an "active transporter." An active transporter simply means that a "carrier" or "transporter" (like a bus) is used to assist the movement of a molecule or substance through a cell membrane wall. An example of this is **insulin**, which is a carrier or transporter of glucose into a cell. Note that this type of activity requires a small amount of energy since this is an active transport, not a passive one. This energy comes from the cell mitochondria in the form of ADP (adenosine diphosphate), which comes from stored ATP (adenosine triphosphate). A carrier or transporter can be a hormone, protein, steroid or mineral.

When you are seeking true healing, health and vitality, therefore, you must think cellularly. **Healing must happen at the cellular level for true, lasting health and vitality to exist.** Spiritually speaking, all life, no matter how small or how large (atoms to universes and everything in between), when manifested physically, must have a mental body (mind portion) and an emotional body (astral portion). This is true for each of your cells, as well as for all plants, all animals, and your entire body. A great example is documented by Christopher Bird and Tom Hopkins in their book *The Secret Life of Plants*, which tells about the ability of plants to feel and remember. These abilities become more obvious in animals, and more so with human beings.

Cells respond to external stimuli not only from hormones, minerals, sugars, proteins and the like; their ability to function is greatly affected by the body's pH factors (acidosis), by congestion, types of foods consumed, and chemical consumption. They also respond to thoughts and emotions (feelings). The types of thoughts and feelings you have, harbor or carry around with you play a major role in cellular functioning. To enjoy a state of total health and vitality it is necessary to clean (detoxify) your body, your mind and your emotions, and thus set yourself free.

As the initial parent cell divides, tissues are formed, then organs and glands, and so on. There are **two types of cell division—meiosis and mitosis**. Through meiosis and mitosis the body grows and repairs itself. Let's now examine the grouping of cells called tissues.

Types of Cell Division

MEIOSIS
A cell divides with only half of the chromosomes of the related somatic or non-reproductive cell. (These cells replace.)

MITOSIS
Cells divide each with the same number of chromosomes as the parent, or somatic cell. (These cells create.)

MODULE 2.4

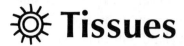 # Tissues

Most of your individual cells are grouped together to form tissues. Then tissues can be grouped together to form organs and glands. There are **four primary types of tissues** that comprise, line, support, protect or control the basic structures of your body.

TYPES OF TISSUES

EPITHELIAL — Covers the surface and linings of the body's cavities or from glands. Found in the digestive tract, lungs, blood vessels, etc.

CONNECTIVE — This type of tissue is supportive and holds all cells, organs and glands together.

MUSCULAR — These tissues support your skeletal structure and are used for movement of various structures, including your limbs.

NERVOUS — These tissues comprise your information highway, the nervous system. These tissues are highly charged and allow electrical transmissions to take place.

Disease is Not Found in Healthy Tissue

When tissues, organs, or glands fail to do their job, this sets up a domino effect throughout your body, causing many different disease symptoms.

Vibrant health = healthy tissue

Tissue regeneration = alkalization + detoxification + nutrition + energy = vibrant health

---

Remember that all your tissues are made up of individual cells, each requiring nutrition, energy and proper elimination.

Now let's examine the tissues called organs and glands in each body system.

MODULE 2.5

The Cardiovascular System and Blood

HEART

Your heart is a four-chamber holding and receiving organ with a system of valves that allow blood in and out. You have two chambers on the right and two chambers on the left. The upper chambers are called **atrials** and the lower, larger chambers are called **ventricles**. Fresh, oxygenated blood comes from the pulmonary arteries into the upper left atrial and moves through the mitral valve into the lower left chamber (left ventricle), then out into the body to feed and oxygenate. This blood comes back around after making its journey through miles of the vascular system, back into the upper right arterial, then down to the right ventricle, and then off to the lungs for more oxygen. Your adrenal glands play a major role in how strongly the heart pumps, and in its rhythm. The heart is said to be a pump, but actually gets its pressure from the lungs.

VASCULAR SYSTEM

Although arteries, capillaries and veins are not organs or glands, they are a link to every cell in your body, including those that form organs and glands. Their job is to carry vital fuels and building materials to all the cells. Your vascular system carries your physical life force, the blood. Blood is used to transport nutrition, hormones, enzymes, oxygen, antioxidants, etc. It works with your lymphatic system in helping remove cellular and metabolic wastes, and can dramatically affect your body temperatures. The health of your cells depends upon the health and strength of your vascular system and the blood that flows through it.

Vessels: Arteries, Capillaries, Veins

ARTERIES — These carry fresh oxygenated blood (which is also "nutrient-rich") from your lungs via the pulmonary arteries, to the heart; then throughout your body to all the cells, tissues, organs and glands.

CAPILLARIES—Capillaries are tiny (minute) vessels that connect the smallest arteries (called **arterioles**) to the beginnings of the smallest veins (called **venules**). Oxygen and other elements are now exchanged for carbon dioxide, other gases and metabolic wastes. These are carried through the venous system back to your lungs, kidneys and colon for elimination. Blood capillary walls consist of only one single layer of squamous cells (**endothelium**).

VEINS — As previously stated, your venous system carries carbon dioxide, cellular wastes and other toxins from the cells and interstitial areas back to the lungs and other eliminative organs to be eliminated. This is a constant cycle that runs night and day, 365 days a year, until death.

An acidic diet, excessive "glue-like" foods (like refined starches), chemicals, heavy metals, minerals, and a lack of calcium utilization (from an underactive thyroid gland), all cause damage to this vital system. Your vascular walls are sensitive to inflammation from acids that are ingested or that are a by-product of metabolism. If this inflammation goes unchecked by steroids (from the adrenal glands), it can cause cholesterol plaquing. This leads to occlusions (blockages) that can cause heart attacks, strokes, tissue death and systemic death.

BLOOD

Blood and chlorophyll are the liquid nectars of life; the life force condensed into nutrients, fuels, building and repair materials, and the like. Without them, plant, animal and human life would come to an end. All creatures in nature have some sort of "blood" or "life force" that sustains their physical body.

Your blood consists of formed elements and plasma. The **formed elements** include red blood cells (erythrocytes), white blood cells (leukocytes) and platelets (thrombocytes). The **plasma** consists of 92 percent water and 8 percent of various substances including nutrients, proteins, ions, gases, metabolic by-products, etc. The chart on the following page will give you an overview of what's in your blood serum.

The blood contains two basic types of cells: **erythrocytes** and **leukocytes**.

Erythrocytes

Erythrocytes are **red blood cells (RBCs)**. They are red because of their **hemoglobin** content. The heme part of the hemoglobin carries one iron atom, which binds to one oxygen molecule, giving it the red color. The globin (a protein) bonds to carbon dioxide. Erythrocytes transport oxygen and carbon dioxide. Combined with its hemoglobin, these cells transport 97 percent of your systemic oxygen and 92 percent systemic

Blood Serum Composition

FORMED ELEMENTS		PLASMA
Water	92%	Erythrocytes — red blood cells (4 to 6 million), carry hemoglobin, which carries oxygen and buffers hydrogen ions (CO_2 conversion); neutralizes carbon monoxide
Proteins	8%	Leukocytes — white blood cells; immune cells (5,000 to 9,000)
albumins	58%	
globulins	38%	
fibrinogen	4%	

		neutrophils	60 to 80%
Other Constituents (solutes)		lymphocytes	20 to 40%
nutrients		eosinophils	1 to 4%
ions		monocytes	3 to 8%
gases		Platelets — (200,000 to 500,000)	
waste by products			
hormones, neurotransmitters			

carbon dioxide. An enzyme called **carbonic anhydrase**, found in erythrocytes, catalyzes (changes) carbon dioxide into hydrogen and bicarbonate ions. This is for transportation purposes, as carbon dioxide lowers the body's pH, making it more acidic. The lungs convert hydrogen and bicarbonic ions back into carbon dioxide. Carbon dioxide now can be exhaled without creating excessive acidosis in the body.

Leukocytes

Leukocytes are **white blood cells (WBCs)**. These are immune cells and are covered under the Immune System section of this chapter. The four types of leukocytes are: **neutrophils, lymphocytes, monocytes (macrophages), eosinophils** and **mast cells**.

Erythrocytes (RBCs) and leukocytes (WBCs) are derived from what are called **stem cells**. Your blood carries many substances that are vital to the health of your body via its cells. It also carries metabolic and cellular wastes and by-products.

Your body is always seeking to maintain an **alkaline/acid balance**. Alkalinity dominates all fluids and tissues, except in the stomach. Your

Fluids of Alkaline Species

FLUID	ACID OR ALKALINE	EFFECTS OF ACIDOSIS
saliva	alkaline	canker sores (herpes)
urine	alkaline	urinary tract infections, kidney or bladder cancer
stomach	acid	ulcers, (gastritis), stomach cancers
intestines	alkaline	ulcers (enteritis and colitis) intestinal cancers
blood	alkaline	death

blood plays a vital role in this balancing process, from breaking down carbon dioxide to supplying electrolytes, steroids (lipids), etc. One of the best examples of this balancing process is the way the red blood cells, through carbonic anhydrase, first convert cellular and systemic carbon dioxide (acidic) into bicarbonate ions (alkaline), and then convert these back to carbon dioxide when these ions reach the lungs.

As stated earlier, humans belong to the frugivore species, which is an alkaline species. The chart on the previous page points out where alkaline fluids predominate in the human body, and the damaging effects of acidosis in these various areas.

When your diet is predominantly acid forming, your hormones become out of balance, your food then ferments and putrefies instead of properly digesting, and excessive mucus and inflammation is produced. Your blood becomes toxic and your lymphatic system becomes clogged. This is called **disease** by many.

Always keep your body alkaline, toxic free, and clean—internally, as well as externally. This creates true health and vitality.

MODULE 2.6

☀ The Digestive System

MOUTH AND SALIVARY GLANDS

The mouth offers the mechanical (teeth) and initial enzyme breakdown of whole food sources into smaller and simpler complexes. The salivary glands secrete **amylase** (ptyalin), which is an alkaline digestive enzyme for starch and carbohydrate breakdown. This enzyme hydrolyzes starch and glycogen to maltose.

STOMACH

The stomach is located between your esophagus and duodenum (first portion of the small bowel). It is below the diaphragm and to the right of the spleen. A portion of the stomach lies under the liver. Foods enter the upper portion of the stomach through the cardiac sphincter valve and leave through the pyloric sphincter valve. The wall of the stomach has four layers. The inner lining or mucosa contains simple tubular glands that secrete your gastric juices. Some secrete pepsinogen and others HCL (hydrochloric acid). There are also cells that secrete mucus.

When we see, smell, or imagine food, this triggers the secretion of gastric juices. The actual presence of food stimulates production of the hormone gastrin from the stomach, which in turn releases more gastric juice.

Protein digestion begins in the stomach when the HCL converts pepsinogen to pepsin, which then breaks down complex protein structures into smaller structures called **peptones**. This is an acid digestive process. If there isn't any protein in the food consumed, the stomach acts as a temporary holding compartment for carbohydrate and fat digestion. These foods start digesting in the mouth with alkaline digestive juices—amylase (ptyalin), etc. If protein is present, then the stomach acids neutralize these enzymes until these foods move into the duodenum where they are reactivated and added to.

The stomach acts like a time-release capsule, allowing your food time to digest (or be broken down) so the body can actually use it properly. The action of your stomach is through nerve and hormonal control. The stomach can absorb mostly alcohol and water, including tinctured herbs and some fruit and vegetable juices.

Spiritually speaking, your stomach reflects the solar plexus, which is the center of the nerve field that feeds the head (upper), mid, and lower extremities of the body. Weaknesses of the stomach can weaken your whole body, affecting emotions (can foster fear), oxygen demands, consciousness, headaches, and other conditions.

SMALL INTESTINES

The small intestines make up the first part of the bowel structure. The small intestines are smaller in diameter than the colon, but are four to six times as long. There are three distinct sections that make up the small intestines, each having its own job to do.

Duodenum

This first section of the small intestine is approximately 8-11 inches long. Through the common bile duct it receives digestive enzymes, alkalizing sodium of bicarbonate from the pancreas, and alkalizing bile from the gallbladder/liver. The major portion of this section of the small intestines is primarily digestive and alka-

---

Duodenum Hormones

PEPTIDE
Stimulates the release of pertidase to finish final protein digestion into amino acids

SECRETIN
Stimulates sodium of bicarbonate and bile for alkalization and fat breakdown

CHOLECYSTOKININ
Stimulates pancreatic enzymes and contracts the gallbladder for bile extraction

Duodenum Enzymes

PEPTIDASE
Completes protein breakdown into amino acids

SUCRASE, MALTASE AND LACTASE
(lactase only to age 3) Change complex sugars into monosaccharides or simple sugars

---

lizing. Hormone secretion is also an aspect of the duodenum.

It is important to understand that the small intestinal walls are made up of circular folds (or **villi**) called plicae circulares. The mucosa folds itself into these villi or microvilli to increase the absorption surface of the intestines. These appear like ripples or waves that allow the body maximum potential for digesting and absorbing its nutrition.

There are glands called **Lieberkuhns** at the base of many of the villi (in the duodenum), which secrete digestive hormones and enzymes.

Jejunum

The second portion of the small intestine is approximately 8 feet long. The duodenum and jejunum make up two-fifths of the small intestines. Digestive enzymes from the duodenum are now acting upon most of the food particles. Absorption of vital nutrients is now taking place as the digestive enzymes break down the food particles to their simplest form.

Ileum

The third portion is approximately 15 to 30 feet long and comprises the lower three-fifths of the small intestine. Most of the by-products of digestion now have become amino acids (building blocks), monosaccharides (fuels), fatty acids (oil and fuel), glycerol, vitamins and minerals. These are now being absorbed or mixed with water to continue on their way out into the colon. This liquid mixture now passes into the first part of the large bowel known as the cecum, which is the first section of the ascending portion.

PANCREAS

The pancreas is both an endocrine gland and an exocrine gland and is located in a horizontal position behind the stomach in front of the first and second lumbar vertebrae. The head of the pancreas is attached to the duodenum (small intestines) and the tail of the pancreas reaches to the spleen.

The body of the pancreas has many exocrine glands, which have their own ducts all leading into the main pancreatic duct, which joins the common bile duct. The common bile duct empties into the duodenum (the first portion of the small intestines). All through the exocrine gland tissue are masses of cells called Islets of Langerhans. These are the endocrine systems of the pancreas.

This endocrine portion of the pancreas will be discussed along with the entire endocrine gland system covered later in this chapter. Since we are considering digestion now, we want to examine the exocrine portion of the pancreas, the ducted portion. These glands supply the bulk of the digestive enzymes needed to break down your food. They also supply sodium bicarbonate, which is an alkalizing substance called **chyme**, which is necessary to alkalize the stomach contents. This chyme is full of HCL (hydrochloric acid) and pepsin. Sodium bicarbonate and bile from the gallbladder join in the duodenum to activate the alkaline digestive enzymes of the pancreas and intestinal wall. If the stomach contents cannot be alkalized, then proper digestion is halted. Your food then ferments and putrefies, causing excessive gas. You then have lost the nutritional value of your foods.

This mixture of enzymes and sodium bicarbonate is called the **pancreatic juice**. Pancreatic juice has a pH of 8.4 to 8.9, which is alkaline. Pancreatic juice is stimulated by two hormones, **secretin** and **cholecystokinin**, which are produced by the duodenal mucosa. This pancreatic juice flows through the main pancreatic duct to the common bile duct and then into the duodenum. Pancreatic juice includes sodium bicarbonate (alkalizer) and the enzymes: **trypsinogen**, **chymotrypsinogen**, **amylase**, and **lipase**.

Your pancreas is one of your vital organs. It is destroyed by acidosis and harmful chemicals. What destroys the liver also destroys the pancreas. Spiritually speaking, your pancreas is tied to your thought processes and how they manifest.

LIVER

Your liver can be compared to a huge chemical factory that supplies a whole city with its functional (metabolic) needs. It has been said that it would require 500 acres of land to build such a factory. Your liver has so many different functions that researchers still haven't discovered them all. It is enough to say that we should take care of this most precious organ.

Pancreatic Juice and its Function

SODIUM BICARBONATE
Alkalizer and enzyme activator (neutralizes stomach acid).

TRYPSINOGEN
An enzyme that is converted into trypsin in the duodenum.

CHYMOTRYPSINOGEN
An enzyme that is converted into chymotrypsin in the duodenum. (Trypsin and chymotrypsin finish protein digestion, converting peptones to peptides. From here, peptides are broken down [from the intestinal wall] by protease into amino acids—the basic building blocks of protein structures.)

AMYLASE
An enzyme which breaks down (hydrolyzes) starch (maltose) or complex sugars (di- and poly-saccharides) into monosaccharides, or simple sugars.

LIPASE
An enzyme that emulsifies (breaks down) fats into fatty acids and glycerol.

The liver is the largest organ in your body and carries on the most functions. It is situated mostly on your right side beneath your diaphragm, level with the bottom of your sternum. The bottom of the liver is concave and covers your stomach, duodenum (the first portion of the small intestines), hepatic flexure of the colon (upper right turn), right adrenal gland, and the upper portion of the right kidney.

Your liver has four lobes and is covered by a thick, tough, fibrous membrane called the **Glisson's capsule**.

All your blood vessels and hepatic ducts enter the liver at the hilus. There are many small intrahepatic bile ducts running through the liver, all leading into the main hepatic duct, which joins the cystic duct from the gallbladder, which then forms the "common bile duct." This common bile duct then enters the upper portion of your small intestine, called the **duodenum**, at the papilla of Vater. This is the main digestive area of the body.

The functional parts of your liver are the liver lobules, consisting of the liver cells (hepatocytes), which are permeated by blood capillaries called sinusoids. The sinusoids are lined with the Kupffer cells (macrophages), which are the immune cells of the liver.

Four Basic Tasks

The liver has four basic tasks, out of which arise a multitude of functions. These tasks are:

STORAGE AND DISTRIBUTION — The liver stores various amino acids obtained from digestion, then reconstructs them for essential body proteins. The liver converts excess glucose into glycogen (stored fat), then converts the stored glycogen back to glucose when the body needs extra fuel. The liver also stores and distributes various vitamins, including Vitamin A, D, E, and K (your fat-soluble vitamins). Your liver also stores various minerals, including iron and copper.

CONVERSIONS, SYNTHESIS, BIOLOGICAL TRANS-MUTATIONS — The liver stores glycogen, and

---

Liver Function

AMINO ACID METABOLISM
- Synthesis of non-essential amino acids.
- Will convert amino acids into glucose (energy) if needed. (It is not recommended to allow your body to get this far in its energy needs.)
- Forms urea from excess amino acids and ammonia.

CARBOHYDRATE METABOLISM
- Converts monosaccharides (other than glucose) into glucose.
- Excessive glucose is converted and stored as glycogen, and vice versa.

FAT METABOLISM
- Cholesterol is synthesized for new cell growth and steroid production.
- Lipo proteins, which are transporters of fat, are synthesized.
- Fatty acids are converted to acetyl groups or ketones, which are used for energy.
- Bile pigments, including bilirubin, are formed from the hemoglobin of old red blood cells.
- Bile is synthesized for fat emulsifying and alkalizing stomach contents.

---

when your blood glucose levels drop, it will convert this stored fat (glycogen) into glucose again. If our glycogen reserves are depleted, it will convert other fats and even stored amino acids into glucose. This shows you that the number one priority of your body is the need for fuels for energy (glucose/fructose).

The liver converts ammonia from excessive protein consumption into urea, which is then excreted by the kidneys. Your liver synthesizes Vitamin K and other various clotting factors, including prothrombin and fibrinogen. It synthesizes non-essential amino acids for growth and repair functions.

Cholesterol is synthesized for use in cell membrane walls, steroid production, and for anti-inflammatory purposes. Various minerals and elements are transmuted into other elements. An example of this is silica, which is transmuted into calcium. The liver also synthesizes albumin and globulin, which are carrier molecules.

SECRETION — Your liver produces and secretes approximately 1 liter of bile per day. Bile is a fat emulsifier and alkalizing agent.

DETOXIFICATION — The liver's immune (Kupffer) cells digest bacteria, viruses and other pathogens within the blood from the digestive tract. A healthy liver can metabolize hormones, chemical drugs, and other chemicals to a certain degree. However, our daily ingestion of these substances is more than most livers can cope with. The liver also produces enzymes to help with the above detoxification process.

You can see from the above functions and processes what your liver does, and how important it is to keep it healthy! Acidosis, alcohol, toxic chemicals, drugs, etc., are all extremely harmful to your liver. Almost all drugs, especially coal tar products like aspirin, severely destroy its tissues. It's your liver—send it love and be good to it!

Your liver is also tied to your mind in ways not yet understood by most people. When the liver is inflamed and impaired in its function, so is your mind. This can create low self-esteem and anger. Remember that your body develops and functions according to how you treat it. Be good to yourself.

GALLBLADDER

Your gallbladder is a pear-shaped sac that is located on the underside of the right lobe of your liver. Your gallbladder is a "holding tank" for bile, which is produced in the liver. As bile is stored in the gallbladder, the body removes water from it, making it concentrated.

As bile is needed for digestive purposes, it moves through a 3-inch duct called the cystic duct into the hepatic duct, which then forms the common bile duct. The hepatic duct then empties into the duodenum (the first portion of the small intestine).

Bile is used as an alkalizer, anti-inflammatory, and emulsifier of fats. It works with pancreatic lipase to break down large fat molecules. Bile contains bilirubin, biliverdin, cholesterol, organic and inorganic substances and salts, lecithin, mucin, etc.

Cholecystokinin (pancreozymin) is a hormone from the intestinal wall (of the duodenum) that causes the gallbladder to contract, releasing bile. Cholecystokinin (pancreozymin) is triggered by fats entering the small bowel.

In Summary

The tissues of the alimentary canal, which is called the digestive tract, are formed from several layers of cells. The first layer is called the mucous membrane; it lines all passages and cavities of the body that have contact with oxygen. This mucous membrane consists of epithelial cells, also referred to as the mucosa, which secretes moisture or mucus to aid in the protection and function of the respective organ. We also have the sub-mucosa or basement membrane. Then the connective and the smooth muscle tissues. Most of the mucus of the mucosa comes from the Brunner's glands, which are located in the sub-mucosa.

We consume food and drink for the very purpose of obtaining fuels, as well as for building and repairing materials. Basically, most elements and compounds are used as energy sources for the body. All foods and drinks must first be broken down from their gross unusable forms into their simplest or nutritional substances so the body can absorb them and use them. Cell membrane walls have microscopic pores so that only the simplest of elements can enter. If not, large particles may enter and cause cellular damage.

Physically, however, most by-products of digestion, if properly broken down into their simplest form, can now be absorbed through the villi into the capillary (blood) bed. The blood now acts as a transporter, carrying the nutrients, building blocks and fuels to the liver, then to the heart, and finally releasing them into the general system for its needs. By-products of digestion include amino acids, monosaccharides (simple sugars), fatty acids, glycerol, vitamins and minerals, etc.

MODULE 2.7

☼ The Eliminative Systems

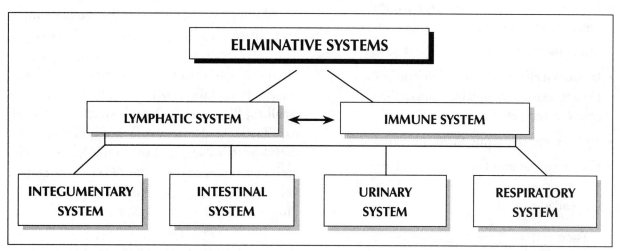

THE LYMPHATIC SYSTEM

The immune and lymphatic systems work together, offering your body both protection and elimination, respectively. Both fall under the category of "Eliminative System," but they are each a separate system unto themselves. Let's examine each of these systems and how they work, both separately and as a team.

The lymphatic system acts as your septic system. It provides not only protection for cells, but serves to remove wastes as well. Cells eat and excrete like you do, only on a much smaller scale. The blood carries the nutrition and fuels to the cells, and your lymph system removes the by-products and wastes caused from metabolizing these nutrients and fuels.

The lymph system consists of the lymph fluid, lymph vessels, lymph nodes, spleen and the thymus gland.

Lymph Fluid

The lymph fluid is an alkaline, translucent fluid that flows from the cells to the venous blood supply via the lymph vessels. Your lymph fluids act as the water that carries the wastes from your toilet to the septic system.

Lymph fluid removes approximately 10 percent of the total fluid supplied by the blood system to a cell. The lymph fluid is the medium or "plasma" that carries a host of substances that need to be removed from cells, as well as substances that are used to protect the cell. These include:

- Excessive unused proteins (including albumin and globulin, etc.)

- Salts and ions

- Gases and toxic, metabolic wastes

- Ureas

- Fats (possible anti-inflammatory compounds)

- Glucose

- Hormones, steroids and enzymes

- Unused nutrients, especially artificial vitamins

- Parasites (bacteria, etc.)

- Chemical toxins, sulfa drugs, chemical medications, etc.

- Minerals (unusable by cells)

- Immune cells, especially lymphocytes (T- and especially B-cells), macrophages (monocytes), etc.

- Dying body cells (due to atrophy or acidosis)

- Fats from the small intestinal tract and liver, which are absorbed through small lymph vessels called **lacteals**.

There is not a "heart" to pump and pressurize your lymph system, so your lymph fluids move by means of the following methods:

- Pressure changes that are reflected through the blood vascular system.

- Contraction of your skeletal muscles, which are activated through movement and exercise.

- Contraction of smooth muscle stimulation.

Low blood pressure (adrenal glands), lack of exercise or inactive lifestyle, impacted bowels, and congested kidneys and skin will all cause your lymph system to back up.

Over-consumption of proteins (many of which are abrasive [foreign] to the body), acids, and mucus-forming substances (milk, complex sugars, etc.) will also burden your lymph system, causing it to become congested and stagnant. **All of this together creates a heavy immune burden and response, and cellular autointoxication leading to cellular hypoactivity and death. In my opinion, this is where cancer originates.**

Lymph Vessels

Lymph vessels extend throughout your body and mimic your blood vessels, except they are larger. The lymph capillaries (and blood capillaries) extend into almost all the interstitial areas of all cells. They are not found in the bone marrow, epidermis (outer layer of skin), in cartilage, or in the central nervous system.

Blood plasma that leaves the blood capillaries nourishes and carries energy factors to cells. The cells' wastes from metabolizing these elements are excreted into what now has become the interstitial fluid, which is collected into the small capillaries of the lymph system. The small capillaries lead into the larger lymph vessels (veins with valves) and off to the lymph nodes and filtering organs, like the spleen, liver, tonsils and appendix, etc. The lymphatic vascular bed moves throughout the body in the same way your blood vessels do.

The thoracic duct, which begins in the abdomen, acts as an enlarged sac, which receives lymph vessels from the lower extremities (limbs) and pelvic areas, including the stomach and intestines. This thoracic duct moves upward through the thorax, picking up lymph vessels from the ribs (intercostal areas), then moves to the left subclavian area (trunk), where it recedes and drains the left upper extremities. The left jugular trunk also drains here, which allows the left side of the head and neck to drain properly. The right side of the head, neck and thorax drain or are connected to the right lymph duct.

As the lymph flows through the lymph vessels toward the subclavian veins, it passes through the lymph nodes, which contain macrophages to phagocytize (consume and destroy) bacteria or other pathogens (antigens). As the lymph fluid is cleaned, neutralized and filtered, it re-enters the blood stream at the internal jugular and the right and left subclavian blood veins.

Lymph Nodes

You have thousands of small septic tanks called lymph nodes throughout your body. Your lymph nodes are bean-shaped holding tanks, or "septic tanks," that are used by your lymph system to filter, neutralize, bond and destroy pathogens (toxins), antigens, etc. They consist of a fibrin net, which serves as a filter for lymph cells. Lymph nodes range in size—from that of a small penny to almost the size of a quarter. The lymph nodes consist of:

- Lymphocytes (including T and B cells)
- Neutrophils
- Plasma cells
- Macrophages (large amounts)
- Antigens
- Antibody molecules

The main network, or grouping, of lymph nodes are in the:

- Neck, upper shoulder and chest area. These serve as filters for the head area (cervical nodes)
- Axilla (arm pits), which filter the thoracic (chest) areas and upper extremities (axillary nodes)
- Groin area for pelvis and legs (lower extremities, inguinal nodes)
- Mesentery or abdominal area (filters the gastrointestinal tract)

When the lymph system becomes overburdened with toxins, parasites, weakened cells from acidosis, mucus, metabolic wastes, etc., your lymph nodes will become enlarged and swollen. Your tonsils are an excellent example of this. Dairy products and refined sugars cause a lot of mucus production from the mucosa, which in turn causes congestive problems (including sinus, throat, bronchi and lungs, etc.). When the tonsils swell from this massive overload, sore throats, inflammation and mucus discharge are some of the symptoms. Colds and flu are another symptom of congestion needing to come out.

When doctors remove tonsils because of a lack of understanding about congestion and the lymphatic system, it sets up a chain reaction. Removing the tonsils causes a burden in the lymphatic system (in the surrounding tissues). This then leads to stiff necks, cervical spine deterioration, pressure build-up in the brain, ears, eyes (glaucoma), etc. Most doctors do not know how to aid the body in ridding itself of this congestion.

Detoxification is the only true answer to this problem. Tissue removal and the treatment of symptoms with sulfa drugs (antibiotics) only add to the problem.

Spleen

Your spleen is an oval-shaped, semi-dark red organ. It is located on your left side (upper left quadrant), to the left of and behind (posterior to) the stomach.

In the embryo stages, the spleen served as a red- and white-blood-cell creator. However, shortly after birth, the spleen produced only lymphocytes and monocytes (WBCs). The spleen is full of the type of lymphocytes called macrophages, which remove pathogens and toxins of all kinds from the blood and lymph.

The spleen acts as a blood reservoir or holding tank where blood is stored for emergencies. The spleen also destroys weakened, toxic and old blood cells, creating bilirubin from their hemoglobin. Bilirubin gives bile its unique color.

Keeping your spleen healthy helps to keep your immune, lymphatic and blood systems healthy. In spiritual circles, the spleen reflects the lower mind (called the "causal mind"), where duality or creation truly starts. Your spleen is the vehicle for the universal mathematics that affect your physical body. Its spiritual color is orange.

Thymus Gland

The thymus gland will be covered later in this chapter, under the Endocrine System. However, it is enough to say that it is a gland that matures and trains B-cells, converting them into T- and helper T-cells, which are a part of your NK (natural killer) cells. These are for cellular-mediated response to pathogens.

Summary: The Lymphatic System

The physical body is a city unto itself. Your immune and lymphatic systems act like a police force and sanitation department, all wrapped into one. The lymphatic system picks up the trash from each house in the city (each cell); trash will vary, of course, depending upon the "lifestyle" within each house/cell. The lymph system, along with its immune cells, has the job of protecting and keeping your body clean.

Many foods that people routinely eat clog and over-burden the lymphatic system. Colds, flu, allergies, sinus congestion, bronchitis, lung issues—including pneumonia and asthma (with adrenal weakness)—along with mumps, tumors, boils, lymphomas, skin rashes, dandruff, etc., are nothing more than an over-burdened, congested lymph system.

All dairy products (pasteurized or raw), refined carbohydrates (complex sugars), irritants (peppers, cola, etc.), toxic chemicals, foreign protein (meat, etc.) cause a lymphatic response of the mucosa, namely excessive mucus production. Furthermore, these substances can be harmful to cells, especially inviting parasitic invasion. Your lymphatic system's job is to try to stop this "terrorist" attack within the tissues of the body. However, once the body becomes over-bombarded with this mucus from the lymph system, the mucus itself then becomes the problem. It can block proper cellular function, causing hypoactivity of the respective organ or gland.

Again, an example of this response is seen in the body's reaction to dairy foods. Their proteins are so abrasive, concentrated and harmful to us that ingesting them creates excessive mucus production. It creates such a chain reaction that you can feel this mucus building up in your sinus cavities, throat and lungs. This causes you to lose your sense of smell, taste and hearing, and impedes your breathing. It also congests your thyroid gland, eventually affecting your whole body in a multitude of ways. It's ironic that we drink milk for calcium when its effects can lead to the body's inability to utilize calcium.

Spiritually speaking, your blood and lymph system is a reflection of spirit. It enhances and nourishes you, but it also cleans and educates you. If it becomes "bottled up" or stagnant, you become bottled up and stagnant. Disease sets in and death can occur.

Clean and open all the pathways within yourself and let spirit (blood and lymph) flow through you unobstructed. This will bring a sense of well-being that's unimaginable.

THE IMMUNE SYSTEM

Your immune system is the police force of your body. It offers protection from invaders (parasites) and toxins. Without your immune system, you would not be able to live on this planet. (Remember the "boy in the bubble" who had no immune system?)

Two Types of Immune Systems

You have two types of immune systems at work. They are the **extracellular immune system** and the **intracellular immune system**.

EXTRACELLULAR IMMUNE SYSTEM—Extracellular immunity protects your internal organs, glands, and tissues. It protects conditions outside of a cell. This type of immunity has been called many names, including "adaptive," "innate," "humoral" or "antibody-mediated" immunity. However, they are really all the same type, mechanically.

Simply put, extracellular immunity starts at conception with the memories genetically passed to cells from the parents, which set the immunity patterns for the child.

This type of immunity is truly adaptive, as your immune system has a mind like you do. It can comprehend, remember, and supply protection from invaders and toxins on a day-to-day basis, creating immunity. It "trains" itself to be ready the next time a similar invasion takes place. This is the beauty of God at work.

INTRACELLULARIMMUNESYSTEM—Intracellular immunity exists inside the cell. This is called "cell-mediated immunity." This type of immunity involves T-cell response to chemicals released by the cell itself.

Immune Cell Response

Each of these two systems of protection (the extracellular and the intracellular) offers a specific type of response.

EXTRACELLULAR RESPONSE — Antibody (humoral) immune response consists of plasma B-cell lymphocytes, which are produced in response to destructive antigens with subsequent antibody formation. This type of response generally creates immunity to the particular type of antigen and is considered an extracellular response.

INTRACELLULAR RESPONSE — Cell-mediated immune response (cellular response) is the production of T-cells by the thymus gland in response to foreign antigens that need to be removed. This is an intracellular immune response.

Your immune system will respond in one of two ways, depending upon the above. The first or **primary response (reaction)** is the initial reaction to an invader. This is a slow, but thorough, response in which T- and B-lymphocyte antibodies are created to attach to the invading or spreading pathogens (microorganisms).

The **secondary response (reaction)** is the immediate response by T- and B-memory cells, which have done battle before with this particular antigen or pathogen. Now these cells can seek out and destroy known invaders, because they are familiar with them and know how to destroy them.

Both of the above responses are designed to neutralize or eliminate destructive cells or pathogens (toxins and parasites). They are determined by the need for either a **non-specific immune response or a specific immune response.**

- *Non-specific Immune Response* — (Inflammation) The response of the tissues and cells to an injury from any source. These sources include chemicals, trauma, invading organisms, etc.

- *Specific Immune Response* — A much stronger response, which takes place when inflammation is not strong enough, or is inadequate to handle the injury or invasion. This response falls directly under T- and B-cell control.

At the bottom line, your immune system rids itself of unwanted invaders in two ways, **phagocytosis** and **inflammation.** Inflammation can be local (cellular) or systemic (in many places throughout the body).

PHAGOCYTOSIS — The ingestion, neutralization or destruction of foreign substances, including microorganisms, their parts, toxins, as well as dead or weakened body cells, and parasitically invaded cells. Cells that create phagocytosis are called **phagocytes. Neutrophils** and **macrophages** make up the bulk of these types of cells.

INFLAMMATION —

- *Local Inflammation* is confined to a specific area. Redness, swelling and heat are experienced from the dilation of the vascular (blood) system. Pain can result in these areas from the swelling and chemical reaction on nerve receptors.

- *Systemic Inflammation* oftentimes goes unnoticed until destruction occurs. Hormone imbalances, high acid-forming diets and heavy chemical ingestion through foods, air and cosmetics create this type of inflammation. Most of the time, this inflammation goes unnoticed until you begin to experience hypoactivity of tissues, glands and organs. As your glands fail to do their job, this creates a domino effect, causing many disease symptoms.

As previously stated, the lymphatic and immune systems work hand-in-hand as if they were one system. The lymphatic tissues, organs and physiological processes are involved in identifying, transporting and eliminating **antigens** or **pathogens**. This system is also responsible for producing the immune response.

There are basically **two lines of defense** that your body has to protect itself from foreign substances, including unwanted microorganisms. They are **mechanical (structural defenses)** and **chemical (mediated defenses)**.

MECHANICAL DEFENSES (STRUCTURAL) — Skin, mucous membrane, tears, saliva, stomach acids, urine. Site-specific protection is affected by the "mucosa immunity system" of the mucosa of the respiratory, genitourinary, and gastrointestinal lining, which have clusters of lymphoid cells, including lymphocytes and macrophages.

CHEMICAL DEFENSES (MEDIATORS) — These chemical catalysts are substances your body uses to bring about an innate immune response. Some chemicals form barriers in the cell membrane wall to stop invasion by parasites. Cells also produce enzymes called lysosomes, which are designed to digest or kill parasitic invaders.

- *Lysozyme* — (enzymes) in tears, sweat and saliva kills various microorganisms.

- *Mucus* — produced by the mucous membrane, coats and supplies WBCs that are designed to phagocytize, neutralize or destroy antigens and pathogens.

- *Histamine* — chemicals (which are released from microorganisms or damaged cells) that attract leukocytes (white blood cells) for emergency aid.

- *Prostaglandins* — a biologically active, carbon-20-based unsaturated fatty acid, metabolized from arachidonic acid. Prostaglandins have a multitude of functions, including vasodilatation and glucose metabolism. They are mediators of many chemical processes.

- *Leukotrienes* — promote inflammation by dilation of the vascular system (capillaries, etc.). They also increase vascular permeability (the ability to secrete blood, nutrition and immune cells through the walls of the capillaries, etc.). Vascular permeability allows fibrinogen and proteins to enter the lymph fluids around a cell. Fibrinogen is converted to fibrin, which is then used to block off the affected areas. Leukotrienes also stimulate phagocytosis by macrophages, as well as attract WBCs for emergency aid.

- *Interferons* — a type of protein that protects cells from viral invasion. They attach themselves to cell walls, and stimulate that cell's production of antiviral properties (proteins).

- *Kinins* — attract WBCs.

- *Complement* — a group of proteins (complement proteins) known to attract WBCs.

To understand autoimmune conditions, let's examine your internal immune system further.

As you have learned, your internal immune system is designed to eliminate weak and parasitically involved cells. Cells have "markers" (antigens) on their surfaces which identify them for what they are. These markers identify them as either a "self" or "non-self" type of cell.

Antigens

Antigens are substances that create an immune response. Antigens are proteins or oligosaccharides (compounds made up of a saccharide). There are two types of antigens: **self-antigens** and **foreign antigens**.

SELF-ANTIGENS — Substances (proteins, etc.) created by your cells to stimulate an immune response. These types of antigens generally are part of a cell membrane wall and act as "markers" or signals for immune cell response. These types of antigens have also been called **auto-antigens**.

FOREIGN ANTIGENS — Substances or parasites that are introduced into the body from the outside world. These include:

- Microorganisms
- Particles (fragments) of microorganisms
- Acids
- Chemicals of all types
- Proteins that are foreign or unusable by the body
- Splinters, wood, glass, etc.

Every single thing in creation is unique. However, there are numerous similarities. Our planet is home to many different races of humans and species of plants and animals, each type identified by various shapes, colorings and markings. The same is true of your cells and their membrane walls (their outer skin), and each cell is unique unto itself.

Cell walls are composed of proteins (chained amino acids), cholesterol (inflammation protection) and phospholipids. When a cell becomes weakened, these proteins and antigens change, which sends a signal for the cell's destruction. The outer body or cell wall changes, just as your skin changes when the cells that comprise it begin to fail.

Immune Cell Response to Antigens (B-Cell Response)

LYMPHOCYTES — To activate a specific immune response, your lymphocytes must be activated. This activation is triggered by an antigen (a signal). Lymphocytes have antigen-binding receptors on their surfaces. These receptors are specific in nature and are designed to bind specific antigens.

INTERLEUKINS — Interleukins, which are produced and released by macrophages and helper T-cells, stimulate lymphocytes to divide after antigens are captured (bound) to the lymphocyte (immune cell). Then:

- The antigen is processed (neutralized and broken down) by macrophages and B-cells.

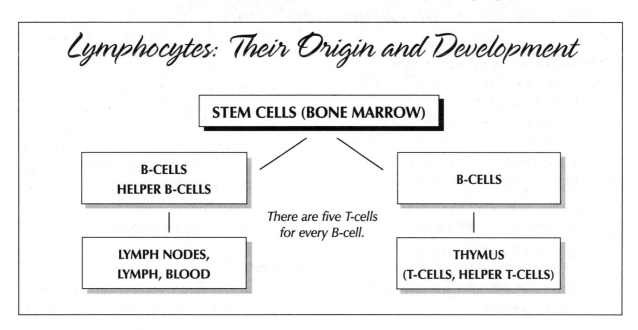

Lymphocytes: Their Origin and Development

STEM CELLS (BONE MARROW)

B-CELLS
HELPER B-CELLS

LYMPH NODES,
LYMPH, BLOOD

There are five T-cells for every B-cell.

B-CELLS

THYMUS
(T-CELLS, HELPER T-CELLS)

- Macrophages present the processed antigen to helper T-cells. Interleukin is released, causing helper T-cells to divide, thus increasing their numbers.
- Helper T-cells combine with the B-cells (that originally processed the antigen), resulting in the formation of cells that produce antibodies against the antigen.

Role of Protein "Markers"

- Identify a cell for type and health (strong and weak).
- Stimulate the production of antibodies by B-lymphocytes to neutralize or destroy the cell.
- Stimulate cytotoxic (chemicals that destroy cells) responses by granulocytes, monocytes, and lymphocytes.

Normal body cells that become damaged or weakened can appear as foreign antigens, inviting an immune response by macrophages, neutrophils, monocytes, etc. This stimulates the production of antibodies by B-lymphocytes to neutralize or destroy the cell if needed. As noted, it also stimulates cytotoxic responses by granulocytes, monocytes and lymphocytes.

This is where the "autoimmune" illusion is first created. When a cell changes its morphology through acidosis, toxic chemical influence, etc., this changes its signal to immune cells (the police), which are now considered foreign antigens or cells that can affect other cells and thus need to be eliminated.

Antibody-Mediated Response

ANTIBODIES — When your body is exposed to an antigen (parasites, toxins, etc.), it activates B-cells, which produce antibodies. These antibodies bind to the antigens and in the process destroy the toxins. Antibodies are found in your body fluids. This is why this type of immunity is called extracellular (outside of the body) immunity. Antibodies can bind to macrophages, basophils and mast cells.

Antibodies are y-shaped **glycoproteins** produced by B-lymphocytes (B-cells) in response to the presence of antigens. Each antibody consists of four polypeptide (two or more amino acids)

Basic Antibodies or Immunoglobulins

ANTIBODY	%	FUNCTION
1gG	80% +	Inactivates/deactivates, or binds antigens together; increases phagocytes; provides immune protection for the fetus; detects complements (proteins).
1gM	10%	Binds antigens together; acts as a binding receptor on B-cells; activates complements. Often first antibody by antigen response.
1gA	15%	Inactivates antigens. Found in saliva, tears, and in mucous membranes. Offers protection on the skin. Also found in colostrum and breast milk.
1gE	1%	Bound to mast cells and basophils to stimulate inflammation.
1gD	1%	Acts as a binding receptor on B-cells.

chains, which create the binding sites for antigen adhesion. They are considered **immunoglobulins** (consisting of many different antibodies). Almost all of your antibodies, except your naturally inherited ones (based on blood types), are created by B-cells bonding with a foreign antigen.

Antibodies are called **gamma globulins**. Large amounts of these are found in plasma (blood) where other proteins, like albumin, etc., exist. Antibodies are also called immunoglobulins (IQ), because they are globulin proteins involved in immunity.

PRIMARY RESPONSE — (takes 3-14 days)

• B-cells are activated by antigen(s).

• B-cells multiply and create B-memory cells. These cells produce antibodies (y-shaped proteins).

SECONDARY RESPONSE — (hours to 3 days)

• Occurs when the body is exposed to familiar antigens. These are antigens that the body has previously battled with and recognizes. These antigens therefore create immediate B-cell response from B-memory cells.

• This rapid response creates even more B-memory cells, therefore increasing further immunity. Memory cells are the basis for adaptive immunity.

ANTIBODIES NEUTRALIZE OR DESTROY ANTIGENS BY:

• initiating lysis (rupturing and breaking down the invader).

• neutralizing toxins of bacterial activity.

• phagocytosis (ingesting, neutralizing and destroying).

• promoting antigen-clumping (agglutination).

• preventing the antigen from adhering to a host cell.

ANTIBODIES DIRECTLY OR INDIRECTLY . . .

• detect antigens or bind them together.

• increase phagocytosis.

• increase inflammation.

• activate complement proteins.

Cell-Mediated Immunity

Cell-mediated immunity refers to T-cell protection of your cells. T-cells protect the inside or intercellular spaces of cells from microorganisms like viruses and some bacteria. T-cells, like B-cells, have antigen-binding receptors on their surfaces, and are very adept at recognizing cellular antigens.

PRIMARY RESPONSE — Antigens activate T-cells, which then begin to divide and create cytotoxin (cytolytic) T-cells. Cytotoxic T-cells produce cytokines, or lymphokines, which are proteins (peptides) that stimulate additional immune response by increasing T-cell formation, macrophage involvement, etc.

T-cells cannot recognize foreign antigens without the help of macrophage processing. This helps a T-cell differentiate between types of antigens. Helper T-cells (called T4s) secrete

Macrophage Processing

PHASE ONE

• Macrophages ingest antigens by endocytosis and break them down into several small pieces.

• Each piece is "stamped" with a protein (major histo-compatibility [MHC] proteins).

• Now these pieces of antigens are ready to bond with helper T-cells.

• B-cell phagocytosis is similar to macrophage phagocytosis.

PHASE TWO

• Macrophage and B-cells process antigens.

• Macrophages secrete interleukin-1.

• Interleukin stimulates helper T-cells to produce interleukin-2.

• Interleukin stimulates helper T-cells to divide.

• Helper T-cells stimulate B-cells.

White Blood Cells

Neutrophils

Definition: Phagocytizes microorganisms and other substances

% of WBCs: 60–80%

Response: Inflammation response

Site of maturation: Red bone marrow

Location of mature cells: Blood, connective and lymphatic tissue

Secretes: Histamine, complement proteins, leukotrienes, kinins and interferon

Type of immunity: Innate (from birth)

Lymphocytes (B-Cells)

Definition: Produces antibodies and other chemicals responsible for destroying microorganisms

% of WBCs: 20–40%

Response: Extracellular (outside) protection from antigens (viruses, bacterial, chemical)

Site of maturation: Red bone marrow, spleen, lymph nodes

Location of mature cells: Blood and lymphatic tissues and nodes

Secretes: Antibodies

Type of immunity: Antibody-mediated

Lymphocytes (T-Cells)

Definition: Produces antibodies and other chemicals responsible for destroying microorganisms

% of WBCs: 0–40%

Response: Intracellular (inside) protection from antigens (parasites, tumors); also known as tumor busters

Site of maturation: Red bone marrow, spleen, lymph nodes

Location of mature cells: Thymus gland

Secretes: Tissues

Type of immunity: Cell-mediated

Eosinophils

Definition: Releases chemicals that reduce inflammation, attacks certain worm-type parasites

% of WBCs: 1–4%

Response: Inflammation response

Site of maturation: Red bone marrow

Location of mature cells: Blood, connective tissues, and lymphatic tissue

Secretes: Histamine, complement proteins, leukotrienes, kinins and interferon

Type of immunity: Innate

Basophils

Definition: Releases histamine, which promotes inflammation; also releases heparin, which prevents clot formation

% of WBCs: 0.5–1%

Response: Inflammation response

Site of maturation: Red bone marrow

Location of mature cells: Blood, connective and lymphatic tissue

Secretes: Histamine, complement proteins, leukotrienes, kinins and interferon

Type of immunity: Innate

Monocytes (Macrophages)

Definition: Phagocytic cell in the blood that becomes a macrophage within tissues, which phagocytizes bacteria, cell fragments, dead cells, weak cells, and other toxins within tissues

% of WBCs: 3–8%

Response: Phagocytosis

Site of maturation: Various tissues of the body

Location of mature cells: Blood, connective and lymphatic tissue

Secretes: Enzymes, lysomes, chemokines, cytokines, O_2 radicals

Type of immunity: Innate

Mast Cells

Definition: Essential to inflammatory response found in connective tissue, under the skin, and in the mucosa of the GI tract and respiratory tissues. Helps promote inflammation through the release of various chemicals. They are mediated by 1gE.

% of WBCs: 0%

Response: Inflammation

Site of maturation: Various tissues within the body

Location of mature cells: Connective tissue, skin, mucosa, and gastrointestinal tissues

Secretes: Histamine, proteinases, prostaglandins, leukotrienes, kinins, interferon, complements

Type of immunity: Innate

interleukin, which stimulates B-cell activity and other T-lymphocytes.

SECONDARY RESPONSE — Your secondary T-cell response comes from T-memory cells. Your T-memory cells work like your B-memory cells in that they "remember" past exposure to antigens and have created "antibodies" to fight them.

Creation of Immune Cells

WHITE BLOOD CELLS (WBCs) — Your immune cells are called white blood cells (WBCs), of which there are many types. Your bone marrow produces your white blood cells as the body's primary internal defense. These cells are then sent through the lymph system to mature or to be converted into larger and more specific cells.

Lymphatic tissues, including the spleen, thymus gland and lymph nodes, are responsible for the growth, maturation and activation of your white blood cells. The growth and function of immune cells are regulated by cytokines, which are protein in nature and act as growth mediators. There are over 100 different types of cytokines produced by your WBCs. These include your interleukins, interferons, tumor necrosis factor, etc.

Let's examine some of the most important immune cells that your body uses to defend itself. **Macrophages** are **monocytes** that have left circulation and have settled and matured in tissues. Macrophages are found in large numbers in the tonsils, spleen, and lymph nodes. Fifty percent or more of the body's macrophages are found in the liver and are called Kupffer cells. However, they are found everywhere, including the brain and blood. They act as scavengers, cleaning as they go. Macrophages and neutrophils are the master phagocytic (ingesting and destroying) cells of your immune system.

Natural killer (NK) cells are a type of lymphocyte processed in the bone marrow, which accounts for 1-5 percent of all lymphocytes. They are considered the masters of the immune

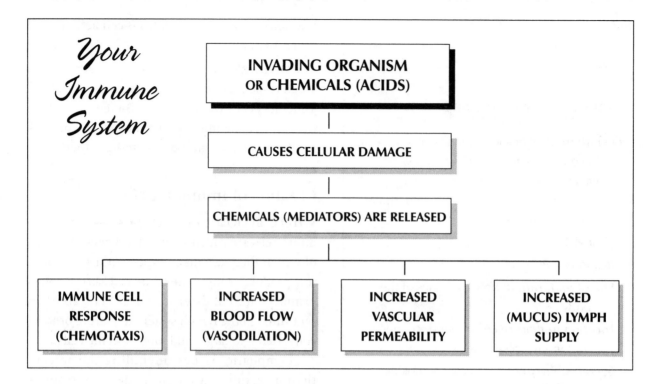

Your Immune System

INVADING ORGANISM OR CHEMICALS (ACIDS)

CAUSES CELLULAR DAMAGE

CHEMICALS (MEDIATORS) ARE RELEASED

IMMUNE CELL RESPONSE (CHEMOTAXIS)

INCREASED BLOOD FLOW (VASODILATION)

INCREASED VASCULAR PERMEABILITY

INCREASED (MUCUS) LYMPH SUPPLY

cells. Their job is to destroy tumor or virus-infected cells. These are a part of your innate immunity because they do not respond to memory, and are not specific in their response. They only recognize a specific class, not a specific type of cell.

Summary: The Immune System

Your body is naturally designed to protect itself from invaders, including parasitic, chemical, etc. Even foods that are harmful when ingested set up an immune and lymphatic response.

Your body as a whole and each cell that comprises it has awareness (consciousness). Your immune system teaches itself to recognize past invaders and stores this information in memory cells. This takes place from conception (memories from parents) and continues on through your exposure to the outside world. Your body and its organs are covered with "skin" or a membrane that is designed to protect it initially (mechanically). From here, immunological (immune) cells and their chemicals are designed to "eat" or destroy these invaders in one way or another.

There are many different types of immune cells, each with its own specific area of expertise. We have and develop our immunity from the following:

• *Active natural* — (nature) one's own innate and adaptive immune response.

• *Active artificial* — (vaccination) immunity created by artificially supplying a pathogen or antigen, so the body can create immunity from the supplied source.

• *Passive natural* — mother to fetus through the placenta. Transferred to a non-immune individual.

• *Passive artificial* — transferred from injected (vaccinated) animals to humans.

Nature does not procreate the weak. If it did, nature would not withstand itself. This is true of your body and the cells that comprise it.

Autoimmune syndromes are nothing more than the strong eliminating the weak. With this in mind, the best course of action in "diseases" or conditions of hypoactivity or weakness is always to strengthen, strengthen and strengthen yourself and your cells. Clean your body of all the chemicals, toxins, pus, stored mucus and parasites (the harmful variety) and get healthy!

INTESTINAL SYSTEM (COLON)

The large intestines, or what is called the colon, are composed of **six sections**. They are the **cecum, ascending, transverse, descending, sigmoid** and finally the **rectum**. The average colon is from five to six feet long. The colon is shaped in somewhat of an upside-down U-shape, extending around the perimeters of your abdomen. It is also made up of circular folds. The colon mainly absorbs water, trace and microtrace minerals, and vitamins.

No digestive enzymes are secreted by the colon. However, some digestion takes place from bacteria. Your food particles and by-products from digestion in the stomach and small intestines are mixed together in the colon, and most of the water is reabsorbed so that a solid mass is formed for elimination from the body. Mucus from the lymphatic system is also dumped into the colon for elimination. The colon has mucus-secreting glands in the sub-mucosa to assist in proper elimination, as well.

The colon has an electrical relationship to all of the major organs and tissues of the body. The contemporary scientific community has not yet discovered this part of the physiology of the colon (or for that matter, the entire intestinal gut tissue and its relationship to all the other tissues of the body).

URINARY SYSTEM

Kidneys

Generally humans have two kidneys. However, I have seen many people who were born with three. Your kidneys are shaped like an ear and are purplish-brown in color. They are situated at the back of the abdominal cavity, one on each side (lateral) of the spine.

The tops of the kidneys are opposite the 12th thoracic vertebra. They weigh approximately 5 ounces each, and are about 4.5 inches long, 3 inches wide, and 1 inch thick. Microscopic nephrons make up the structural and functional aspects of the kidneys.

As in most organs, and especially in glands, you find an outer portion—called the cortex and an inner portion—the medulla. Urine is formed in the nephrons, which are made up of a renal corpuscle and a venal tubule. These look like long pyramids. The cortex (outer) portion of the kidney houses most of the small capillary beds that are the filtering tissue between the blood and the nephron. This area is involved in filtration and reabsorption.

Urine consists of many by-products of metabolism, like ureas, ammonia, hydrogen ions, creatinine, chemical toxins, medications, synthetic vitamins, and minerals, etc.

These wastes (urine) travel down this pyramid (nephron tubules) into the inner portion (or medulla), where they enter into common ducts called papillary ducts, which empty into the kidney reservoirs (calyces). From here the urine moves down through the ureter to the bladder.

As you can see, the kidneys are a part of your elimination system. They form urine from blood plasma. They play a major role in the regulation of your blood, and thus all bodily fluids. They help eliminate your metabolic and toxic wastes.

Kidneys are very sensitive to acidosis from meats, teas, coffees, chocolates and carbonated soda drinks. Most people consume these types of "foods" (toxins) that, after a while, yield them discomfort and pain in the mid- to lower back.

Ureters

Tubes from your kidneys to the bladder.

Bladder

Your bladder is mainly a holding, collecting tank, or sac, for urine on its way out from the kidneys.

The elimination of urine from the bladder is called "micturition," "voiding" or "urination."

Urethra

The tube that leads from the bladder to the outside of your body.

INTEGUMENTARY SYSTEM (SKIN)

Your skin is the largest organ of the body. It is also the largest eliminative organ, eliminating as much bodily wastes each day as your kidneys, bowels and lungs. The skin is obviously your body's outer covering. It offers protection from the outer environment and parasitic conditions.

Your skin has two major divisions, or separate layers. The first division is the beginning, or first innermost, layer and is called the dermis. The subcutaneous tissues lay just below the dermis, which houses the bulk of the main arteries, veins, nerves and glands that feed the skin.

The second gland division or layer is the epidermis, or outermost portion. This portion (or division) has four to five different layers, depending upon the location. Your hands and feet have thick skin because of the activity these portions encounter. You've heard the sayings, "He has thick skin," or "She has thin skin." Now you know where this reference comes from. The following is a quick rundown of the epidermis, starting with the outermost layer of your skin.

- stratum corneum (a few cells to 50 cells deep)
- stratum lucidum
- stratum granulosum
- stratum spinosum
- stratum germinativum

Your skin consists of cells that are called keratinocytes, because they create a hard substance called keratin, which is found in your finger nails, hair and any horny tissue. Keratinocytes are germinated (begin their journey) in the stratum germinativum layers of the epidermis, moving and maturing through the various layers until they reach their final days in the outermost layer, the stratum corneum.

Your skin has many functions, including the regulation of body temperature. This is accomplished through the arterioles (blood vessels) and sweat glands. The skin is also the largest sensory organ, expressing both internal and external sensations.

Spiritually speaking, your skin is tied to your ego, or ethnic body. It gives you individuality. It is tied to your liver, which reflects the mind. Both work hand-in-hand, affecting the thought processes of the individual.

In detoxification, always clean out the liver to clean the skin. Always keep your skin clean, as this will serve its function as one of your eliminative organs. Besides, clean skin makes you feel clean.

Disease is not the presence of something evil, but rather the lack of the presence of something essential.

— Dr. Bernard Jensen

☀ The Endocrine Glandular System

The Endocrine Glandular System is the most overlooked system in the body, even though it is the "master computer" of your body. It tells your cells what to do, and how much to function, through the release of hormones like steroids, neurotransmitters, serotonins, enzymes and the like.

Basically, you have two types of glands: (1) **endocrine glands**, which are ductless glands that produce internal secretions (hormones, etc.), and discharge these directly into the blood or lymph system to be circulated throughout the body; and (2) **exocrine glands**, like the salivary glands, which produce external secretions that then reach your epithelial cells directly, or through a duct. It is difficult to say which is the most important gland we have because all tissues in the body are interrelated. However, approximately 75 percent of all "disease" symptoms can be attributed to the failure of the endocrine gland system. This can include a lack of proper calcium utilization, causing scoliosis, depression, connective tissue weaknesses, varicose veins, hemorrhoids, hernias and aneurysms, as well as lower steroid production that leads to fibrocystic issues, fibromyalgia, fibroids, cysts, cholesterol plaquing and other conditions.

Your principal endocrine glands are the adrenal glands, pancreas, thymus, thyroid/parathyroid, the testes, ovaries and the great master gland, the pituitary. Up until the last ten to twenty-five years, we mostly found chronic and/or degenerative conditions in the elderly from the failure of these glands. Today, because of our lifestyles, diets, and especially because of genetic weaknesses, these glands have become weakened to the point where even infants have chronic and

degenerative conditions. Let's examine each of your endocrine glands and their functions.

PITUITARY GLAND

The pituitary is the "master gland" one of the main computers of the body. It releases hormone-like substances that stimulate other endocrine glands and tissues to produce or release specific hormones, steroids, neurotransmitters and the like. The structure of the pituitary is divided into two parts: the posterior lobe, which is an outgrowth from part of the brain, and the anterior lobe, being an outgrowth from the pharynx. The pituitary is attached and lives under the hypothalamus portion of your brain (behind the eyes in the middle of the head).

The pituitary, being the master gland, controls some of the functions of most other glands. When the pituitary becomes weakened it can affect the whole body, causing a chain reaction, thereby producing multiple symptoms. The pituitary gland can affect the thyroid or adrenal glands in a positive or negative way. It is important to understand these reflex possibilities to help you address your weaknesses properly and to gain more successful results.

Some of the far-reaching effects of a weakened pituitary gland include neurological weaknesses such as: multiple sclerosis, Parkinson's, and cerebral palsy (from lack of adrenal cortex stimulation), as well as hypothyroidism, hypofunction of the ovaries, underactive or overactive tissue or cell growth, rapid aging, diabetes, and lactation problems.

The middle of the transverse colon (large intestine) has a relationship to the pituitary and brain. Oftentimes this part of the bowel becomes impacted, toxic and weakened, thereby feeding toxins directly to the pituitary gland. Being one of the first areas of the body formed in the embryo stages of life, the GI tract is linked to all tissues in the body in ways we do not yet understand. We do know that in the embryo stages the spinal cord and the gut tissues are the first manifestation from the head area. As the embryo cell opens up, this gut tissue now becomes the source of most of our organs and glands. **This gut tissue in the fetus later becomes the GI tract**, thus creating a dynamic relationship between the GI tract and the rest of the body. Because of this, it is vital that you clean and strengthen the GI tract in your detoxification program, that is, if you wish to have true success at regenerating your glands, as well as your whole body.

PINEAL GLAND

The pineal gland is a small, flattened, cone-shaped gland located behind and just above the eyebrows (connected to the roof of the 3rd ventricle of the brain). Scientific research hasn't revealed much about this endocrine gland as of yet. We know that it synthesizes melatonin, which is a hormone that relaxes you and aids in the sleep process. Melatonin may affect skin and hair pigmentation. Melatonin is inhibited by light striking the retina. The pineal gland is regulated by light (internal and external).

In spiritual circles the pineal gland is called the "third eye," "tisra til," or the "10th door." It is considered the window into the heavens —the eye of heaven—and is a point focused on in meditation.

THYROID AND PARATHYROID GLANDS

The thyroid consists of two lobes in the anterior portion (front) of the neck. The parathyroid consists of four or more small glands on the back of the thyroid.

Since many people choose to consume "cooked" dairy products and refined sugars (highly mucus-forming), they develop congestion throughout the sinus cavities, head area, throat, bronchi and lungs. The thyroid/parathyroid, since it is located in the throat area, also becomes congested and either becomes hyperactive (overactive) or, as in most cases, hypoactive (underactive). From clinical observation, blood tests that show levels of thyroid hormones T4s, T3s and TSHs are very inaccurate at determining thyroid function. I have included the **Basal Temperature Test** in Appendix A because it is a better overall indicator of thyroid function.

The job of the thyroid/parathyroid glands includes increasing and/or decreasing the following: metabolism; the ability of cells to absorb and use glucose; protein metabolism for growth; the use of fats; rate and strength of the heart beat; rate and depth of respiration; and the rate of calcium absorption from blood, intestines, bones and kidneys. The thyroid/parathyroid also has an interrelationship with other glands, not quite understood at this time.

The symptoms of hypothyroidism (low thyroid function) include: bone loss, improper bone growth, brittle and ridged fingernails, hair loss, cold hands and feet, a dislike of cold weather, heart arrhythmias, heart attacks, depression, connective tissue weaknesses, scoliosis of the spine, arthritis, fatigue, slow metabolism, obesity, hot flashes, cramping, spasms, myxedemas and growth issues.

The symptoms of hyperthyroidism (overactive thyroid) include goiter, protruding eyes, hyperactivity, thyrotoxicosis, and excessive-growth issues.

Since the thyroid/parathyroid affects the body's ability to utilize calcium, we find that bone problems, depressive disorders and connective tissue weaknesses can be eliminated by regenerating the thyroid/parathyroid glands. Hyperthyroidism is easy to overcome through detoxification. Never allow any doctor to destroy or remove the thyroid gland because of hyperactivity. The thyroid/parathyroid gland is vital to your well-being in a multitude of ways that greatly affect your quality of life.

THYMUS

The thymus gland consists of two pinkish/gray, flat-looking, symmetrical lobes and is located in the middle of your sternum (mediastinal) in front of (anterior to) and above your heart. Each lobe of the thymus gland has several lobules. However, as in many glands, there is a cortex (outer portion) and a medulla (inner portion). The outer portion is full of lymphoid tissues containing many cells called thymocytes. The medulla has some thymocytes but mostly contains large corpuscles (Hassall's).

The thymus gland is considered the master gland of the immune system. It is large in children, but becomes much smaller with age. Because of diet and lifestyle, the thymus can be almost completely atrophied by the time of old age.

Your thymus gland is essential to the maturation (maturing) of thymic lymphoid cells called T-cells. T-cells are small-to-medium-sized lymphocytes (white blood cells) that are a part of a class of immune cells called NK or natural killer cells. These cells, along with the B-cells (bone marrow cells), are the Marine and Navy Seals of your body's police force. These are vital, as they are the source of cell-mediated immunity, meaning not controlled by antibodies. Cell-mediated immunity is vital in helping the body fight the invasion of molds, yeasts, fungus, bacteria, viruses and the like. Keep your thymus and the rest of your body always healthy. Remember, the strong survive, the weak perish.

ADRENAL GLANDS

An adrenal gland is located on top of each kidney, and, except for the pituitary gland, the adrenal glands are possibly the most important glands in the body. The reason for this is two-fold. First, they produce neurotransmitters, which are essential for brain and nerve function. These neurotransmitters include epinephrine (adrenaline), norepinephrine and dopamine, which affect the sympathetic and parasympathetic nervous system, turning nerve responses on or off. This affects almost all tissues in the body, including the heart, vascular system, intestines, skin and kidneys. The sympathetic and parasympathetic nervous systems comprise the two divisions of the autonomic nervous system (ANS). This system regulates your unconscious (involuntary) tissue actions like pupil dilation and constriction, heartbeat and breathing.

Low blood pressure (systolic under 118) is always an indicator of adrenal weakness, and at least 50 percent of high blood pressure cases reflect adrenal (medulla) weakness as well. **A healthy blood pressure is 120–130 systolic (top number) over 60–70 diastolic (bottom number).** Long-term effects of adrenal medulla weakness include, but are not limited to: asthma, multiple sclerosis, Parkinson's, cerebral palsy, panic attacks, shyness and impatience.

The second reason for the importance of the adrenal glands is the cortex (or outer portion) that produces cortical-type steroids or hormones. These hormones include glucocorticoids (cortisol and cortisone for carbohydrate utilization); aldosterone (regulating our electrolytes, sodium and potassium); estradiol (an estrogen); and progestins (including progesterone). Many of these steroids act as anti-inflammatory compounds, which are vital to combating inflammatory processes within the body. These steroids affect muscle, nerve, gastrointestinal and cardiovascular tissues.

Cortisol, for example, is a catabolic hormone (steroid) that initiates change and activates breakdown. Cortisol also aids in the conversion of fat and protein to glucose. Cortisol is one of the adrenal gland's (glucocorticoid) steroids that mediates inflammation. Catabolic (breakdown) processes in the body generally cause acidosis, hence inflammation. This process can produce a great amount of inflammation and tissue damage. This damage stimulates the adrenal glands to increase cortisol production, which can cause further inflammation.

Also, excess production of cortisol from the adrenal glands can affect blood pressure by increasing or reducing the loss of sodium in the urine, because cortisol increases protein breakdown and decreases protein synthesis. It affects all the other tissues in the body. Especially hard hit is your muscle tissue. All this is initiated by acidosis and heads one down the road to disease and degeneration. It affects the aging of the skin, promotes osteoporosis by reducing TSHs, which reduces the production of thyroid hormone, which eventually leads to hypothyroidism. Remember, the thyroid gland is responsible for the body's calcium utilization. Caffeine, soda, and tea can also enhance the production of excessive cortisol.

All these steroid-type hormones are synthesized from cholesterol, which also acts like or is used by the body as an anti-inflammatory agent or lipid. All things happen for a reason. If your cholesterol is building up on vascular walls or in tissues, what does that tell you? Remember that cholesterol is an anti-inflammatory agent or lipid. If it is building up in your body, or if your liver is producing too much of it, this tells you that you have too much inflammation in your body.

Since most people choose to eat a predominantly acid-forming diet, over-acidic (acidosis) conditions of the body (both systemic and cellular) begin to take place. Acidosis and inflammation are virtually the same thing. Added to acidic diets are the acid-type hormones. Females produce testosterone and a lot of estrogen, which are acid-type hormones. Each month ovarian estrogen is produced in large amounts, which breaks down the inner lining of the uterine wall, causing the monthly menstruation cycle. Men

Adrenal Gland Weakness

- Low adrenal gland (*medulla*) function causes low blood pressure from insufficient neurotransmitters and starts a process of nerve disorders, breathing problems, and heart arrhythmias.

- Low adrenal gland (*cortex*) function causes insufficient steroid production leading to acidosis and inflammation.

This causes—

IN FEMALES:
- Ovarian cancer, breast cancer, cervial cancer, uterine cancer
- Ovarian cysts
- Conception problems
- Miscarriage problems
- Menstrual bleeding problems
- Uterine fibroids
- Endometriosis
- Fibromyalgia
- Fibrocystic breasts
- Osteoporosis
- Unchecked inflammation

IN MALES:
- Prostate cancer
- Erection problems
- Testosterone dominance
- Prostatitis

IN FEMALES AND MALES:
- Scleroderma
- Bursitis and arthritis
- Spinal and pelvic inflammation
- Lower back weakness
- Sciatica
- Diabetes
- Kidney and bladder weakness

also produce the acidic hormones testosterone and androsterone. These are aggressive-type hormones. They effect many different cellular changes from the breakdown of tissue to the increased growth of tissue . . . all types of tissue, from hair (pubic, facial, etc.) to muscle tissue. These hormones affect sexual behavior, increase blood flow and cause erections. These acid-type hormones in men and women are naturally counterbalanced by the body with the production of progesterone and other steroids, which are anti-inflammatory and produced in the adrenal glands. When these acid-type hormones are over-produced, or not balanced by steroids, they can cause inflammation in tissues.

You can begin to see how inflammation is developed in the body through diet and hormone imbalance (from glandular weaknesses). This inflammation leads to tissue failure and death. This is why it is essential that our endocrine gland system functions properly and remains in balance. When the endocrine glands become hypo- (under) or hyper- (over) active, this creates many disease symptoms.

As you can see, when inflammation goes unchecked by proper steroid activity, this inflammation begins to harden and destroy tissue. Long-term inflammation leads to devastation of tissues, leading to tissue (cellular) death.

Another extremely important factor, as previously stated, is the inflammation in the vascular system (vasculitis, phlebitis, etc.) from over-acidic diets. When the adrenals do not produce enough steroids to fight the inflammation, we find that the body will use cholesterol directly. This causes our vascular system to become occluded (blocked) from plaqued cholesterol.

PANCREAS

(Also see The Digestive System, previously covered in Module 2.6)

Your pancreas is both an endocrine and an exocrine gland, meaning that it produces hormones (insulin) that are secreted directly into the blood (endocrine), and other substances (enzymes, etc.) that are secreted by ducts (exocrine).

- The endocrine portion consists of cells called **islets of Langerhans**, which secrete various hormone-like substances that assist the body in utilization and energy factors. The various cells that comprise the islets of Langerhans are as follows:

- **Alpha cells** secrete glucagon, which increases blood glucose levels by stimulating the liver to convert stored glycogen to glucose. Glucagon also increases the use of fats and excess amino acids, for use as energy.

- **Beta cells** secrete insulin, which decreases blood glucose levels. Insulin acts as a "driver" that transports glucose through cell membrane walls. It facilitates the conversion of glucose to glycogen and is thought to be involved in amino acid synthesis.

- **Delta cells** secrete somatostatin, which inhibits:
  - the secretion of glucagon
  - the secretion of insulin
  - a growth hormone from the anterior portion of the pituitary gland
  - the secretion of gastrin from the stomach

OVARIES

The ovaries are two almond-shaped glands found in the female of a species. The ovaries have two functions. One is to produce the reproductive cell (ovum) and the other is to produce hormones. In humans, the ovaries are found on each side of the pelvic cavity, each attached to the uterus. Each ovary consists of two parts: the cortex (or outer portion) and the medulla (or inner portion).

The cortex (outer portion) consists of mainly various types of follicles (small sacs). Each follicle (or sac) has an ovum (egg) and a small, yellow endocrine gland (corpus luteum).

This gland (corpus luteum) secretes both estrogen and progesterone. It should be noted that pro-hormones from the adrenal glands are necessary for proper progesterone production in the corpus luteum. The FSH (Follicle Stimulating Hormone) from the hypothalamus induces the

---

Hormones

One of the major problems that you or your healthcare practitioner face is how to make tissues (including organs and glands) respond after they have become hypoactive, especially to the point of chronic or degenerative states. This is a question that all practitioners should ask themselves. The one thing that you do not want to do is to treat the symptoms that are the effect of this underactivity, especially by supplementing the by-product (hormones, enzymes, steroids, neurotransmitters, etc.) that the tissue (gland) makes and provides for your body.

Examples of this are hormones like estrogen (ovarian) or thyroxine (thyroid). When you supplement what your body naturally supplies, you stop that particular tissue from producing it. I learned that when you take synthroid (a synthetic form of thyroxine), it makes your thyroid glands even weaker. This is true of all the hormones, including DHEA, melatonin, etc. You do not want to supply a hormone (or substance) that your body needs to produce. Again, this will shut down your body's ability to produce these substances. This is because your body sees no need to produce these catalysts if they are already present. This eventually makes the respective gland even weaker.

---

release of the ovum (egg). The estrogen-releasing hormone—the LH (Luteinizing Hormone)—comes from the anterior portion of the pituitary gland. Both of these are vital to proper ovulation.

Estrogen is an acid-type hormone that stimulates tissues in many different ways. The most notable way is the stimulating of the inner lining of the uterus to bleed each month, causing menstruation. It is also used for development and maintenance of secondary sexual characteristics, like breast size and shape. Estrogen affects the shape of the female body. A female also produces a form of estrogen in her liver, fat cells and adrenal glands.

Estrogen must always be counterbalanced by a steroid called progesterone. Progesterone is a steroid produced in the ovaries and the adrenal glands. Progesterone needs a pro-hormone, DHEA, produced in the adrenal glands, to be properly produced. Therefore, when the adrenal glands are hypoactive, this can affect the production and release of progesterone, leaving a woman estrogen dominant. This causes a domino effect, creating extensive cellular acidosis, and leads to ovarian cysts, uterine fibroids, fibrocystic issues, female cancers and other conditions.

Always keep your glands healthy, as these are the regulators of most of your bodily functions.

TESTES/TESTICLES (GONADS)

A male has two oval-shaped testicles located in the scrotum. These are the male reproductive glands and are a part of the endocrine gland system. Reproductive cells called spermatozoa are produced in the testes. These glands also produce testosterone and inhibin.

Testosterone is secreted by the interstitial cells called "Cells of Leydig," and inhibin is secreted by the sustentacular cells. It should be said here that testosterone (steroid) is like estrogen in its aggressive nature in creating cellular changes. Progesterone is a cortical-type steroid produced in the adrenal glands that counterbalances estrogen and testosterone, especially when they create inflammation. Testosterone is also produced in the cortex of the adrenal glands of both males and females.

Testosterone accelerates growth and cellular function, as well as stimulates the flow of blood. It has similar characteristics to estrogen in affecting secondary sexual characteristics. It also affects:

- erections
- proper growth and development of male sexual organs
- deepening of the voice
- greater muscle development
- development of pubic, facial and excess body hair
- distribution of fat
- many metabolic relationships

Summary: The Endocrine Glandular System

All of the endocrine glands are vital to the health and well-being of the physical body. It is enough to say that every tissue in your body interacts with every other tissue. This is why we should look at the body as a whole entity, working as one for the well-being of itself. All that it does is for self-survival.

Study and learn about the functions of your endocrine glands. This will help you a great deal. We must learn the ways and secrets of this incredible, conscious machine that can perform like a new car if kept clean and fed properly with the correct building materials and fuels. Look to nature for your answers, not science. Use science to try to fill in what pieces of information you might need to understand how things work.

However, always step back and try to get a picture of your body as a whole and how it would function in nature. There is an old saying that exemplifies this: "Sometimes you can't see the forest for the trees." If you're always looking at the trees, you sometimes miss the beautiful forest. The whole is far greater than its parts (and yet, its parts make up the whole). That is to say, forget what you think you know about health and observe nature and how it works. You will learn a lot more about the truth of things, especially on how to get healthy.

As previously noted, 75 percent of all diseases have an endocrine gland involvement. Through generations of toxic and acid food consumption we have weakened our glandular system to the point of atrophy in many cases.

Most humans do not think of strengthening their cells, so they keep passing down genetically weakened tissue generation after generation. The problem here is that each generation is weaker than the last. Look around and observe the conditions of our children. They're coming into this world with chronic and degenerative glandular weaknesses. No medicine on earth can stop this. Health is the only answer!

As previously stated, your glands are the bosses (or controllers and regulators) of the cells, tissues and organs of the body. When they become hyper- (over) active or hypo- (under) active, it can create many cellular changes. This can have a highly acidic effect upon tissues, leading to lymphatic and immune responses. This is especially true with estrogen, testosterone and aldosterone. Long-term exposure without cortisone and progesterone buffers can lead to fibrocystic conditions of tissues, as well as tissue atrophy (destruction) and cancers.

Glandular Hormones and Their Functions

The following is an overview of your endocrine glands and the hormones, steroids and neurotransmitters they produce. Hormones, steroids and neurotransmitters are the commanders of how, what , where and why certain interactions go on between constituents and cells. They are also catalysts and can act as anti-inflammatories and cellular proliferators. Some are catabolic and affect tissue and nutrient breakdown, while others are anabolic or rebuilding, effecting utilization issues. Learn about your body and how it functions. Keep it simple. Think for yourself and always ask: "Why and what happens if glands fail to do their jobs? What will the effect be?"

Gland	Hormone	Function
Pituitary Anterior-front position	GH (STH)—growth hormone	Increases protein synthesis, blood glucose levels and releases fatty acids from cells. Regulates cell division.
Pituitary Anterior-front position	TSH (TTH)—thyroid-stimulating hormone (Thyrotrophic)	Increases thyroid hormone secretion (thyroxin and triiodothyronine).
Pituitary Anterior-front position	ACTH—adreno-corticotropic hormone	Increases the secretion of glucocorticoids (steroid-type hormones) from the adrenal cortex. Affects skin pigmentation changes, etc.
Pituitary Anterior-front position	MSH—melanocyte-stimulating hormone	Increases melanin production of melanocytes (controls skin color).
Pituitary Anterior-front position	LH—Luteinizing hormone	Promotes ovulation and the secretion of progesterone and estrogen by the corpus luteum in the ovaries.
Pituitary Anterior-front position	LH (ICSH)—Luteinizing hormone	Promotes testosterone synthesis and sperm cell production in the testes.
Pituitary Anterior-front position	FSH—follicle-stimulating hormone	Promotes estrogen secretion in the ovaries. Promotes sperm cell production in testes.
Pituitary Anterior-front position	Prolactin (lactogenic)	Stimulates milk production and secretion.
Pituitary Posterior-back position	ADH—antidiuretic hormone	Increases the reabsorption of water from the kidneys.

GLAND	HORMONE	FUNCTION
Pituitary Posterior-back position	Oxytocin	Increases uterine contractions, milk production and availability from the mammary glands.
Thyroid Gland	Thyroxine (T4) and Triiodothyronine (T3)	Increases metabolic rate (digestive, oxidative, etc.) Affects normal growth and development.
Thyroid Gland	Calcitonin	Affects calcium utilization, preventing bone breakdown (osteoporosis).
Parathyroid Glands	PTH—parathormone	Essential for normal blood calcium levels (increases bone breakdown to maintain blood calcium, phosphorous metabolism, and vitamin D synthesis).
Adrenal Glands Medulla	Neurotransmitters— Epinephrine, Norepinephrine, Dopamine, Acetylcholine	Produces and secretes neurotransmitters, which increases or decreases cardiac output, blood flow to tissues, neuro response, (affects muscular, skeletal and nerve cells). They increase glucose and fatty acid availability in the blood, all to increase systemic and cellular energy.
Adrenal Glands Cortex	Mineralocorticoids (aldosterone)	Regulates electrolytes, increases rate of sodium transport, increases rate of potassium excretion (elimination). Can affect H_2O retention, sweat glands, intestines, and salivary glands.
Adrenal Glands Cortex	Glucocorticoids— cortisol, hydrocortisone, corticosterone	Important in water, muscle, CNS, bone, GI tract, cardiovascular and hematological metabolism. Acting principally on carbo-hydrate metabolism, controls amino acid and fat metabolism. Anti-inflammatory, inhibits immune response.
Adrenal Glands Cortex	Androgens— testosterone, adrenosterone (masculinization)	A masculine steroid, which affects reproduction, increases sex drive and sex characteristics (pubic hair, size, etc.) Catabolic in nature.
Adrenal Glands Cortex	Estrogens—estradiol, estrone (female characteristics)	Induces estrus, develops female sex characteristics. A catabolic steroid that induces tissue changes.

Gland	Hormone	Function
Adrenal Glands Cortex	Progestins—progesterone	Anabolic steroids that aid tissue repair. Anti-inflammatory and antispasmodic in nature. Heavily found in the placenta.
Pancreas	Insulin	Increases cellular transport and use of glucose. Affects sugar, amino acids and fat metabolism. Facilitates conversion of excess glucose to glycogen.
Pineal Gland	Melatonin	Influences sleep/wake cycles, influences the life force within the body. Possibly affects reproduction and pigmentation (melanocytes).
Ovaries	Estrogen—estradiol	Aids in uterine development, cleansing (menstruation) and function, sexual characteristics and behavior.
Ovaries	Progesterone	Used as an anti-inflammatory after menstruation and in the placenta. Also used for tissue repair.
Testes	Androgens—testosterone and inhibin	Sexual characteristics and behavior; aids in sperm cell production. Affects energy and metabolism.
Thymus Gland	Thymosin	Matures and promotes T-cell production.

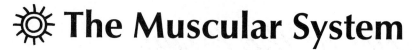 The Muscular System

CONNECTIVE TISSUE

Connective tissue is a strong tissue, composed of collagen (protein) fibers, that forms organs, glands, tissues (muscles), etc. Connective tissue offers support, strength and form to cells and their respective tissues. Calcium is one of the main components, besides protein, that affects the strength of connective tissues. When the thyroid gland is weak, you lose your ability to utilize calcium. This can create a variety of effects, including: hemorrhoids, varicose/spider veins, prolapsed conditions of organs (bladder, uterus, skin, etc.), fingernail ridging and weaknesses, and hair loss.

TENDONS

Tendons are composed of fibrous connective tissue and serve as fasteners or attachments of muscles to bones and other parts.

MUSCLES

Muscles are tissues that consist primarily of contractile cells. These tissues (muscles) serve to produce movement. They also serve as structural support. An example of this would be the spine, where all the muscles on each side of the vertebrae serve as supports. If one side becomes weaker through toxicity and inflammation, the strong side will pull the spine out of place.

There are three basic types of muscles in your body: **involuntary** (or **smooth muscles**), **voluntary** (or **striated muscles**), and **cardiac muscles**.

INVOLUNTARY (OR SMOOTH MUSCLES) — Fall under the autonomic nervous system (without conscious control). Smooth muscles are composed of spindle-shaped cells and have no cross fibers or sections (unstriated). Involuntary muscles mainly comprise internal organs, including the GI (gastrointestinal) tract, urinary tract and respiratory passages.

VOLUNTARY (OR STRIATED) — Found mainly as skeletal muscles, but also can be found in the throat (esophagus, etc.). Voluntary muscles fall under the voluntary nervous system (CNS) for conscious control. These muscles have fibers grouped into bundles and are surrounded by connective tissue formed into cylinders. These are stronger muscles, designed for heavier activity (pulling, stretching, etc.).

CARDIAC MUSCLES — Similar to striated muscles in that they are made up of tissues that are like long cylinders. Cardiac muscles form a continuous network of cylinder fibers with intervals of intercalated disks or cross-type fibers called Purkinje fibers. Purkinje fibers create the impulse-conducting system of the heart.

Muscles come in many shapes and sizes. They include:

- Strap or flat type
- Striated, which have cross-over sections in their fibers for added strength
- Unstriated, which have no cross-sections. They are called smooth muscles.
- Spindle-shaped (triangular) muscles with a "fleshy" body and tapering at one end like a "top"
- Papillary muscles which are like columns supporting valves (heart)
- Sphincter muscles—circular-type muscles which make up various sphincters, including the stomach. Sphincter muscles also encircle various ducts and orifices (anus, etc.).

Muscles of the Body

ANTIGRAVITY MUSCLES
Muscles that help support posture

AGONIST MUSCLES
Muscles that are the prime central movers

ANTAGONISTIC MUSCLES
Muscles that create opposing actions

BIPENNATE MUSCLES
Muscles with tendons

CARDIAC MUSCLES
Muscles of the heart

EXTENSOR MUSCLES
Muscles that extend a part

EXTRINSIC MUSCLES
Muscles located outside an organ that
help hold its position

FIXATION MUSCLES
Muscle that holds (steadies) a part, so
that more precise movements in a related
structure can take place

FLEXOR MUSCLES
Muscles that help to flex or bend parts

HAMSTRING MUSCLES
Muscles (3) located in the back of the
thigh

INTRINSIC MUSCLES
Muscles that have both ends tied within
a structure

INVOLUNTARY MUSCLES
Smooth muscles that respond by way of
the autonomic nervous system

SKELETAL MUSCLES
Muscles that are attached to bones and are
considered of the voluntary type

SMOOTH MUSCLES
(Unstriated) Involuntary muscles which are
unstriated (have no cross-section tissues),
such as the intestinal tract, etc.

STRAP MUSCLES
Muscles which are flat in nature (thyroid
cartilage, etc.)

STRIATED MUSCLES
Muscles that have cross-sections of tissue
in their fibers for added strength

SYNERGISTIC MUSCLES
Muscles that assist other muscles with their
actions

VOLUNTARY MUSCLES
Muscles that respond to the voluntary
nervous system (CNS)

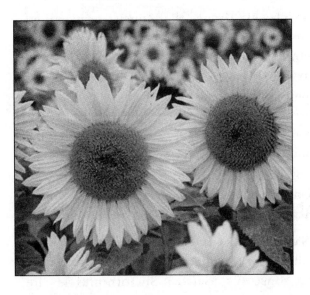

MODULE 2.10

☼ The Nervous System

CENTRAL NERVOUS SYSTEM (CNS)

The central nervous system (CNS) consists of the brain and spinal cord. These tissues consist of gray and white matter. The white matter transmits impulses throughout the CNS.

The brain is made up of nerve tissue and is contained within the cranial cavity of the cranium. It has three parts to it: the **cerebrum, cerebellum**, and the **brainstem** (medulla, pons and midbrain). There are five lobes that make up these three parts. These five lobes are the **frontal, parietal, occipital, temporal** and the **insular**.

The brain and spinal cord are the centers of communication, regulation, coordination and sensory evaluation of the body.

The medulla area of the brain lies at the base of the skull, atop the axis at the spine. The medulla has many jobs and functions, including influencing blood pressure, heart rate, metabolic rate and rate of glandular secretions. It also affects mineral utilization (thus pH factors), and controls oxygen supply and water retention. The medulla is also considered the equilibrium center. This area of the brain is greatly affected by congestion from dairy products and refined sugars. You especially see this when the tonsils (lymph nodes) have been removed. This causes poor lymphatic drainage of the cerebral areas, leading to poor circulation and elimination within these tissues and to a host of other conditions including dizziness, equilibrium problems and blood pressure issues.

AUTONOMIC NERVOUS SYSTEM (ANS)

The autonomic nervous system is self-controlling (somewhat automatic) or independent of our outward consciousness. It controls the involuntary bodily functions.

Two Branches

SYMPATHETIC NERVOUS SYSTEM

- The sympathetic nervous system is called the *thoracolumbar division* as it relates to the thoracic and lumbar regions of the body.

- The sympathetic nervous system dominates during stressful situations. It causes the fight-or-flight sensation in the presence of fear and danger.

PARASYMPATHETIC NERVOUS SYSTEM

- The parasympathetic nervous system is called the *craniosacral division,* as it relates to the cranial and sacral spine regions (upper spine and brain).

- The parasympathic nervous system dominates during non-stressful times.

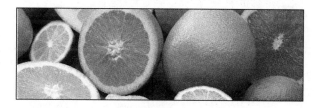

SYMPATHETIC IMPULSES AFFECT:
(Fight-or-flight response)

- vasodilatation in skeletal muscle
- vasoconstriction in the skin
- increase of heart rate and force
- dilation of bronchioles
- stimulation of liver to change glycogen to glucose
- activation of sweat glands

- decrease in peristalsis and intestinal secretions
- dilation of pupils
- increase in thickness of saliva from salivary glands
- creation of goose flesh (hair stands on end)
- slowing of the digestive process
- release norepinephrine

PARASYMPATHETIC IMPULSES AFFECT:

- slowing of a fast (tachycardia) heart rate
- normalization of bronchioles
- increase of peristalsis and normalization of digestive juices
- constriction of the pupils
- normalization of urinary function
- release acetylcholine as a transmitter

MODULE 2.11

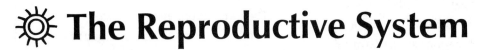 # The Reproductive System

PROSTATE GLAND

The prostate gland is part of the male reproductive system. It is clam-shaped and consists of three lobes, which surround the neck of the bladder and urethra. It is partly muscular tissue and partly glandular tissue. The glands are exocrine and have ducts that open into the prostate portion of the urethra (the tube or canal that urine flows through from the bladder to the outside of the body). In men the semen is discharged through the urethra.

The prostate gland secretes a thin, semi-clear, alkaline fluid, which makes up 30 percent of the seminal fluid. This fluid is used primarily for lubrication, but also stimulates active sperm movement. Prostatitis (inflammation of the prostate gland) occurs from acidosis. The most common contributing factor, however, is hypoactive adrenal glands. This creates low steroid production to counterbalance aggressive male hormones. This leads to prostate over-stimulation and inflammation.

TESTES

See Glandular System Module 2.8

OVARIES

See Glandular System Module 2.8

UTERUS

The uterus is a muscular, ear-shaped sac (or cavity) that becomes a "house" for a fertilized egg. This hollow sac becomes the home for the embryo, as it unfolds into the fetus, on its journey to become the newborn infant.

A mucous membrane called the **endometrium** lines the uterus. The uterus is divided into three parts: the main body (or the upper portion), called the **fundus**; the center (constrictive) or central area, called the **isthmus**; and finally, the lower portion that unites with the vagina, which is called the **cervix**.

The uterus lies in the mid-pelvic area, between the sacrum and the symphysis pubis. The lower portion of the fundus has two tubes that extend one to each ovary. These are called the **fallopian tubes**. The fallopian tubes are the pathway the ovum (egg) takes on its journey from the ovaries to the uterus.

Menstruation is a monthly ovulation cycle where estrogen (an acid hormone) triggers cellular bleeding in the uterus. This is God's way of "cleaning the house" each month. In this way, if the ovum (egg) becomes fertilized, its home will have been cleaned and prepared. It should be noted here the importance of progesterone, which is a steroid produced in the ovaries and in the adrenal glands. Adrenal progesterone (or DHEA-induced ovarian prog-esterone) is essential to stop the action of estrogen and its effect upon the uterine tissue. If progesterone (anti-inflammatory steroid) is not being properly produced because of a hypo-function of tissue, a woman will develop ovarian cysts, uterine fibroids, bleeding problems, A-typical cell formation, endometrioses and cancers.

MODULE 2.12

☀ The Respiratory System

LUNGS

We each come with a set of lungs located in the pleural cavity—one on each side of the sternum and reaching down from the upper chest (above first rib) to the diaphragm. The lungs are cone-shaped "spongy" organs, which allow outside air (food) to be brought into your body, and toxic gases and by-products to be exhaled or eliminated.

The upper part of the lungs is connected to the pharynx (nasal cavity) by way of the larynx (voice area) and trachea. The lungs are made up of lobes, lobules, bronchi, bronchioles, alveoli and a pleural sac (covering).

Your lungs are both a digesting organ and an eliminative organ. The lungs are a digestive organ in the sense that we consume (via breathing) vital elements, including oxygen, hydrogen, nitrogen, and carbon into the body to be used as catalysts, fuels and the like.

Your lungs also act as one of your four major eliminative organs (colon, kidneys, skin and lungs). As you inhale oxygen and other elements, these are exchanged through the alveoli into the pulmonary arterial capillaries of the lungs, which then send these elements through the heart and off into the entire system. The by-products of these elements are carbon dioxide and other gases, which act as a filter for all the "other" debris and toxins that you inhale (dust, chemicals, gases, etc.). These are then eliminated through the lymphatic capillaries and vascular system, or are expectorated by coughing and spitting the mucus that trapped these toxins.

Anatomy of the Lungs

LOBES (CHAMBERS)

- Right lung has 3 lobes and the left lung has 2 lobes (this allows room for the heart).
- Each lobe consists of respirator bronchiole, alveolar ducts, alveolar sacs, and alveoli.

LOBULES

- Small divisions of the 5 basic large lobes.

BRONCHI

- Two tubes that extend from your trachea (one on each side), into each lung. These two main tubes then break off into smaller bronchi.

BRONCHIOLES

- There are 50 to 85 in each lobe of each lung.
- Each divides into 2 to 11 alveolar ducts.
- Small fingers (extensions) of the main bronchial tubes that bring air into your lungs. This allows for greater air distribution. Theses divide into alveoli ducts, which lead to the alveoli.

ALVEOLI (AIR SACS)

- Only a thin, single-celled membrane which separates air from blood.
- Your lungs contain over 300,000,000 alveoli (or air sacs) that allow over 2,500 gallons of air to pass into your blood stream each day.
- There is over 750 sq. ft. of pulmonary capillary surface area for the exchange of oxygen.

PHARYNX

The pharynx is a muscular tube that connects the nasal cavity to the larynx. It also connects the mouth with the esophagus. It extends from the base of your skull to your sixth cervical vertebra. There it divides into anterior (behind), which becomes the esophagus, and inferior (in front), which becomes the larynx.

LARYNX

The larynx consists of nine cartilages, bound together by an elastic membrane and controlled by muscles. It connects with the epiglottis, hyoid bone, thyroid cartilage, vocal cords and cricoid cartilage at one end, and the trachea at the other.

TRACHEA (WINDPIPE)

Your trachea is a 4.5-inch-long cartilaginous tube. The trachea bridges the larynx to the primary or main bronchi. It extends from the sixth cervical to the fifth dorsal (thoracic) vertebra. At this point it divides into two main bronchi, one leading to each lung. The mucosa is made of ciliated epithelia that sweep mucus, trapped dust and pathogens upward.

MODULE 2.13

☀ The Skeletal System

Your skeletal system comprises all the bones, cartilage, tendons and ligaments that make up your physical body. "Skeleton" is a Greek word meaning "dried-up" body.

Bones, cartilage, tendons and ligaments are forms of connective tissue. Bones consist of **osteocytes** or **bone cells**, which are embedded in calcified extracellular compounds and substances called a matrix. This bed or matrix contains the minerals of calcium phosphate and calcium carbonate, as well as collagen (tough rope-like protein) fibers.

As previously stated, bones are formed from fibrous connective tissue. You especially see this in the beginning stages of life (embryonic). As the fetus develops, this connective tissue becomes dense and hardens, becoming the skeletal system. Bones serve as protection for vital organs, and as structural supports and functions.

Your physical body is composed of 206 bones (more or less):

- Head—29
- Upper extremities—64
- Trunk—51
- Lower extremities—62

TYPES OF BONES

Bones are classified by their shape and size, e.g., long bones, short bones, flat or irregular bones.

LONG BONES — Longer than they are wide. Bones of the extremities (arms, legs)

SHORT BONES — Somewhat as wide as they are long (e.g., ankle, wrist)

FLAT BONES — Flat bones are thin bones (e.g., skull, sternum, ribs)

IRREGULAR BONES — These bones come in different shapes and sizes (e.g., facial, vertebrae)

The outer surface (or portion) of bones is more dense or compact than the inner portion. The inner structure (or portion) of a bone is more spongy or cancellous.

The long bones are hollow, with dense or compact bone surrounding a canal (marrow) that houses **bone marrow**. Bone marrow is the soft tissue in the marrow cavities of many bones, especially the larger ones. You have two types of bone marrow.

Bone Terminology

BODY SHAFT
The main portion of a bone.

CANAL
A passage through a bone, also called meatus.

FORAMEN
A hole in a bone, generally for vessels or nerves.

PROCESS
An extension or projection from a bone.

TUBERCLE
A lump or hump in a bone.

HEAD
The end of a bone—enlarged and often rounded.

NECK
The tapered portion of a bone between the head and the shaft (body).

CREST
The prominent ridge of a bone.

RED BONE MARROW — Produces your red blood cells and B-lymphocytes and other immune cells.

YELLOW BONE MARROW — Predominately fat that is stored for energy needs.

BONE STRUCTURES

COMPACT BONE — Which consist mainly of solid matrix (mineral matter) and cells. The **dense** or **compact** portion of bones is made up of osteocytes, blood vessels, lymph and lymph vessels. It is through canals in this portion of the bone that nutrition and wastes are carried from bone cells. **Compact bone** is found in long bones and the thinner surface of all other bones.

CANCELLOUS BONE — Which is more honeycomb (spongy), with small marrow-filled spaces. Cancellous bone is located in the end (epiphyses) of long bones and forms the center of all other bones. The honeycomb or spongy look comes from interconnecting rods or plates of bone called **tradeculae**.

BONE GROWTH AND REPAIR

Bone growth and repair takes place through hormone stimulation from the thyroid/parathyroid glands. This is why when the thyroid becomes underactive you develop bone/connective tissue weaknesses that affect all the organs, glands, bones and the vascular system.

Ossification is a word used for the formation of bone by **osteoblasts** (cells that become osteocytes or bone cells). There are **two types of ossification**. Both types of ossification involve compact and cancellous bone.

INTRAMEMBRANOUS OSSIFICATION — Bone formation within connective tissue.

ENDOCHONDRAL OSSIFICATION — Bone formation that takes place inside cartilage.

When injury (or lifestyle) weakens bone cells, **osteoclasts** (bone-eating cells) remove them, making room for **osteoblasts** to rebuild the bone or cartilage.

The importance of an alkaline diet with proper glandular (thyroid/parathyroid, pituitary, adrenal and pancreatic) function cannot be overstressed. Acidosis stimulates osteoclasts and the formation of calcium deposits. Calcium is ionized (hardened) in the presence of acids (anionic). The regulation of ionic calcium in the body's fluid is essential to the proper growth and repair of bones.

This, as previously stated, is greatly influenced by diet, lifestyle, hormones and steroids.

Bones, as any tissues, organs and glands of your body, are composed of cells. All cells in your body require an energy source (nutrition) and a way to eliminate (lymphatic system, kidneys, skin, lungs and bowels).

Make all the cells in your body healthy. **Detoxify** (clean), **alkalize** and **regenerate**. Every cell in your body will thank you.

First understand Nature, then copy it.
— V. Schauberger

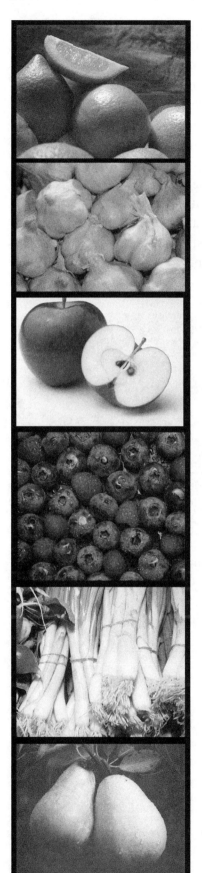

CHAPTER THREE

The Foods We Eat

Now that we have learned what species we belong to, how our body works, and something about its systems (including organs and glands), we will examine the proper foods that God designed for our species.

What is so important about the types of foods we eat?

I have heard many doctors say that it doesn't matter *what* we eat. On the other hand, The American Dietetics Association, considered by many to be the authority on the correct foods to eat for health, has been making specific dietary recommendations for years. Still, cancer is reportedly in every other (or every third) person, and statistics for the incidence of diabetes as well as multiple sclerosis, Parkinson's disease and every other disease you can name (and some that you can't) are soaring. Why?

It's All About Energy

Energy is the number one factor (or constituent) needed for life to exist, and the basis for creation itself. Energy is determined by the movement and interaction of the atoms that comprise all life. Even carbon, the basis of all life on this planet, could not exist without the movement and interplay of atoms. Atoms (energy) cannot be created or destroyed, however they can be changed. Energy can be increased or decreased.

Energy levels (frequencies) can be low or high (represented by broad or short waves), and these levels are determined by the molecular composition of the initiating force. Energy is also classified as being kinetic or potential. **Kinetic energy** is energy at work. **Potential energy** is stored energy—it has potential for use. The chemical energy in food is potential to a certain degree, until released via enzyme and other chemical activators. Then this potential energy becomes kinetic, or more active, electrifying and creating activity in its wake.

A great example of the difference between potential and kinetic energy is found in comparing **cooked foods** with **raw foods**. The electromagnetic energy (combined molecular energy) of cooked foods is dramatically lower than that of raw foods. The reason is that when heat is applied to a compound its molecular structure changes somewhat, as electrons are altered. Think about what happens to water when you heat it—its form changes from liquid to vapor. With heat, unsaturated fats become saturated (as water-soluble constituents are destroyed, leaving only some of the elements that comprise them), and many dangerous and carcinogenic compounds are created when foods are cooked. Heat also destroys the enzymes in food, which are absolutely necessary as catalysts. The bottom line is that the more energy your cells have, the healthier your body is. The less energy a cell has, the closer to destruction (by the immune system or parasitic response) it comes.

Carbon, hydrogen, oxygen and nitrogen are the basic elements of all organic matter on earth. All foods and their constituents (like proteins, carbohydrates and fats) are mostly created from these basic elements, which are the building blocks that determine to what category molecules or compounds, etc., belong. These categories of molecular structures (such as sugars, starches, proteins, fats) make up the foods that sustain life on this planet.

This chapter will view food and the process of eating from the perspective of chemistry and physics, and set it in the context of some overviews from God and nature. Let's first examine some of the most important constituents that your body requires to sustain, clean and repair itself.

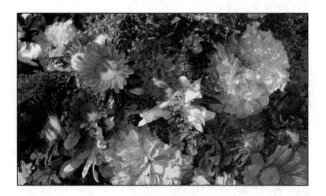

There is among the Indians a heresy of those who philosophize among the Brahmins, who live a self-sufficient life, abstaining from eating living creatures and all cooked food.

— Hippolytus, Rome, 225 A.D.

☀ Carbohydrates and Sugars and their Metabolism

In Chapter Two we learned that a cell is like a self-sustaining city, but that it basically requires two outside factors. First, it needs an energy source. Just as our car needs fuel, so do our cells. Secondly, they must be able to eliminate the by-products of these burned fuels. These by-products must be carried away from the cells, much like the plumbing and septic systems work in your house.

Carbohydrates refer to a group of chemical substances made up of carbon, oxygen and hydrogen (carbon and water). They include starches, sugars, glycogen, dextrins and celluloses. Carbohydrates are classified or grouped by the number of carbon atoms they contain and by the combinations of sugars. Since organic carbon compounds supply the main energy source for cells, these carbohydrates are used by your body for its primary energy supply.

All green plants use the sun's energy (photosynthesis) to combine carbon dioxide and water to form carbohydrates. Cellulose, the chief constituent of the cell walls of plants, is a type of carbohydrate. When consumed by humans, cellulose acts as an intestinal broom and energizer to the cells of the intestinal walls.

SUGARS

A sugar is a carbohydrate belonging to the saccharide family. **Simple sugars** (also called monosaccharides) are the main fuels for your body. Sugars are as essential to your body as gasoline is to your automobile. It helps run your machine (your body) via the cells. However, there are several important distinctions to understand about sugars.

Glucose (simple sugar) and its initial compounds, such as starch and cellulose, make up the most abundant organic chemical compounds on earth. Since your body can only use substances in their simplest forms, all complex sugars (di- and polysaccharides) must first be broken down into simple sugars (monosaccharides). This is one aspect of the process of digestion.

After digestion breaks down complex sugars to glucose, this glucose is then absorbed into the blood from the intestinal tract. Glucose is then transported to cells where it is reduced to carbon and is oxidized for energy and heat. Part of this carbon is stored for future energy needs (the way a battery stores energy). Some excess carbon, which is not used, is stored as **ATP (adenosine triphosphate)** or converted to fat and/or stored as glycogen. **Glycogen** is stored mainly in the liver and muscle tissue, but can also be stored in many other places. When the body is deprived of glucose or fructose, it will start to use its glycogen reserves. Glycogen is then converted back into glucose. Remember that the body *must* have a fuel source, as does your car.

When refined or complex sugars (several glucose and fructose complexes bonded together) are consumed, this creates a glucose overload, which in turn creates excess carbon molecules. This excess carbon is converted into **carbon dioxide** and **carbonic acid**. **Carbon dioxide** is eliminated via lungs, kidneys and skin. **Carbonic acid** requires oxidation or transmutation via oxygen or mineral salts, respectively. Both of these substances are **acid-forming** and must be neutralized and removed by the body, as they are strong contributors to acidosis.

Sugar (glucose) overload is common in our society. We consume a great deal of refined and complex carbohydrates and sugars. This keeps a high demand upon the pancreas to produce insulin, and upon the liver and kidneys to convert or eliminate the excess. Add to this excess the problems created by protein and fat consumption and you can begin to form a picture of why people today have so many health problems.

Raw fruits and vegetables are balanced in their simple sugars, amino acids and fatty acids.

The Danger of High-Protein Diets

Some substances are not fuel sources, but are building materials. Proteins, for example, are non-fuel substances that are used by the body as building materials, as immune factors, as catalysts or carriers, etc. Just as the body must convert a carbohydrate into a simple sugar before it can be utilized, all proteins must first be broken down into amino acids before the body can use them to build and repair itself; in much the same way that a carpenter would use two-by-fours or two-by-sixes in building or repairing a structure. However, if the body needs to, it will convert amino acids to glucose.

The grave mistake made by many who want to lose weight is in making the body burn protein for fuel. When the body is deprived of sugars, it will go to stored fat or break down its own tissues for energy. This leads to muscle, liver, pancreatic and kidney damage.

In Chapter 4 we will discuss the "Protein Myth" more thoroughly.

This is another reason that I call them "God-foods" designed for humans.

Most artificial sweeteners have been linked to cancer. Nutrasweet® or aspartame is an example of an artificial sugar. Aspartame is a neurotoxin that breaks down into formaldehyde, and Americans use over 7000 tons of this a year.

It is a myth that natural, simple sugars "feed" (i.e., encourage) cancer. Quite the contrary. Simple sugars strengthen and energize cells, which is a *must* in successful cancer treatment, as cancer cells are normal cells that have lost their vitality and health through acidosis. **Remember, a simple sugar (glucose in particular) is the proper fuel for cells.** Protein and fats should never be used for fuel unless it is absolutely necessary, because cellular damage can result.

Fructose is the highest energetic form of a monosaccharide or simple sugar. Neurons (nerve cells) especially attract fructose molecules. Fructose enters a cell through diffusion instead of via active transport, which its counterpart glucose uses. Diffusion saves energy for the body and cells.

Any activity requires energy, including the activity of transporting nutrients across cell walls. Most nutrients also require a helper or carrier to assist in this movement through the cell wall into the cell. As ATP (adenosine triphosphate) is a cell's stored energy, it is used in active transport (the assisted transportation of nutrients across cell membrane walls). Glucose needs insulin to a certain degree as a "utilization hormone" for this active transport. Fructose, on the other hand, requires no ATP or insulin and is simply pulled or absorbed through the cell wall by diffusion.

For diabetics, fructose is perfect, especially if they remove complex sugars from their diets. Complex sugars create excessive glucose levels in the blood, which then creates more insulin demand.

Raw fruits and vegetables are always your best sources of simple sugars. This is one reason why your body becomes stronger and more

Carbohydrate Metabolism

> **FOOD CARBOHYDRATES**
> grains, vegetables, starches, sugar

> **IN THE MOUTH**
> Salivary Enzyme Amylase *(Ptyalin)* reduces cooked starch to maltose and dextrin

> **IN THE PANCREAS**
> Pancreatic Enzyme Amylase *(Amylopsin)* converts starches to maltose and dextrin

> **IN THE INTESTINES**
> Intestinal Enzyme Sucrase converts sucrose to glucose and fructose.
>
> Intestinal Enzyme Maltase converts maltose to glucose.
>
> Intestinal Enzyme Lactase converts lactose to glucose and galactose.

energetic on these foods. Foods high in protein and low in sugars, or foods high in complex-sugars, rob your body of vital energy, create acidosis and elevate blood sugars.

Simple sugars also aid alkalization of the tissues, which is vital for tissue regeneration and vitality. As stated, fructose is the highest electrical sugar in nature and is superb for brain and nerve regeneration.

COMPLEX SUGARS

Complex sugars are of two types—polysaccharides and disaccharides.

POLYSACCHARIDES — A chain or series of linked monosaccharides or disaccharides. They can consist of a few or many saccharide bonds.

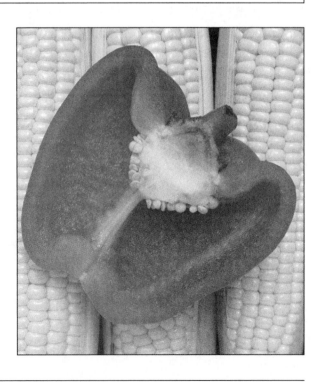

Digestive and Metabolic By-Products of Carbohydrates

NUTRITIVE PRODUCTS

Glucose = energy

Fructose = energy

Galactose = energy (infancy)

Glycogen = stored fat for future energy needs

Water

Fatty acids = secondary response

Amino acids = secondary response

TOXIC BY-PRODUCTS

Pyretic acid

Lactic acid

Carbon dioxide

CARBON CAUSED ACIDOSIS ELIMINATION

- oxidized by oxygen
- bonded to various mineral salts to form non-acid compounds
- carbon dioxide conversion to bicarbonate

Polysaccharides, when hydrolyzed, yield over twenty monosaccharides. Polysaccharides include two groups, **starch** and **cellulose**.

- *Starch:* starch, glycogen, dextrin, insulin
- *Cellulose:* cellulose, hemicelluloses (pentosaniek)

DISACCHARIDES — Complex sugars having two monosaccharides linked together. Disaccharides include three groups, maltose, lactose, sucrose.

- *Maltose* — from malt grains (germinated grains and seeds); 2 glucose molecules
- *Lactose* — from milk and dairy products; 1 glucose and 1 galactose molecule
- *Sucrose* — from refined beets, sugar cane, inverted or refined sugars; 1 glucose and 1 fructose molecule

Disaccharides are converted to monosaccharides ($C_6H_{12}O_6$) or simple sugars.

SIMPLE SUGARS

There are five types of monosaccharides or simple sugars.

- *Glucose* — from vegetables; contain 6 carbon bonds called hexoses
- *Fructose* — from fruits; contain 6 carbon bonds called hexoses
- *Galactose* — from milk (infants only); contain 6 carbon bonds called hexoses
- *Ribose (RNA)* — from fruits and vegetables; contain 5 carbon bonds called pentoses
- *Deoxyribose (DNA)* — from fruits and vegetables; contain 5 carbon bonds called pentoses.

☀ Proteins and their Metabolism

The term "protein" is used to designate a structure created from chained amino acids. We tend to use this word in general when defining the needs of the body, but is important to understand that your body is not designed to use and metabolize "structures." Since your body is designed to use only the simplest of compounds and bio-available elements, it must break down (digest) these "structures" into the elements that comprise them, and then use these simpler compounds for its own needs.

Proteins are made up of amino acids, which are made up of carbon, hydrogen, oxygen, lots of nitrogen, phosphorus, sulfur and iron. As noted above, your body cannot use a "protein" structure. Therefore, part of your digestive process will break these structures down into their simplest form—into amino acids, the basic building blocks or material that your body uses to build its own protein structures. Amino acids are used to make repairs, to create new structures, to enhance immune response, to act as transporters and to serve a multitude of other purposes.

PROTEIN DIGESTION

IN THE STOMACH VIA GASTRIC JUICES — HCL (hydrochloric acid) causes the conversion of pepsinogens to pepsin, which breaks down complex protein structures to proteoses and peptones.

IN THE PANCREAS — Pancreatic enzymes trypsin and chymotrypsin convert peptones to polypeptides.

IN THE INTESTINES — Intestinal enzyme peptidase converts peptones, polypeptides and dipeptides into amino acids.

Digestive and Metabolic By-Products of Protein

NUTRITIVE PRODUCTS

Amino acids = for building, repair, immunity, hormone production, transport, etc.

Water

Carbohydrates = secondary response

Fatty acids = secondary response

TOXIC BY-PRODUCTS

Nitrogen compounds (nitrates, etc.)

Ammonia

Purines, pyrimidine, etc.

Uric acid, uratinim, etc.

Phosphoric acid

Sulfuric acid

Glucogenic acids

Ketogenic acids

Carbon dioxide

☀ Fats (Lipids) and their Metabolism

Fats are one of the "Big Three" componants that all foods have to some degree. **Proteins** (amino acids), **carbohydrates** (sugars) and **fats** (essential fatty acids) are the main building blocks, fuels and carriers that your body requires to keep itself healthy. Fats are vital to your body in numerous ways:

- Fats are used as storage units for energy (triglycerides).

- Fats provide "padding" or "cushioning" as protection for your internal organs.

- Fats assist with the utilization of fat-soluble vitamins (including A, D and E).

- Fats are used as part of your body's mechanism to insulate your internal components and vital organs from environmental conditions (like cold weather).

- Fats guard against internal heat loss.

- Fats combine with certain proteins creating diglyceride phospholipids, which are a part of every cell membrane wall.

- Fats serve as anti-inflammatory mediators.

As we noted earlier, all components of life, including all foods, are made up of the four basic elements of oxygen, hydrogen, carbon and nitrogen. Each component will contain varying amounts of some or all four of these elements. Water—H_2O—for example, has two atoms of hydrogen (H_2) combined with one atom of oxygen (O). Fats are comprised of mainly carbon (C), hydrogen (H) and oxygen (O), and are insoluble in water but soluble in ether and other solvents. Fats are divided up into two basic types, **saturated** and **unsaturated**, and are comprised of **fatty acids** and **glycerol** (an alcohol).

Fatty acids are the building blocks of fats, just as amino acids are the building blocks of proteins. Fatty acids form "chains" through their carbon bonding. These carbon chains attract hydrogen to them. When each bonding site of a carbon chain has been bonded with a hydrogen atom, the chain—or fat—is considered **saturated**. These are generally considered long-chain fatty acids and because of their more complete, or "full," bonding they become harder and have a higher melting point. In other words, the more saturated a fat is, the more it stays hard at room temperature. **Unsaturated fats**, on the other hand, have less hydrogen bonding. When two or more adjacent carbon atoms are free of hydrogen bonding they are considered **monounsaturated fatty acids**. When two or more pairs or "sets" of carbon atoms within the chain are unbonded to hydrogen, we call these **polyunsaturated fatty acids**.

Three of the most common fatty acid chains found in human tissues are oleic acid ($C_{18}H_{34}O_2$),

---

Fat Composition

Fat molecules consist of 3 molecules of fatty acids and 1 molecule of glycerol. Three fatty acids constitute most of the fats found in your body.

Fatty Acid	+ Glycerol	= Type of Fat
1-Stearic Acid	+ Glycerol	= Tristearin
Palmitic Acid	+ Glycerol	= Tripalmitin
Oleic Acid	+ Glycerol	= Triolein

---

stearic acid ($C_{18}H_{36}O_2$), and palmitic acid ($C_{16}H_{32}O_2$). These three fatty acids when combined with glycerol form the three basic fats found in our foods, and are called **triolein**, **tristearin** and **tripalmitin**.

ESSENTIAL FATTY ACIDS

The fatty acids that are essential to your body, but not naturally synthesized within the body, must therefore be obtained from your diet. These are known as essential fatty acids, and there are three basic ones: **linoleic acid**, **linolenic acid** and **arachidonic acid**. Linoleic acid is the most vital of the three as it can be converted into linolenic and arachidonic acids. In my opinion, humanity (through the medium of science) is in its infancy in understanding the true needs of our homo sapien bodies. Types of essential fatty acids include:

LINOLEIC ACID—Promotes healthy skin and hair and is the main essential fatty acid.

LINOLENIC ACID — Promotes nerve and brain function.

ARACHIDONIC ACID — Promotes formation of prostaglandins, thromboxanes, prostacylins and leukotrienes.

The Role of Essential Fatty Acids

- Used in the production of cholesterol, an anti-inflammatory lipid used to make steroids and phospholipids. Cholesterol is involved in the synthesis of vitamin D.
- Used to produce phospholipids, which are used in cell membrane walls.
- Involved in the production of prostaglandins, which serve as anti-inflammatories and are involved in proper blood clotting. They increase immune response and function, especially of T-lymphocytes.
- Inhibits thromboxane, which is involved in platelet agitation.

Fats are . . .

OXIDIZED
To carbon dioxide and water to produce energy

STORED
For future energy

CHANGED
To phospholipids for cell membrane walls. To acetyl groups for the synthesis of cholesterol and to make secretions, mucus, sebum, etc.

- Promote healing.
- Strengthen nerve tissues and nerve response.
- Involved in the manufacture of hemoglobin. Thus involved indirectly in oxygen transport and the increase of oxygenation to tissues.
- Assist cell wall permeability.
- Nourish and protect the skin, essential fatty acids and the utilization of vitamins A and E which help promote skin and hair health.
- Increase the body's ability to burn fat.
- Affect regulation of the nerve response in the heart, thus affecting its rhythm.
- Involved in maintaining proper body temperature.
- Used with bile salts to emulsify fats and make them ready for hydrolyzing.
- Used in the development and function of the brain.

SOURCES OF FATS

The human body receives fatty acids in two ways: from foods—dietary fats—which are absorbed through the intestinal wall, and through the conversion of excess amino acids (proteins and carbohydrates (sugars) into stored fats (glycogen and triglycerides). The following highlights two essential fatty acids (oils in liquid form) found in nature:

OMEGA-3 — These are "long-chained" metabolic by-products of the metabolism of linolenic acid. These oils are found mainly in flesh foods, especially fish oils. These oils tend to stay liquid at room temperature and are comprised of Eicosapentaenioic Acid (EPA), and Docosahexaenoic Acid (DHA) and Alpha-Linolenic Acid (ALA).

OMEGA-6 — A plant-based form of essential fats of which Gamma-Linolenic Acid (GLA) is the most commonly known and researched. Vegetables, fruits, nuts and seeds are nature's sources of omega-6 fatty acids.

Top Food Sources of Omega-6 Oils

The following foods are rich in linolenic acid which metabolizes into Omega-3 fatty acids.

FLAX SEED OIL — Also known as linseed oil. Has been used for over 5,000 years for many purposes. High in Linolenic Acid and Gamma-Linolenic Acid.

BLACK CURRENT SEED OIL — Known for its rich oils high in Linoleic Acid and Gamma-Linolenic Acid.

BORAGE OIL — The borage plant is known as "the adrenal" herb. The adrenal glands supply your body's steroids, which are manufactured from cholesterol, one of the main products of essential fatty acids.

EVENING PRIMROSE OIL — This flower is also known as Evening Star and Night Willow. I have used Evening Primrose Oil in cases of Multiple Sclerosis (MS) with great results. A rich source of Linoleic and Linolenic Acids.

A note of caution about oils: Never use cheap, refined, commercial or processed oils found in clear glass or clear plastic bottles. These oils are mostly rancid and full of solvents, pesticides and chemical preservatives, like BHA, BHT, methyl silicone, and others. These oils are "super-cooked" which means that most of their nutrition is lost, changed or bonded, causing body acidosis, and liver and kidney damage.

AN EXAMPLE OF FAT METABOLISM

As stated earlier, your body is not designed to absorb or use "structures." Like proteins, fats are structures. They consist of chained or bonded fatty acids. Since your body and its cells can only use simple compounds for activity and sustenance, fats that are consumed from foods must be broken down into the fatty acids that comprise them, much the same way that proteins are broken down into amino acids. This digestive action takes place in the first part of the small intestine with the assistance of bile from the liver/gallbladder. The following describes the process of fat digestion and metabolism:

1. **Bile Salts** emulsify fats and make them water-soluble so that pancreatic and intestinal lipase can convert them to fatty acids and glycerol.

2. **Gastric juices**—enzyme gastric lipase—converts (emulsifies) fats into fatty acids and glycerol (an alcohol).

3. **Intestinal (duodenum)** enzyme steapsin—a lipase from the pancreas—converts fats into fatty acids and glycerol (an alcohol).

4. **Fatty acids and glycerol** bind to form neutral fats, which then bond to various proteins to form chylomicrons. Fats in this form are absorbed and carried throughout the lymphatic system and the blood system where they are dispersed to the tissues of the body. Fatty acids cannot be converted to glucose. However, they can enter the Krebs (energy) Cycle through acetyl groups.

5. **Adipose (fatty) tissue** is created for the body's energy reserve and factors for cellular health and immunity.

Digestive and Metabolic By-Products of Fats

NUTRITIONAL PRODUCTS
- Essential fatty acids
- Fatty acids
- Glycerol (an alcohol)
- Glycerides
- Water

TOXIC BY-PRODUCTS
- Acetate (Acetone) (Ketone)
- Aceto acetate (Acetoacetic acid) (Ketone)
- Carbon dioxide
- Betahydroxybutyric acid (Ketone)

Conclusion

When fats are oxidized into water and carbon dioxide, several by-products (ketones) are formed. These include acetone, acetoacetic acid and betahydroxybutyric acid. When these ketones are produced in excess, either through incomplete oxidation or excessive break down of body fats from high protein diets, a condition occurs called **ketosis**, which results in **acidosis**. This leads to tissue damage and hypo-function of cells (organs and glands). Ketosis can also occur in hyperthyroidism, starvation, fevers, and various toxemias.

Keep it simple. All the substances that your body requires, including fats, are found in organic fruits, nuts, seeds and vegetables. If it's not in them, you don't need it! Science has lost touch with the simplicity of health. Animals intuitively eat the food assigned for their particular species. So should you. However, there are chronic and degenerative cases where the supplementation of a small amount of plant oil, like Evening Primrose, will help tremendously. This is especially true in any neurological condition, such as M.S., Parkinson's, and Lou Gehrig's Disease.

☼ Enzymes: The Biocatalysts

Putting the puzzle of health together would not be complete without the understanding of enzymes. The physical world, on all levels, is in a continual process of consumption. One living structure consumes another for part of its energy source. The consumption of food by animals and humans is just one small example of this. There is a chemical and biochemical interplay among all aspects of life. Elements and compounds are constantly being transmuted (changed) into other compounds or elements. As a rule, the "complex" is broken down to the "simple." One example of this would be protein structures—complex structures that are broken down through digestion (by enzyme action) into amino acids. Amino acids are simple compounds or basic building materials used by the body for growth and repair. In another example, complex-sugars like maltose and sucrose are broken down into a simple sugar, glucose. These processes are all essential for proper utilization. However, each life form is unique and will utilize these building materials in a variety of ways to suit its uniqueness.

Enzymes are the catalysts of all these chemical and biochemical processes. No chemical or biochemical process can take place without an enzyme present to initiate this process; whether this process is **catabolic** (tearing down) or **anabolic** (building up). An example of catabolic action would be digestion (the process described above), where the structures are broken down into building materials. We also have anabolic building and rebuilding processes going on in our bodies, such as cellular birth and cellular repair.

All body processes including liver function, kidney function, immune and lymphatic response, and the grand communication of the nervous system, depend upon enzymes to function. Enzymes have been called the "workforce" of life. They are the laborers, the builders, the construction workers. They make life happen.

Enzymes are organic catalysts produced by living cells, which act upon what are called "substrates." They form a temporary bond with these substrates and are then referred to as "enzyme substrate complexes." Enzymes are like magnets, promoting the formation or destruction of elements or their substrates to produce the desired product. We need and use thousands of enzymes throughout the body. Metabolism alone requires several thousand enzymes. Enzymes can act like some proteins, which means they can be carriers for nutrients. But they are mainly used as catalysts, required anytime a chemical action or reaction needs to take place. They also can affect the rate of this action or reaction. In a healthy body, enzymes can be used over and over again.

It is important to note that the pH of the body, as well as dehydration (water levels), radiation, toxicity and body temperatures can impair, destroy or stimulate enzyme factors. This can lead to hypo- or hyperactivity of tissues, lack of proper digestion, poor nerve response and breathing issues, just to name a few conditions.

Enzymes have a consciousness all their own, as each living thing does. Each has a specific job to do and knows it. Some speed things up and others slow things down. It does not matter what the process is; an enzyme must be present.

There are basically two types of enzymes in humans. First, our **systemic enzymes**, which are responsible for running the machinery (e.g., immune, kidney, bowel, nerve functions). There are hundreds of enzymes used in metabolism (running the body) and cellular growth and repair, including DNA replication. Blood clotting, oxygen exchange and the transport of carbon dioxide, all require enzymes. Cellular respiration (the way cells eat and excrete) is as vital a process for cells, as it is for the body as a whole; both respiration processes need enzyme action.

Second, our **digestive enzymes** are used to break down the structures we consume into building materials. Cells cannot eat structures; they need building materials. In constructing a house, a builder will often tear down a structure to get whatever materials he can save, and then use those materials to create a new structure. Our body has to do the same thing. It needs to break down the "structures" we eat into the simplest of compounds or elements for building, repairing, or for fuel. Enzymes are needed in this entire process.

Digestive enzymes are called **hydrolytic enzymes** because they bond (catalyze) water molecules to larger food particles, to split them into smaller compounds or elements. We have digestive enzymes starting in the mouth, such as **amylase** and **ptyalin**, which break down sugars and starches. We also have digestive enzymes in the stomach. These enzymes are called **inactive enzymes** or **pro-enzymes** because they must be activated before they can catalyze or affect a change. **Pepsinogen** is an example of a pro-enzyme that is changed into pepsin by the action of HCL (hydrochloric acid). **Pepsin** is acidic in nature and is designed primarily for initial protein breakdown.

The stomach chyme, enriched with pro-enzymes (although some are dormant from the acid action of HCL), is dropped from the stomach into the duodenum (the first part of the small bowel), and alkaline digestive enzymes (such as amylase, lipase, protease, and cellulose) are then released from the pancreas. **Amylase** breaks down starch, **lipase** works on fat, **protease** handles protein, and **cellulose** digestive enzymes attend to cellulose. The pancreas also produces **trypsin** and **chymotrypsin** as well as **peptidase**, which are a part of the protease family. These are alkaline enzymes that finish protein digestion or break down peptides and polypeptides into amino acids.

It is essential for the pancreas to produce sodium bicarbonate (bicarbonate ions) and for the liver/gallbladder to produce bile, as both of these substances alkalize and sanitize the predigested food particles from the stomach. If the tissues of these organs are congested, weak, or impaired in such a way that these alkalizing principles are restricted or blocked from entry to the small bowel, the duodenum stays overly acidic, and inflammation and ulceration of the duodenum are the result. An over-acidic environment also destroys or neutralizes the alkaline digestive enzymes of the pancreas, virtually stopping proper digestion. This leads to starvation at the cellular level as other enzymes and parasites become involved, because fermentation and putrefaction now takes over the digestive process.

Studies undertaken at Yale University and other research facilities have shown that enzymes, including digestive enzymes, are produced by many cells in the body (not just the saliva, stomach and pancreas). It has been demonstrated, for example, that white blood cells can supply amylase as well as proteolytic-type enzymes. What an incredibly intelligent machine your body is! I say "machine" with all due respect to the fact that each and every cell is an individual part of God, with its own individuality and consciousness.

We have been talking about **endogenous enzymes**, those produced in the body. However, we also must consider a second category of enzymes essential to life—the **exogenous enzymes** that are external to the body, and found in foods. Exogenous enzymes play a vital role in assisting the body in breaking down these foods into useable building materials.

Food enzymes are vital to the health of the physical body. Without them health begins to decline. Man still does not understand why these food enzymes are so important when we have our own digestive enzymes. But the body must have the support of these food enzymes for the process of digestion and utilization to properly take place.

Enzymes are destroyed when subjected to temperatures starting from 110–130 degrees Fahrenheit and above. Lower temperatures can also destroy enzymes if the food is cooked for long periods of time. When we cook our foods, we are destroying the life-giving properties within them, including the enzymes. Remember: no other animal on this planet cooks its food before eating it. If we feed animals cooked foods they become sick and die, and veterinarians will tell you to never feed your animals from the table because they will get the same diseases we do.

SUPPLEMENTING WITH DIGESTIVE ENZYMES?

The sale of digestive enzyme supplements is big business these days, and there are companies that support their use by advocating live blood-cell analysis and other diagnostic tools. We all have digestive weaknesses to some extent, and especially if the pancreas is weak. If you are thin and can't put on weight; or you have diabetes or hypoglycemia; or you see undigested foods in your stools (except corn); then you should consult with your healthcare practitioner about regenerating your pancreas.

Relying on supplemented digestive enzymes on a regular basis can eventually shut down your pancreas. Nonetheless, in some extreme or chronic conditions, it may be advisable to take digestive enzymes with **every other meal or every third or fourth meal**. Only take them for short periods of time, until you can restore normal pancreatic and intestinal function. Definitely stop taking them when you eat raw, uncooked foods. Wean yourself from them until you are only using them with cooked, hard-to-digest foods. Then stop entirely. If you are eating all cooked, acidic foods, you may need to add *occasional* digestive enzymes, since cooking your food destroys its enzymes and puts the total burden of digestion upon your body. Consuming your foods *juiced* and/or eating them *raw* will help tremendously in revitalizing your pancreas and yourself.

It is beyond the scope of this book to explore further on the subject of enzymes as biocatalysts. However, it is enough to reiterate that life begets life and death begets death. Without enzymes we have death.

Enjoy the natural flavors of fresh, whole, ripe and raw foods. God has given us a smorgasbord of foods and the ability to obtain them. Seek out organic, fresh and raw, enzyme-rich foods, as enzymes are the keys to life.

No matter from which angle we view health and disease, we cannot escape from being entangled in the conclusion that intractable disease is as old as cookery. Disease and cookery originated simultaneously.

— Dr. Edward Howell, *Enzyme Nutrition*

☼ Vitamins (Co-Enzymes)

From the beginning, humans ate primarily whole foods or so-called "natural" foods, which underwent no processing. **The nutrient content of food is decreased when it is processed.** Intensive animal rearing, manipulation of crop production, and food processing have altered the qualitative and quantitative balance of nutrients of foods consumed by the Western world. This change is possibly one of the reasons that chronic, debilitating diseases are rampant in our modern culture. Modern research suggests that simply taking a synthetic multi-vitamin/mineral formula does not change this. Research from around the globe asserts that vitamins in their naturally-balanced state are essential for better assimilation, synergistic action, and maximum biological effect. And yet most consumers buy vitamins and minerals that are synthetic, which their bodies usually can't assimilate properly. The U.S. National Academy of Science, Food and Nutrition Board, recommends that people meet their daily nutritional needs through a varied diet rather than through vitamin and mineral supplementation. Vitamin and mineral supplements—even those with 100% of the Recommended Dietary Allowances (RDAs) for vitamins and minerals—cannot provide all the other nutrients that the body gets from a well-balanced diet.

About Vitamins

- Too much vitamin supplementation causes acidosis.
- Vitamin C is acidic, leaches out calcium, and lowers beneficial cholesterol.
- Do not megadose anything, especially oil soluble vitamins.
- Supplementation of separated constituents can lead to imbalances in your body's chemistry.

- Artificial vitamins accumulate in your tissues causing obstructions and toxicity.

Vitamin A

Other names: beta-carotene, retinol, anti-ophthalmic

Actions: Boost immune system. Builds resistance to infections. Keeps tissue in good health. Vitamin A and B2 work together to help keep mucous membranes in the gastrointestinal tract healthy.

Best sources: Tomatoes, carrots, kale, turnip greens, spinach, broccoli, squash, yams, endive, watermelon, asparagus, apples, apricots, prunes, papaya, avocados, paprika, pumpkin and lemon grass.

Vitamin B1

Other names: thiamin, thiamine chloride

Actions: Nervous system. Keeps digestive system functioning well. Helps produce hydrochloric acid needed for proper digestion.

Best sources: Peas, lentils, seeds, nuts, beans, beets, potatoes, oranges, leafy green vegetables, blackstrap molasses, okra, sunflower seeds, Brazil nuts, rice bran and brown rice.

Vitamin B2

Other names: riboflavin, vitamin G

Actions: Boosts immune system. Essential for growth, eyes, skin, nails, hair. Helps metabolize proteins and carbohydrates.

Best sources: Green vegetables, rice bran, avocados, grains, wheat germ, almonds, sunflower seeds, Brussels sprouts, prunes, tops of beets and turnips, apples, bananas, carrots, grapefruit, kelp, coconut.

Vitamin B3

Other names: Niacin, nicotinic acid

Actions: Proper circulation and healthy nervous system. Gastrointestinal tract.

Best sources: Wheat germ, nuts, brown rice, sunflower seeds, potatoes, green vegetables, almonds, rhubarb, whole barley, rice bran.

Vitamin B5

Other names: Pantothenic acid, calcium pantothenate

Actions: Regulates metabolization of fats and carbohydrates. Adrenal glands, increases production of cortisone. Good for anti-stress.

Best sources: Peas, royal jelly, green vegetables, avocados, bananas, broccoli, collard greens, oranges, beans, molasses.

Vitamin B6

Other names: Pyridoxine, pyridoxine HCL, niacinamide, pyridoxal phosphate

Actions: Helps metabolize fats and carbohydrates. Proper DNA and RNA action, nervous system, brain. It plays an important part in metabolizing unsaturated fatty acids to vitamin F. Helps keep blood healthy, promotes red cell formation and supports normal hemoglobin levels. Essential to cell respiration.

Best sources: Green leafy vegetables, bananas, avocados, wheat germ, walnuts, blackstrap, molasses, cantaloupe, cabbage, green peppers, carrots, brown rice, honey, prunes, hazelnuts (filberts), potatoes, sunflower seeds.

Vitamin B9

Other names: Folic acid, pteroylglutamic acid, folacin

Actions: Forms red blood cells. Production of DNA and RNA. Amino acid metabolism.

Best sources: Green leafy vegetables, broccoli, asparagus, lima beans, Irish potatoes, nuts, beets, sprouts, avocados, spinach, cabbage, lettuce, bananas, mushrooms, Brussels sprouts, dates, cantaloupe.

Vitamin B12

Other names: Cobalamin, cyanocobalamin

Actions: Essential for growth, production and regeneration of red blood cells.

Best sources: Sunflower seeds, comfrey leaves, kelp, bananas, concord grapes.

Vitamin B13

Other names: Orotic acid

Best sources: Calcium, orotic acid.

Vitamin B15

Other names: Pangamic acid, calcium panmanate

Actions: Increases tolerance to hypoxia (insufficient oxygen to tissues and cells).

Best sources: Seeds, nuts, brown rice.

Vitamin B17

Other names: Nitrilosides, amygdalin, laetrile

Actions: Preventive and anti-cancer effect.

Best sources: Raspberries, cranberries, apricots and especially apricot pits, blackberries, mung beans, lima beans, garbanzo beans, flax seed, peach or plum pits.

Vitamin C

Other names: Ascorbic acid, L-dehydroascorbic acid

Actions: Activates growth and repair in tissues, boosts immune system, antioxidant, all organs and glands, connective tissues. Promotes healing in every situation of ill health. Can lower beneficial cholesterol and triglyceride levels. Also, synthesis of collagen for healthy skin and mucous membranes.

Best sources: All fruits and vegetables, especially strawberries, blackberries, citrus fruits, tomatoes, peppers, apples, persimmons, guavas, mangos, acerola, cherries, potatoes, cabbage, kale, papayas, spinach, broccoli, turnip greens, green bell peppers, red peppers, avocados, bananas, collards, black currants, parsley, rose hips, etc.

Vitamin D

Other names: Ergosterol, viosterol, calciferol

Actions: Absorption of calcium. Regulates and boosts resistance to infections. Essential for the formation of teeth and bones.

Best sources: Sprouted seeds, alfalfa, mushrooms, sunflower seeds, sunshine, wheat germ.

Vitamin E

Other names: Tocopherols, Tocotrienols

Actions: Oxygenates tissues, reduces need for oxygen intake, reproductive organs, heart. Protects cell membranes.

Best sources: Unprocessed and unrefined vegetable oils, raw and sprouted seeds, nuts, green leafy vegetables, brown rice, wheat germ, peas, lettuce, spinach, broccoli, asparagus, avocados.

Vitamin F

Other names: none

Actions: Lowers blood cholesterol. Helps lower risk of heart disease. Helps adrenal glands.

Best sources: Unprocessed and unrefined vegetable oils, flaxseed, linseed, safflower and sunflower oil, nuts, olive oil, wheat germ.

Vitamin H

Other names: Biotin

Actions: Metabolism of fats, carbohydrates, proteins and amino acids. Antiseptic.

Best sources: Almonds, oat bran, walnuts, tomatoes, green peas, bananas, some mushrooms.

Vitamin K

Other names: Phytonadione, menadiol, menadione

Actions: Intervenes with the blood coagulation mechanism. Helps liver. Metabolizes calcium (bones).

Best sources: Spinach, cabbage, asparagus, broccoli, cauliflower, tomatoes, carrots, kelp, alfalfa, blackstrap molasses, turnip greens, green vegetables, chlorophyll.

Vitamin P

Other names: Bioflavonoids

Actions: Blood vessel wall and capillary maintenance. Connective tissue. Strengthens capillary walls, anti-coagulant for capillaries, protects vitamin C.

Best sources: Apricots, cherries, paprika, grapefruit, lemons. Fresh fruits and vegetables, especially citrus, green peppers, grapes, strawberries, black currants, prunes.

Vitamin T

Actions: Platelet integrity in blood.

Best sources: Sesame seeds, tahini.

Vitamin U

Actions: Promotes healing in peptic ulcers, duodenal ulcers.

Best sources: Raw cabbage juice, fresh cabbage.

Choline

Other names: Acetylcholine

Actions: Aids in digestion and absorption. A part of phospholipids, like lecithin.

Best sources: Wheat, green leafy vegetables, cabbage, cauliflower, chickpeas, lentils, peanuts, legumes.

Inositol

Other names: Hexahydroxycyclohexane

Actions: Hair growth, heart; part of B-complex.

Best sources: Most fruits and green leafy vegetables.

PABA

Other names: Para-amino benzoic acid, vitamin Bx

Actions: Promotes growth. Good for skin, hair.

Best sources: Molasses, bran, brown rice, sunflower seeds, wheat germ.

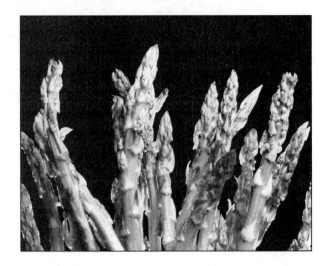

MODULE 3.6

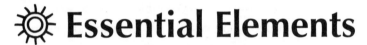

☀ Essential Elements

MAJOR MINERALS, TRACE MINERALS AND TISSUE SALTS

The human body reduced to its simplest form is a small pile of ashes. The carbon, hydrogen, oxygen and nitrogen from protein-rich tissues and carbohydrate (or fat stores) have dissolved into the air or evaporated as water, leaving only the minerals. These "mineral ashes," weighing approximately five pounds, might be small in quantity, but they would represent a vital role played out in all body tissues.

Minerals are involved in a variety of functions. They are necessary to promote growth and regulate body processes. They provide structure to bones and participate in muscle contraction, blood formation, protein building, energy production, and lots of other bodily processes. They are found in soil and water and are ingested via food and drink.

There are at least twenty-two minerals essential to human health (over sixty-five minerals have been found in the body), and these nutrients are divided into two categories: **major minerals** and **trace minerals**. Major minerals are present in the body in amounts greater than a teaspoon, while a trace mineral can total less than a teaspoon. The terms "major" and "trace" do not reflect the importance of a mineral in maintaining optimal health, as a deficiency of either major or trace minerals produces equally harmful effects. Henry Schroeder, M.D., Ph.D., of Dartmouth College has said, "Your mineral needs are even more important than your vitamin needs, since your body cannot make minerals."

Minerals work either together or against each other. Some minerals compete for absorption, so a large intake of one mineral can produce a deficiency of another. This is especially true of the trace minerals, such as copper, iron and zinc. In other cases, some minerals enhance the absorption of other minerals. For example, the proper proportion of calcium, magnesium and phosphorus in the diet enhances the absorption and use of all three minerals. Absorption is also dependent on body needs. A person who is deficient in a mineral will absorb more of it than someone who is adequately nourished. The three minerals that tend to be low in the average Western-world diet are calcium (utilization may be the big problem here), iron and zinc.

Commercial food processing definitely reduces the nutrient content of food and can be dangerous to human health. The refining of whole grains (including wheat, rice and corn) has resulted in a dramatic reduction of their natural-food-complex nutrition. The milling of wheat to white flour reduces the natural-food-complex vitamin and mineral content by 40-60 percent. Food refining appears to reduce trace minerals such as manganese, zinc and chromium, as well as various macro-minerals (magnesium). The treatment of canned or frozen vegetables with EDTA (a preservative) can strip much of the zinc from foods. High rates of calcium-metabolism disorders suggest that the forms of calcium many are consuming simply do not agree with the body, or are not assimilated properly, resulting in calcium loss.

Organically-grown produce contains higher levels of some essential minerals than does conventionally (non-organically) grown produce, and appears to contain lower levels of toxic heavy metals. Even if modern food practices did not affect nutrition (which they do), all minerals that humans need for optimal health do not exist uniformly in soils. Soils that are deficient in certain minerals can result in low concentrations of major or trace minerals in drinking water and plant crops, which contribute to marginal or deficient dietary intake. Luckily, we are able to draw from a wide variety of fruits, vegetables, nuts and herbs from all parts of the world.

MAJOR MINERALS

Calcium (Ca)

Acid/Alkaline: Alkaline-forming

Types: protein bound Ca. 46%; diffusable Ca. 6.5%; ionized Ca. 47.5%

Food sources: Kelp, sesame seeds, dark leafy green vegetables, carrots, oranges, almonds, broccoli, papaya, sunflower seeds, walnuts, cashews, Brazil nuts, tofu, bone meal, brown rice, and most fruits and vegetables.

Note: Coffee, commercial teas, carbonated drinks, (soda pops, etc.), marijuana, excess salt, cigarettes, refined sugars, alcohol, and chemical diuretics all inhibit or "pull" calcium out of bone and tissues.

Uses in the body: Calcium is the most abundant mineral (metal) in your body. Necessary for bone, cartilage, tendons and connective tissue strength. (Used in bone matrix.) Assists the actuation of many enzymes including pancreatic. Works with neuro-transmissions. Used in ATP,

---

Calcium Utilization

- Bone, nerve and connective tissue weakness can be a direct result of poor calcium utilization. This results in: hemorrhoids, varicose veins and spider veins, wrinkles, hernias, aneurysms, prolapsed conditions of bladder, uterus, bowels, etc.

- Thyroid/parathyroid weakness (hypo–activity) lowers or blocks proper calcium utilization.

- Phosphorus, calcium and magnesium must be in balance with each other for proper tissue function, growth and repair.

- High calcium supplementation will push out or deplete your phosphorus levels.

- Calcium cannot be properly utilized without parathyroid hormones. Stone formation, including bone spurs, will result if you supplement anything but plant calcium, especially when the parathyroid is weak.

Adenosine Triphosphate release (cell energy reserves). 99% of the body's Ca is located in the bones and teeth. Plays a role in blood clotting. One of many cellular transporters.

Deficiencies: A lack of utilization is epidemic. Utilization requires parathyroid/thyroid hormones and alkalization.

Short term deficiencies: Muscle cramping and spasms, pounding heartbeat, loss of sleep, irritability, tooth decay, periodontal disease, softened bones, nervousness, back and leg cramps, brittle bones, connective tissue weakness including varicose and spider veins, hemorrhoids, prolapsed conditions of organs and skin, petechiae, hot flashes, hot and cold syndrome, and heart arrhythmias. Plays a role in muscular contraction. Use is regulated by parathyroid hormone and vitamin D. Builds bones and teeth. Normalizes heart action, nerve irritability, blood coagulation, normalizes metabolism. Calcium neutralizes excessive serum histamines. Increased calcium consumption can increase calcitonin production by the thyroid gland (C-cells). This actually inhibits bone reabsorption, thus creating the opposite effect of rebuilding your bones. Lead interferes with calcium utilization.

Long term deficiencies: Osteoporosis, scoliosis, rickets and diseases involving the loss of calcium from the bones or the failure of growing bones to have enough calcium for strength and proper growth. Stunted growth. Also, arthritis and depression.

Toxicity: Acidosis, bone spurs, kidney stones, stenosis issues, and calcium deposits in tissues. Also possibly hypertension, confusion, nausea and vomiting.

Carbon (C)

Acid/Alkaline: Acid-forming

Food sources: Air, carbohydrates, sugars, fruits and vegetables, nuts, olives and avocados.

Uses in the body: Main source of energy. A component of carbohydrates and building blocks of fats and amino acids. Necessary for teeth, connective tissue, skin, hair and nails.

Chlorine (Chloride) (Cl)

Acid/Alkaline: Acid-forming

Food sources: Most fruits and vegetables: coconut, avocados, dates, turnips, lettuces, kale, kelp/dulse, celery, tomatoes, potatoes, apricots, orange juice, pineapple, watercress, raw white cabbage, spinach, asparagus, cucumbers, parsnips, carrots, onions. In cooked dried beans and peas, and sea salt, etc.

Toxic sources: Water supplies

Uses in the body: An electrolyte, along with sodium and potassium. Affects blood, nerves, epithelium. Aids digestion and elimination, normalizes osmotic pressure in blood and tissues. Helps maintain normal heart function, acid-base balance and water balance. Increases capacity of blood to carry carbon dioxide to lungs for excretion. Helps to cleanse both the intestines and body of toxins. Produces the normal acid environment in stomach. (This aids in absorption of iron and vitamin B12.)

Deficiency: Disturbed digestion, water retention issues, weight loss.

Toxicity: Very toxic in even slightly higher amounts. Symptoms are weakness, confusion and coma.

Hydrogen (H)

Acid/Alkaline: Alkaline-forming

Food sources: All foods, especially carbohydrates and fats. Sugars, fruits and vegetables (especially carrots, celery, spinach, tomatoes and cabbage).

Uses in the body: Blood; all cells.

Magnesium (Mg)

Acid/Alkaline: Alkaline-forming

Food sources: All fruits and vegetables, especially dark leafy greens, seaweeds, nuts, seeds, dried fruits, potatoes, sesame seeds, alfalfa, figs, brown rice, kelp, pineapple, honey, celery, whole-grain products, almonds, avocados, bananas, apples, peaches, lima beans, black-eyed peas, wheat germ, brown rice.

Toxic sources: Water

Uses in the body: Strengthens muscles and nerve tissues. Activates many enzymes, especially in carbohydrate metabolism. Needed for proper bone and teeth formation. Conditions liver and glands. Stimulates elimination. May help combat stress, maintain muscle contractions and aid in adaptation to cold, and regulation of normal heart rhythm. May reduce effects of lead poisoning and reduce kidney stones. Also, blood albumen.

Note: Alcohol, diuretics, emotional or physical stress, diarrhea, zinc, and fluoride increase the need for magnesium.

Deficiency: Symptoms may include diarrhea, fatigue, calcium depletion, and heart arrhythmias. Also, soft and porous bones, poor digestion, GI upsets, fatigue, sleep disturbances, irritability, confusion, cramping and spasms, tachycardia, nervousness, kidney stones, convulsions, poor complexion. A severe magnesium deficiency may result in coronary heart disease, mental confusion, and blood clot formation.

Toxicity: Severe nausea and vomiting, extremely low blood pressure, extreme muscle weakness, difficulty breathing and heartbeat irregularity.

Nitrogen (N)

Acid/Alkaline: Acid-forming

Food sources: Proteins (Amino Acids). Dominating foods: nuts, seeds, alfalfa, green leafy vegetables.

Toxic sources: Meats

Uses in the body: Acts like and is the main element of a protein and the mineral phosphorus. Muscles, cartilage, tissue, tendons, ligaments, lean flesh.

Deficiency: Abnormal growth, thinness, neuromuscular issues, and death.

Toxicity: Acidosis

Oxygen (O)

Acid/Alkaline: Alkaline-forming

Food sources: Fresh air

Toxic sources: Pollution

Uses in the body: Creates oxidation. Needed for bones, teeth, skin, red blood cells, circulation and optimism!

Deficiency: Lack of oxygen causes death.

Phosphorus (P)

Acid/Alkaline: Acid-forming

Food sources: present in nearly all foods, especially peas, seeds, corn, mushrooms, carrots, nuts (pecans, almonds, etc.), whole grain products, dried fruit, legumes.

Toxic sources: Meat, grains, intestinal products and wastes, phosphate mining, soaps, phosphate additives in carbonated drinks, etc.

Uses in the body: Phosphorus is essential for calcification of bone (85% of your body's pH is in your skeletal system). Used in many enzyme processes including metabolism. Controls the activities of most hormones and many vitamins. A factor in carbohydrate, fat and protein metabolism. Organic phosphates are a part of all cellular structures and many of their functions. Part of ATP (Adenosine Triphosphate), which is a cell's power company. Used in the oxidation of sugars for the formation of ATP.

Builds bones, teeth, blood, brain and hair. Metabolism of fats and carbohydrates. Transporter of fatty acids.

Deficiency: Leads to bone pain and poor bone formation, osteoporosis, poor memory, tissue weakness, prolapsed conditions, fatigue, irritability, poor growth, rickets, skin sensitivity, decreased appetite and weight. General weakness. Excessive amounts of phosphorus can occur from prolonged and excessive intake of non-absorbable antacids, high consumption of soft drinks, canned and processed foods.

Toxicity: Rarely toxic. Symptoms may include brittle bones related to loss of calcium (osteoporosis), seizures, heartbeat irregularities and shortness of breath.

Potassium (K)

Acid/Alkaline: Alkaline-forming

Food sources: All fruits and vegetables, especially dark green leafy ones. Kelp, dulse, seeds, figs, celery, mushrooms, dried fruits, potatoes, avocados, broccoli, legumes, papaya, raisins, brown rice, Brussels sprouts, bananas, and watermelon.

Toxic sources: Prescription drugs, especially some diuretics, can cause excessive potassium loss from the body. Also, chronic diarrhea and diabetic acidosis.

Note: Excess Vitamin D can contribute to potassium loss and the suppression of thyroid function. Same with PABA supplementation. Also, potassium deficiency (or loss) is also affected by magnesium, zinc, and iron deficiency.

Deficiency: Heart arrhythmias, shortness of breath, weakness in muscles, poor digestion and utilization. Slowed growth, paralysis, sterility, mental apathy and confusion, kidney damage. Dry skin, acne, chills, insomnia, decreased reflex response, glucose intolerance. Potassium deficiency can occur with chronic diarrhea, vomiting, diabetic acidosis, kidney disease, or prolonged use of laxatives or diuretics.

Uses in the body: Balances body fluids, regulates nervous and muscular irritability. Aids in formation of glycogen from glucose, fats from glycogen, proteins from peptones and proteases. May cure acne, allergies, alcoholism, heart disease and help to heal burns.

Toxicity: Excess intake of potassium can cause high concentration of the element in blood, disturbances in heart and kidney function, and alterations in fluid balance. Fatalities may result when high levels of potassium in the bloodstream cause heart attacks.

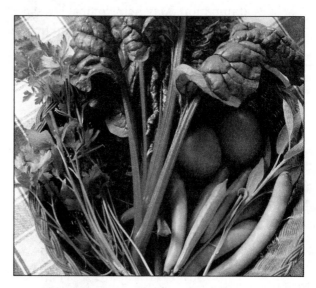

Sodium (Na)

Acid/Alkaline: Alkaline-forming

Food sources: All fruits and vegetables, especially dark green leafy ones, carrots, celery, watermelon, strawberries, apples, huckleberries, gooseberries, cauliflower, asparagus, salt (all types), cucumbers, beets, okra, pumpkin, string beans, kelp/dulse.

Toxic sources: Most processed foods, water supplies.

Note: Diuretic drugs are the chief offenders in throwing off excess sodium from the body.

Excessive sweating can reduce sodium in the body to low levels. Also, low sodium may be indicative of reduced adrenal cortex function. Sodium has a strong affinity for Oxygen.

Uses in the body: An essential body electrolyte. A principle cation (positively charged ion) for intra- (inter) cellular activities and homeostasis. Plays a major role in the osmotic pressure of a cell, thus affecting water and nutritional utilization by cells. Involved in muscular contraction. Plays a role in carbohydrate and protein metabolism; plays a role in glucose catabolism (breakdown) and glycogen formation (glucose storage); plays a role in neuro- (electrical) transmission through the nervous system (affecting conductivity of a cell); and plays a role in normal heart rhythms.

Deficiency: Sodium deficiency symptoms include muscle weakness and muscle shrinkage, twitching, fatigue, poor concentration, memory loss, loss of appetite, nausea, diarrhea, arthritis, nerve pain, digestive distress, poor adrenal function, and weight loss. These are usually a result of starvation or severe fasting, vomiting, dry skin, allergies, low blood pressure, constipation, perspiration or diarrhea. A severe deficiency of sodium chloride could cause dehydration and death.

Toxicity: A diet high in sodium is linked to hypertension (and restriction of sodium lowers blood pressure). Diets in the U.S. contain excessive amounts of sodium (as much as 15 times the recommended daily intake).

Sulfur (S)

Acid/Alkaline: Acid-forming

Food sources: Kale, turnip, Brussels sprouts, dried beans, cabbage, cauliflower, garlic, onions, raspberry, kelp, broccoli, lettuce, wheat germ, etc.

Toxic sources: Hair permanents, straighteners, some conditioners can affect sulfur levels.

Note: Sulfur is known to protect cells from the toxic effects of heavy metals. Also, tobacco decreases absorption.

Uses in the body: Sulfur disinfects the blood, helps the body to resist bacteria, and protects the protoplasm of cells. It aids in necessary oxidation reactions in the body, stimulates bile secretion, and protects against toxic substances. Because of its ability to protect against the harmful effects of radiation and pollution, sulfur slows down the aging process. It is needed for the synthesis of collagen, a principal protein that gives the skin its structural integrity. Needed for hair, nails, insulin, cartilage, and blood. Aids digestion and elimination. Oxidizing agent in hemoglobin.

Note: Sulfur is the key substance that makes garlic the "king of herbs."

Deficiency: Restricted growth, eczema, dermatitis, poor growth of nails and hair or brittle hair and nails.

Toxicity: Increased cardiac risk. Unlikely to threaten life.

ABOUT TRACE MINERALS

Trace elements are minerals needed in small amounts by plants, animals and human beings. There are trace amounts of over sixty-five minerals in our bodies, including: aluminum, arsenic, barium, bismuth, beryllium, bromine, cadmium, chromium, copper, folic acid, fluorine, gallium, germanium, gold, iodine, iron, lead, lithium, manganese, mercury, molybdenum, quinine, selenium, silicon, silver, strontium, tin, titanium, tungsten, vanadium and zinc. They play a major role in health and are essential in the assimilation and utilization of vitamins and other nutrients. They aid in digestion and provide the catalyst for many hormones, enzymes and essential body functions and reactions. They also aid in replacing electrolytes lost through heavy perspiration or extended diarrhea and protect against toxic reactions and heavy metal poisoning. Current research now proves that human beings should get the required trace elements from their food in a balanced diet, especially fresh fruits and vegetables.

The late Dr. Henry Schroeder stated that trace elements (minerals) "are more important than are the vitamins, in that they cannot be synthesized by living matter. Thus they are the spark-plugs in the chemistry of life, on which the exchanges of energy in the combustion of foods and the building of living tissues depend."

There are many factors that can contribute to mineral imbalances. This means that the minerals we think we are consuming do not necessarily wind up doing their work in our bodies. What are some of the barriers to mineral absorption?

Diet

A major factor contributing to a mineral imbalance is improper eating habits, including excessive intake of refined carbohydrates, alcohol, and fad diets. Even the mineral content of a "healthy" diet can be inadequate, depending upon the soil in which the food was grown or the method in which it was prepared.

Stress

Both physical and emotional stress can lead to mineral imbalances. Certain nutrients such as the mineral zinc and the B-complex vitamins are lost in greater quantities due to increased stress. Nutrient absorption can also decrease when the body is under stress.

Medications

Medications can deplete the body store of nutrient minerals or increase the levels of toxic metals. The well-known effects of diuretics include not only sodium loss, but in many cases, a potassium and magnesium loss. Antacids, aspirin, and oral contraceptive agents can lead to vitamin and mineral deficiencies as well as toxic metal excesses.

Pollution

Toxic metals such as lead, mercury and cadmium can interfere with mineral absorption and increase mineral excretion. All our lives we are continually exposed to a variety of toxic metal sources such as cigarette smoke (cadmium), copper and aluminum cookware, hair dyes (lead), lead based cosmetics, hydrogenated oils (nickel), antiperspirants (aluminum), and dental amalgams (mercury and cadmium). These are just a few of the many sources of metal pollution an individual may be exposed to every day.

Nutritional supplements

Vitamin and mineral supplements can also cause imbalances. Calcium absorption is decreased in the presence of phosphorus. Vitamin C is required for iron absorption, but in excess amounts it can cause a copper deficiency. Vitamin D enhances calcium absorption, but, in excess amounts, can produce a magnesium deficiency or other conditions.

TRACE MINERALS/ MICRO-TRACE MINERALS

Arsenic (As)

Acid/Alkaline: Acid-forming

Food sources: Water, air and soil.

Toxic sources: Fish, grains and cereals, coal burning, pesticides, insecticides (via a chemical called arsenoxide), herbicides, defoliants, metal work, manufacture of glass and mirrors, tobacco smoke, dental compounds for root canal fillings. Also, breathing sawdust or burning smoke from wood treated with arsenic, living near uncontrolled hazardous waste sites, eating food, drinking water, or breathing air containing arsenic. Inorganic arsenic compounds are used to preserve wood.

Uses in the body: The role of arsenic in the body is unknown. In animal studies, arsenic was essential for growth, development, and reproduction, possibly because of its role in the metabolism of methionine, an amino acid involved in growth. Has a "garlic" odor when burned. Stored mostly in the liver. Excreted in urine. Possible uses in the body: skin, hair, nails, thyroid gland and brain.

Deficiency: Arsenic settles in the muscles and the brain (dislodging phosphorus). Sweet metallic taste, garlicky odor to breath and stools, constriction of throat, constant backache (causes chiropractic adjustments not to hold), fatigue, low vitality, difficulties in swallowing, burning sensation (inflammation) in eyes, throat and chest, enlargement of tonsils, muscle spasms, pain in muscles of the back, listlessness, loss of pain sensation, loss of body hair, skin color changes (dark spots) gastroenteritis.

Toxicity: Metabolic inhibitor (reduces energy production efficiency), cellular and enzyme poison. Constricts the throat and causes muscle spasms. An extreme "nerve" toxin. Anorexia. Ingesting high levels can result in death. Breathing high levels of inorganic arsenic can give you a sore throat or irritated lungs. Also, nausea, vomiting, decreased production of red and white blood cells, abnormal heart rhythm, damage to blood vessels, and a sensation of "pins and needles" in hands and feet. Also, constant backache.

Beryllium (Be)

Food sources: Water, air and soil.

Toxic sources: Industrial exposure, mining, metal working, burning coal, copper processing, and possibly paints, colors, cosmetics.

Uses in the body: There is currently no information regarding whether beryllium is essential for optimum biochemical function.

Deficiency: Dyspnea, weight loss, cough, fatigue, chest pain, anorexia, and weakness.

Toxicity: Effects the lungs, liver, kidneys and heart. Enzyme inhibitor, including ATP, DNA and several hepatic enzymes; cell death in all tissues.

Boron (B)

Acid/Alkaline: Acid-forming

Found in: Volcanic springs in Tuscany, as borates in hernite, and as colemanite in California.

Food sources: Water supply. Fresh fruits: apples, carrots, grapes, pears, leafy vegetables, nuts and grains.

Toxic sources: Soaps, cements, some cleaners, glass, ceramics.

Deficiency: Poor dietary intake of boron causes bone changes similar to those noted in osteoporotic women. Boron deficiency results in decreased blood levels of ionized calcium and calcitonin, elevated levels of total calcium and urinary excretion of calcium. In animals, it causes depressed growth rates. Boron and magnesium metabolism might be related, since a combined deficiency of these two minerals exacerbates the osteo-condition, suppresses bone anabolism, and results in decreased magnesium concentrations in bones. In contrast, boron supplementation elevates serum concentrations of beta-estradiol and testosterone and produces changes consistent with the prevention of calcium loss and bone demineralization.

Toxicity: Nausea, diarrhea, skin rashes, arthritis, and fatigue. Limited research on animals shows that excessive boron intake might suppress growth and immunity.

Cadmium (Cd)

Food sources: Water, air and soil.

Toxic sources: Cigarette smoke, air from battery manufacturing, metal soldering, welding and electroplating, pipes, water supplies, mining, the air near zinc refineries, burning of fossil fuels or municipal waste, dentures, paints, galvanized pipes, contaminated shellfish.

Foods that help to detox cadmium: Vegetables from the cabbage family, paprika, fruits.

Uses in the body: An environmental poison found in water, on our food and in the air. It's found in processed grains, dairy products, meats, fish, fertilizers, auto exhaust, cigarette smoke, batteries, solder and dentures. It disrupts the absorption of other minerals and tends to settle in the heart and right kidney and affects proper functioning of several enzymes.

Deficiency: Anemia, muscle deterioration, hypertension, liver and kidney damage, zinc deficiency, arthritis, pneumonitis, vomiting, diarrhea, loss of calcium in bones, deterioration of heart and blood vessel structures, prostration, emphysema.

Toxicity: Cadmium is not excreted from the body and can accumulate over time to toxic levels. Excessive intake occurs when soft water leaches cadmium from pipes. Hypertension, kidney damage, loss of sense of smell (anosmia). Studies show that alcohol increases the retention of heavy metals such as cadmium.

Chromium (Cr)

Acid/Alkaline: Acid-forming

Food Sources: Natural water sources, mushrooms, sugar cane, brewer's yeast, molasses, spices and herbs.

Toxic sources: Industry leather tanning processes, raw cement and wood finishing.

Note: Scientists estimate that 90% of Americans don't get enough chromium and that 60% are diabetic or hypoglycemic.

Uses in the body: Master regulator of insulin. The average body contains about 600 mcg. of chromium with the highest concentration occurring during infancy. The main function of chromium is as a component of glucose tolerance factor (GTF), a substance that works with insulin to facilitate the uptake of blood sugar (glucose) into the cells. Needed for energy, thyroid, spleen. Aids carbohydrate metabolism. Works with insulin in glucose utilization and energy release. Chromium deficient diseases are aggravated by vanadium deficiency.

Deficiency: Hypoglycemia, diabetes. Possible sleep and dream disturbances, anxiety, fatigue, shortened life span. Industrial chromium has carcinogenic effects upon the lungs and can cause bronchial inflammation, skin ulcerations, and conditions have been observed in cerebral hemorrhage and thrombosis.

Toxicity: Excess intake or tissue accumulation of chromium can inhibit rather than enhance the effectiveness of insulin. At extremely high levels, it may encourage the growth of cancer. Kidney and liver impairment.

Cobalt (Co)

Food sources: All green leafy vegetables. Also, various fruits, vegetables and herbs.

Toxic Sources: Cobalt is used as an anti-foaming agent in the processing of some beer. Consumption of large amounts of this beer could cause polycythemia and heart disorders.

Uses in the body: Aids in normal growth and appetite, pancreas. The only known function of cobalt is as a constituent of vitamin B12. In this capacity, cobalt aids in the formation of normal red blood cells, maintenance of nerve tissue, and normal formation of cells.

Deficiency: A deficiency of cobalt is equivalent to a deficiency of vitamin B12, and can cause anemia, nerve disorders, and abnormalities in cell formation. Also, "scaly" skin and atrophy.

Toxicity: Rare. Large doses of inorganic cobalt (not combined with vitamin B12) might stimulate thyroid and bone marrow function, resulting in excess production of red blood cells (polycythemia).

Copper (Cu)

Acid/Alkaline: Alkaline-forming

Food sources: Dark green leafy vegetables, raisins, radishes, nuts (especially almonds) oranges, blackstrap molasses, avocados, and broccoli.

Toxic sources: Copper water pipes and cooking utensils.

Note: Long-term uses of oral contraceptives can upset the balance of copper in the body causing excessively high cholesterol levels.

Uses in the body: Liver, gallbladder, blood, lungs, heart. Absorption and metabolism of iron. Oxidation of fatty acids, of tyrosine to melanin pigments. Metabolism of ascorbic acid (vitamin C). A catalyst used in the manufacture of hemoglobin. Essential to catecholamine synthesis. Copper is a component of the antioxidant enzyme: superoxide dismutase, and might protect cell membranes from potential damage by highly reactive oxygen fragments. In this antioxidant role, copper might function to prevent the development of cancer.

Deficiency: Copper settles in brain and ovaries. Can cause chronic diarrhea, burning sensation in throat and tonsils, malabsorption problems, or iron-deficiency anemia. Also loss of color from skin and hair (inability of body to manufacture collagen), baldness, heart disease, Menkes' Syndrome, nervous system impairment, low resistance to infection, scoliosis, poor tissue formation, impaired respiration, skin sores, retardation.

Toxicity: Symptoms can include ulcerative colitis, Wilson's Disease. Mental and emotional problems.

Note: Daily intake of more than 20 mg. can cause nausea and vomiting.

Fluorine/Fluoride (F)

Acid/Alkaline: Acid-forming

Food sources: Carrots, turnip and beet greens, dandelion, sunflower seeds, garlic, spinach, green leafy vegetables, nuts (especially almonds), dandelions.

Toxic sources: Fluoride is added to many water supplies and to food processed in areas containing high levels of fluoride. It is added to most toothpastes and may be added to the soil in certain fertilizers. Also found in seafood and oats.

Uses in the body: Stronger tooth enamel and bones, fewer cavities, fewer bone fractures, less osteoporosis in older women, higher birth weights and higher rates of growth in children, reduces loss of hearing if caused by otospongiosis of the inner ear. Also needed for blood, skin, hair and nails.

Deficiency: Decay of teeth, curvature of the spine, weak eyesight.

Toxicity: Fluoride remains in the body for a long time, because it is incorporated into the bones. Even just a little over the recommended levels can cause painful and aching bones, stiffness, weakness, chalky white areas on the teeth, brown or pitted teeth, knots on the bones, rapid aging, increased rates of cancer, high death rate (up to three times higher in areas of high fluoride concentration in water supply), sagging and wrinkled skin, scleroderma (hard patches of skin). People in India sometimes suffer from the bone deformities (i.e., hunchback) of skeletal fluorosis even when the fluoride concentration in the water is only 1½ times the RDA. Hot weather, drinking lots of water, and low protein diets increase fluoride intake and side effects. Large doses of fluoride are extremely poisonous.

Iron (Fe)

Acid/Alkaline: Acid-forming

Food sources: Fruits and vegetables, especially dark green leafy vegetables, nuts (including almonds, hazelnuts, etc.), oranges, grapes, bananas, kelp/dulse, raisins, figs, beets, carrots, tomato juice, asparagus, parsley, lima beans, cucumbers, Brussels sprouts, winter squash, broccoli, watercress, blackberries, whole grain products, root vegetables, spinach, raw broccoli, green peas, avocados, prunes, raisins, sesame and pumpkin seeds.

Toxic sources: Industry, old plumbing pipes, water supplies, environmental sources, including air, cast-iron pots and pans.

Uses in the body: Essential for the formation of hemoglobin, myoglobin and many enzymes, necessary for the formation of red blood cells, and helps fight stress and disease. Iron affects the release of the adrenal hormone aldosterone. Aldosterone increases sodium levels. This aids alkalization and balances potassium. Works with glucose and fructose as well as with some vitamins (E, C, etc.) and some amino acids. Iron strengthens the immune system and increases resistance to colds, infections and disease. It is the oxygen-carrying component of the blood. Other possible uses in body: growth, reproduction, teeth, skeletal, liver, lipids, cholesterol.

Vitamin E and zinc, taken in large doses, interfere with the absorption of iron. Caffeine from coffee, tea or soft drinks interferes with the absorption of iron. Excessive phosphorus consumption in people who eat lots of canned food or in people who drink many soft drinks may block absorption. Excessive sweating, or rapid food transit time through the intestines can reduce iron. Low iron builds high lead and visa versa. Lead interferes with hemoglobin formation and can create iron deficiency anemia.

Deficiency: Slight iron deficiency (that does not affect red blood cell counts) may cause tiredness, headache, slower running times in competitive runners, weakness, difficult menstruation, irritability, depression and sleeplessness or troubled sleep. Severe iron deficiency may cause anemia or low red blood cell counts, constipation, mouth soreness, brittle nails, pale skin or difficulty in breathing. Other possible symptoms could be food cravings for "nonfood items" such as ice, clay or starch, heart disease, impaired mental skills. Can affect job performance, mood and memory. Increases intestinal irritation and inflammation.

Toxicity: Taking too much iron can cause unhealthy iron deposits in the body, and can lead to the production of free radicals. The buildup of iron in the tissues has been associated with a rare disease known as hemochromatosis. Overdoses can cause bleeding from the stomach or intestines, a drop in blood pressure, liver damage, reduced resistance to infections, and could be fatal for young children.

Lead (Pb)

Acid/Alkaline: Acid-forming

Food sources: Food and plants grown in soil contaminated with lead.

Toxic sources: Lead is ingested from a variety of

sources including fresh and canned food, water, lead-based paint, lead-glazed pottery, hair dyes, air pollution, car exhaust, tobacco smoke, on the solder of tin cans, fumes from gasoline vapors while filling your gas tanks are full of lead. Lead is a protoplasmic poison found in bleached white sugar.

Foods that help to detox lead: Pumpkin seeds, okra, rhubarb root, cayenne pepper, peppermint, dulse, leafy greens and fruits.

Note: Watch out for copper and aluminum cookware and storing acid-foods in metal containers.

Uses in the body: Unknown. Lead interferes with hemoglobin formation and can create iron deficiency anemia. Lead is a protoplasmic poison, which means it interferes with the proper life-energy enzyme exchange in the living body.

Deficiency: Lead is one of the most common and persistent neurotoxins in the environment. Causes damage even at low levels. Lack of will power, fatigue, lack of abstract thinking, allergies, anemia, headaches, weakness, hyperactivity in children, brain dysfunction, causes behavioral and learning problems, especially in children. Lead settles in the brain, nerves, bones and the right kidney.

Toxicity: Impaired nervous system (which can result in behavioral problems such as hyperactivity in children), anemia, weakness, muscle deterioration, lethargy, mental impairment, abdominal discomfort, constipation, lack of will power, lack of abstract thinking, lack of mental capacity, tooth decay, allergic reactions to food and environment, increases in diabetes and multiple sclerosis.

Lithium (Li)

Acid//Alkaline: Alkaline-forming

Food sources: Kelp/dulse, whole grain foods, seeds.

Uses in the body: Reduces aggressiveness, violence and self-destruction.

Deficiency: Depression, manic depressive disorders, mania, suicide, spousal and child abuse.

Toxicity: Tremors, drowsiness, headaches, confusion, restlessness, dizziness, psychomotor retardation, lethargy, coma.

Manganese (Mn)

Acid/Alkaline: Alkaline-binding

Food sources: All dark leafy green vegetables, spinach, bananas, beets, blueberries, oranges, grapefruit, apricots, peas, kelp and other seaweed, celery, legumes, nuts, grains, asparagus, pineapples.

Toxic sources: Industrially inhaled manganese has been linked to psychiatric and nervous disorders!

Uses in the body: Thyroxine formation, formation of urea, lipotropic activity of choline. Utilization of thiamine. Metabolism of carbohydrates, strengthens tissues and bones, kidneys, liver, pancreas, spleen, brain, heart and lymph. Works with neurotransmitters and energy metabolism. Component of bone and cartilage formation. Activates many enzymes including pyruvate, carboxylase, mitochondrial superoxide, arginase and dismutase. Essential to catecholamine synthesis. Helps fertility and reproduction, helps growth and sex hormone production, helps regulate blood sugar and helps the body use proteins and carbohydrates.

Deficiency: Rare. Atherosclerosis, confusion, tremors, impaired vision and hearing, skin rash, elevated cholesterol, increased blood pressure, irritability, pancreatic damage, sweating, increased heart rate, mental impairment, grinding of teeth, fatigue and low endurance. Weak bone, hair and finger-nails. Skin conditions. Conception issues and weight loss. Glandular disorders, weak tissue respiration, defective reproduction functions, seizures and convulsions, possible cramping, paralysis. However, calcium deficiency is the reason for cramping.

Toxicity: Known to be highly toxic when inhaled or taken intravenously. Excess symptoms are CID or the human equivalent of Mad Cow Disease.

Mercury (Hg)

Food sources: Many types of fish, especially tuna

Toxic sources: Contaminated fish, dental amalgams, water supplies, thermometers, some batteries, manufacture and delivery of petroleum products, fungicides (for grains and cereals), florescent lamps, hair dyes, cosmetics, combustion of fossil fuels, fertilizers, pharmaceutical preparations (diuretics and hemorrhoidal, etc.). This source of mercury might suppress the immune system and the body's natural defense against infection and disease.

Uses in the body: Mercury salts are used in medicine, agriculture, and industry and accumulation of toxic levels is possible. Mercury alters the shape and function of enzymes. The body accumulates mercury in the kidneys, nerves, blood, liver, bone marrow, spleen, brain, heart, skin and muscles. The developing infant is very susceptible to mercury toxicity during pregnancy. While pregnant and/or breast-feeding, eat in moderation any fish that tends to be high in mercury.

Deficiency: Mercury settles in liver, spleen, kidneys, intestinal wall, heart, skeletal muscles, lungs and bones. Immediate gastro-intestinal disturbances, loss of appetite and weight, inflammation of gums, difficulty chewing and swallowing, metallic taste in mouth, thirst, nausea, vomiting, pain in the abdomen, bloody diarrhea.

Toxicity: Excess mercury suppresses selenium, causes severe emotional disturbances, cell destruction, blocked transport of sugars (energy at cellular level), increased permeability of potassium, loss of appetite, depression, tremors, decreases senses, peripheral numbness, poor memory and especially neuro-muscular conductors. Has been linked to MS and Parkinson's. Has been associated with heart attacks (MIs).

Molybdenum (Mo)

Food sources: Brown rice, millet, dark green leafy vegetables, peas, legumes, beans, whole grains.

Toxic sources: Tap water

Uses in the body: Regulates calcium, magnesium, copper metabolism. Conversion of purines to uric acid. It's a component of the enzyme xanthine oxidase that aids in the formation of uric acid (a normal breakdown product of metabolism). It is important in the mobilization of iron from storage, and is necessary for normal growth and development.

Deficiency: Copper deficiency. Increased heart rate, mouth and gum disorders, anemia, loss of appetite, weight loss, impotence in older males, increased respiratory rate, night blindness, stunted growth.

Toxicity: Generally considered non-toxic. However, prolonged intake of more than 10 mg. is associated with gout-like symptoms, such as pain and swelling of the joints.

Nickel (Ni)

Food sources: Found in trace amounts in all foods.

Toxic sources: Is used in industry as a catalyst in the hydrogenation of oils and fats (hardened fats). Commonly found in all brands of margarine, as well as oils and fats labeled "hydrogenated," meaning hardened vegetable oil (also in breads, chips, cookies, candies, etc.). Found in steel and other metal manufacturing industries, cigarettes, and in dyes and hair treatments.

Note: Poppy Seeds remove nickel deposits!

Foods that help to detoxify nickel: The best dietary sources that assist the body to remove excess or toxic amounts of nickel and other metals are fruits and green leafy vegetables.

Uses in the body: No established role for nickel has been identified, although the mineral is found in association with the genetic code within each cell and might help activate certain enzymes. Some say pancreas and insulin. It is probably involved in the activity of hormones, cell membranes and enzymes. Low blood levels of Ni are observed in people with vitamin B6 deficiency, cirrhosis of the liver, and kidney failure. The significance of these blood levels is not known. In contrast, elevated blood levels of nickel are associated with the development of cancer, heart attack, thyroid disorders, psoriasis and eczema.

Deficiency: Nickel settles in sinus, joints, and spinal column. Can be a nephro-toxin, effecting the urinary tract, especially the kidneys. It is found to bind with blood fungus causing tumors. Can paralyze the spinal column and bring on epilepsy. Can cause dermatitis and other skin conditions, allergic reactions and chronic rhinitis. Inflammation of lungs and liver, leading to necrosis and carcinoma.

Toxicity: Leads to paralysis, overflow of blood to brain, and epilepsy. In excess, can be a carcinogenic. Can rob the body of oxygen. Every tumor needs nickel to hold it together!

Selenium (Se)

Acid/Alkaline: Acid-forming

Food sources: Kelp/dulse, garlic, mushrooms, organic vegetables, grains, broccoli, onions, brazil nuts. Most foods.

Toxic sources: Soil. Also, the refining of flour removes much of the selenium that is concentrated in the germ and bran. It is important to eat whole-grain products, since the selenium is not added back into "enriched" flour.

Uses in the body: The most important known function of selenium is as a component of the antioxidant enzyme glutathione peroxidase. Selenium is a co-factor in an enzyme that protects body tissues (especially cell membranes) from oxidation by unstable free radicals. Selenium also works closely with the antioxidant vitamin E. Protects all membranes, reduces risk of cancer, enhances immune system, antioxidant. Lowers requirement for B12.

Deficiency: Muscle weakness, linked to cancer and heart disease, fatigue, dandruff, loose skin, growth retardation, elevated cholesterol levels, susceptibility to infection, sterility, and liver damage. Down's Syndrome, fibrocystic breast disease, Cystic Fibrosis, Muscular Dystrophy.

Toxicity: May include "garlic" breath, loss of hair, fingernails and toenails, irritability, liver and kidney impairment, metallic taste in mouth, dermatitis and jaundice. Large overdoses can cause death.

Silica or Silicon (Si)

Acid/Alkaline: Alkaline-forming

Food sources: Alfalfa, kelp, dark green leafy vegetables, horsetail, nettle, flaxseed, many fruits including apples, grapes, etc. Nuts, seeds, onions, berries (including strawberries), lettuce, figs, dandelion, cucumbers, cooked, dried beans and peas, sunflower seeds, tomatoes.

Uses in the body: Blood, muscles, skin, nerves, nails, hair, connective tissue, pancreas, tooth enamel, and thymus (has an antiseptic action). Silicon levels are high in people with atherosclerosis, but we're not sure whether or not the mineral is related to the development or progression of cardiovascular disease. The daily diet contains ample amounts of silicon and the mineral is well absorbed.

Deficiency: Silicon's primary function is in the development and maintenance of bone. A silicon deficiency causes weak and malformed bones of the arms, legs and head. Si is also important in the formation of connective tissue (the protein webwork in bone in which calcium is embedded). Reduces resistance to infectious diseases. Rapid aging, tendonitis, bone decalcification, cardiovascular disease, abnormal skeletal formation, artherosclerosis.

Tin (Sn)

Food sources: Water, air and soil.

Toxic sources: Leakage of the metal cans into canned foods.

Uses in the body: Supports hair growth and can enhance reflexes.

Deficiency: Tin absorption is poor and it's not clear how much of the daily intake of 1.5 to 3.5 mg. actually crosses the intestinal lining and enters the blood. Deficiency can cause symmetrical baldness, reduced response to noise.

Toxicity: High intakes of tin might destroy red blood cells.

Vanadium (V)

Food sources: Vanadium in foods is found in an organic form.

Toxic sources: Used in alloy steels, making rubber, plastics, ceramics and other chemicals. Can also be found in air, food and water supplies.

Uses in the body: Required for glucose tolerance factor. Vanadium forms compounds with other biological substances. The average human body contains 20 mg. of vanadium, which probably is involved in cholesterol metabolism and hormone production. Preliminary reports show that vanadium might protect against the development of breast cancer and might slow down the growth of tumors.

Deficiency: Hypoglycemia, diabetes, increased dental cavities, elevated triglycerides, elevated cholesterol, chest pain, coughing, wheezing, runny nose and sore throat. In animal studies, a deficiency caused growth retardation, bone deformities and infertility.

Toxicity: Extremely harmful to lungs, throat and eyes in high levels. Leads ultimately to death.

Zinc (Zn)

Acid/Alkaline: Acid-forming

Food sources: Pumpkin seeds, seaweed (c.a. kelp and dulse, etc.), nuts, green leafy vegetables, mushrooms, onions, wheat germ.

Uses in the body: Enhances immune system and thymus. Protects against birth defects. Involved in many enzyme systems and in the synthesis of nucleic acid (DNA and RNA), so it is directly related to growth and repair of the body. Brain, genital organs, thyroid, liver and kidneys. Effects transfer of carbon dioxide from tissue to lungs. Constituent of digestive enzyme for hydrolysis of proteins. Aids in healing wounds.

Deficiency: Lack of intestinal absorption. Restrictive growth. Loss of appetite, poor skin color and appearance, white spots on fingernails, slow wound healing, infertility, diabetes, loss of taste, poor night vision, birth defects, stretch marks, behavioral disturbances, failure of the testes or ovaries to develop, and dwarfism. Chronic diarrhea, cirrhosis of the liver, diabetes and kidney disease are prone to zinc deficiency.

Toxicity: High doses can produce liver disease with lethargy, pain in the stomach and fever. Also, increased colon and breast cancer.

TISSUE SALTS IN BIOCHEMISTRY

Tissue salts in biochemistry are the inorganic elements of the body. In 1665 an Englishman named Robert Hooke discovered what was called "the cell." In 1838 and 1839 the German scientists Matthias Schleiden and Theodore Schwann, respectively, unfolded the cell theory. In 1850, Virchow unfolded his own version of the biochemical theory of cellular treatment. Moleschott of Rome and W.H. Schuessler of Oldenburg (Germany) focused upon what they called inorganic chemistry, or biochemic treatment of disease through tissue salts.

Tissue salts, known as **cell salts**, are considered the workers and builders of the body, and are found mostly in the blood and tissues. Water and organic substances are the inert matter used by salts (ions) in building and maintaining the cells of the body.

The actions of cell salts inspire fluids, cells and tissues to respond, causing polarization or depolarization. This leads to the building (anabolism) and/or tearing down (catabolism) of cells. Plants take up elemental minerals and metals like calcium, sodium and sulfur from the earth through their root systems. Then, through plant physiology (mainly by photosynthesis) they convert these basic elements into salts so that the human body can absorb them and use them.

BASIC TISSUE SALTS

The following are the basic twelve tissue or cell salts set forth in W.H. Schussler's biochemical theories of the 1870s.

Chloride of potash

Other names: *Kali muriaticum,* kali. mur., potassium chloride

Found in these tissues: Fibrin, unites with hydrogen to form HCL (hydrochloric acid); aids in the production and promotion of bile; alkalizer; aids in digestive enzyme formation.

Deficiency: Digestive problems, excessive thinness, weakened tissues, congestive and excessive mucus production, swellings, granulation of eyelids, nose, etc., sluggish liver, and jaundice.

Chloride of soda

Other names: *Natrum muriaticum,* nat. mur., sodium chloride

Found in these tissues: Found in all tissues and fluids of the body, especially extracellular. An alkalizer found in gastric juices.

Deficiency: Fluid regulation, acidosis, dehydration, elevated carbon dioxide and cellular carbonic acid, constipation, heat stroke, ulcers, heart palpitations.

Fluoride of lime

Other names: *Calcarea fluorica,* calc. fluor., calcium fluoride

Found in these tissues: Connective tissue (which covers all tissues, organs, and glands), and is the main component of bones and teeth.

Deficiency: Prolapsed conditions, including varicose veins and spider veins, hemorrhoids, bladder and uterus (prolapsed), etc.

Phosphate of iron

Other names: *ferrum phosphoricum,* ferr. phos., iron phosphate

Found in these tissues: Hair cells, muscular membranes of blood and lymph vessels, strengthens and enhances the blood. Use in the first stages of injury or illnesses.

Deficiency: Used in blood or bleeding syndromes (disorders), affects oxygen and carbon dioxide transportation, congestive conditions, insomnia, inflammatory conditions, debility.

Phosphate of lime

Other names: *Calcarea phosphorica,* calc. phos., calcium phosphate

Found in these tissues: All cells and fluids of the body. Combines with albumen to build new RBCs, gastric juices, bones and teeth. Promotes growth.

Deficiency: Development issues, wasting conditions, debility, malabsorption, cancers, exhaustion, slow healing, muscle cramps and spasms, epilepsy and the like, circulation weakness or blockage.

Phosphate of potash

Other names: *Kali phosphoricum,* kali. phos., potassium phosphate

Found in these tissues: Skin and mucosa of the body, oxygen transport, used in detoxification by the lymphatic system and liver, use during inflammatory processes.

Deficiency: Skin conditions, lymphatic congestion (or inactivity), low immune response, low oxidative issues (including acidosis), asthma, rheumatism, fatigue and "laziness," debility, heavy "mucus" conditions and pain.

Phosphate of magnesia

Other names: *Magnesia phosphorica,* mag. phos., magnesium phosphate

Found in these tissues: Blood cells, bones, teeth, brain, nervous system, and muscle, essential to motor nerve function, antispasmodic.

Deficiency: Spasms, cramping, convulsions, etc., motor nerve syndromes, lockjaw, palpitations of the heart, nerve pain, hypertrophy of glands and organs, paralysis.

Phosphate of soda

Other names: *Natrum phosphoricum,* nat. phos., sodium phosphate

Found in these tissues: Fluids of the body, bonds to uric acid.

Deficiency: Breaks down lactic acid, gallstones and liver stones, sluggish gallbladder (promotes bile flow), gout and rheumatism, nausea, acid stomach, acidosis.

Silicic acid

Other names: *Silicea,* silicea

Found in these tissues: Connective tissues, esp. the bones, hair, nails. Brain and nerve tissues, transmuted into calcium, alkalizes.

Deficiency: Nerve weakness, skeletal weakness, connective tissue weakness, prolapsed conditions, depression, inflammation, memory loss ("brain cloud"), arthritis, rheumatism, etc., low perspiration, night sweats, tumors.

Sulphate of lime

Other names: *Calcarea sulphurica,* calc. sulph., calcium sulphate, plaster of Paris

Found in these tissues: Connective tissue, cells of the liver, attracts water, aids in the catabolism process of cells.

Deficiency: Abscesses, pimples, skin conditions, lymphatic swelling, inflammation (immune response with edema), some headaches.

Sulphate of potash

Other names: *Kali sulphuricum,* kali. sulph., potassium sulphate

Found in these tissues: Found in all tissues, especially in brain and nerve tissue, muscle and blood cells, metabolism. Antiseptic in nature.

Deficiency: Diabetes, especially in low brain and nerve function, low vitality and endurance, low metabolism syndromes, microbial overgrowths (like Candida albicans), intestinal, etc., putrefactive conditions, poor memory, Alzheimer's, low adrenal function affecting neuro-transmitters.

Sulphate of soda

Other names: *Natrum sulphuricum,* nat. sulph., sodium sulphate

Found in these tissues: Intercellular fluids, works with sodium chloride in balancing the body's intercellular and extracellular fluids, acts as a stimulant to the nervous system, pancreas, liver, intestines, etc. Promotes digestion through pancreatic function.

Deficiency: Dehydration, malabsorption, starvation, constipation, sluggish digestion, diabetes, sluggish liver and gallbladder (jaundice, etc.) asthma, vertigo and nausea.

MODULE 3.7

☼ Phytochemicals

"Phyto" means "plant." Phytochemicals refer to the thousands of compounds naturally contained within plants and fruits. This module will list and explain some of these, but keep in mind that this is only a partial list. New ones are being found every day, as humans will forever be discovering God.

The chemistry of food is somewhat complex when you realize that many compounds work synergistically, while many biotransmute (change) into other constituents and simpler compounds. Most people focus mainly on the vitamin and mineral content of a food, ignoring this long list of other properties and elements that are just as vital to the health of the body.

Plant amino acids are more energetic and easy for your body to break down and use, which is why raw foodists who eat a balanced variety of fruits, vegetables and nuts are never deficient in amino acids necessary for health. Meat, on the other hand, requires a more radical and energy-robbing digestive process to obtain the amino acids that comprise it. The other important factor here is that meat protein leaves an acid reaction in the body creating more acidosis, whereas vegetables leave an alkaline reaction in your body curing acidosis. Your body requires live foods, full of phytochemicals, to make it alive.

Some phytochemicals are noteworthy for their antioxidant properties, other phytochemicals are valuable as astringents. Because of the importance of these two properties in detoxification we will look at them a bit more closely.

PHYTOCHEMICAL ANTIOXIDANTS

Antioxidants include beta-carotene, lycopene, chlorogenic acid, gamma-terpinenes, quercetin, lutein, proanthosyanidins, rutin, hesperidin, vitamin A and vitamin E (tocopherols), to name a few.

These agents protect cells from highly oxidative free radicals. Free radicals are highly reactive and destructive compounds, which are by-products of metabolism, radiation therapy, tissue infractions, chemicals and foreign protein ingestion. Oxidative free radicals can damage cell membrane walls, cellular mitochondria and cellular proteins. This affects energy transport and the DNA itself, leading to cellular mutations. Free radicals also destroy enzymes, the key to all chemistry changes. Many vitamins act as coenzymes and antioxidants, attaching themselves to, or absorbing, free radicals. Proanthocyanidins are a popular form of antioxidant. They are found in fruits, especially grapes and grape seeds. These antioxidants are now sold in stores worldwide under the name of pycnogenol. Other antioxidants are also available in supplemental form from health food stores. These include vitamin A, vitamin E, CoQ10 and beta-carotene.

After thirty years of clinical observation, it is my opinion that obtaining your antioxidants from your raw, unprocessed foods is far superior to buying extracted, nonsynergistic types. This is because antioxidants work with astringent and other biochemical properties in a synergistic manner, which increases their effectiveness. One needs many antioxidants to achieve vitality, and each one plays a major role in the process.

PHYTOCHEMICAL ASTRINGENTS

Astringents pull and constrict tissue, pulling toxicity and congestion (mucus) out. At the same time these foods stimulate the lymphatic and blood flow within the body, allowing the body to get rid of these toxins and mucus. Some astringents can release trapped, foreign proteins, bind them together and then carry them away to be eliminated. The lemon is one of the best examples of a highly astringent food. You can feel the membranes in your mouth pucker or constrict when you eat them. This astringent action takes place throughout the body. Grapes have a similar action. Both are excellent tumor busters. In other words, foods high in astringents (namely fruits) begin detoxification—the process of internal cleansing of the body.

Tannic acid and various mineral salts, including zinc oxide, are the most common astringent elements in foods. Eat your foods ripe, fresh and raw, and you will not need to worry about their chemistry, only their power to clean and heal.

Eating foods that are biologically suited for our species keeps us clean and healthy inside.

Only then can we become vital and dynamic. Never underestimate the power of fruits to clean and sustain you. (Remember, it all started with the apple.) Food has always been one of the main focuses for humans, as it is for all animals. I quote an old naturopath, Hippocrates, "Let your food be your medicine and your medicine be your food."

OTHER PHYTOCHEMICAL COMPOUNDS IN PLANTS

Acids

Acids are compounds that are low in pH, and corrosive and inflammatory to your body. However, they serve a vital purpose in oxidation and ionization of other nutrients and minerals within the body. They have a stimulating effect upon cells and tissues. There are hundreds of acids. Many play a role in protein, carbohydrate and fat synthesis. Acids react with metals to form salts, which help to maintain body homeostasis. Acids liberate hydrogen ions causing metabolic changes and utilization issues, much the same way that ascorbic acid affects calcium and its utilization. Acids come in the form of basic elements like nitrogen, phosphorus and sulfur. When the root of a plant takes in these basic elements, the plant transmutes these basic elements into salts which then can be accepted by the human intestinal tract. Other plant acids are found as alkaloids, ascorbic acid, and many other compounds. Some hormones, steroids and digestive enzymes act as acids in your body. Estrogen is an "acid-type" of a steroid, which dilates the capillaries and creates bleeding in the uterus. As you can see, acids initiate change and activity. They are also the byproducts of digestion and metabolism. An acid we're all familiar with is phosphoric acid, which is what makes soda pop burn your mouth when you drink it.

Alcohols (see Essential Oils)

Alkaloids

Alkaloids are alkaline substances that react with acids to form salts. Some alkaloids include morphine and nicotine. However, there are many others, each with a vital role within the physiological and metabolic functions of the body. Some alkaloids suppress tissue functions while others stimulate it.

Bitter Principles

These are compounds that are bitter to the taste. They are stimulating to hepatic (liver), intestinal, as well as pancreatic tissue. They aid the secretion of digestive enzymes as well as bile and bicarbonate for alkalization. They include the terpenes, cotters and iridoids. Recent research has discovered that many bitter principles have antibiotic, antifungal and anti-tumor activities. Gentian Root, Valerian Root and Golden Seal Root are examples of herbs with high amounts of bitter principles.

Coumarins

These constituents tend to fall under the aromatic category. They have anti-clotting effects in low dosages and are used as a poison in high dosages. Coumarin glycosides are very fragrant and have shown to have antifungal, anti-microbial, anti-tumor and hemorrhagic effects.

Essential Oils

All foods and plant life have their essential oils, also called volatile oils or essences. These are concentrated compounds comprised of organic substances including alcohols, ketones, phenols, acids, ethers, esters, aldehydes and oxides. Essential oils give the aroma to a plant, flower or food. They play a vital role in the health of your nervous system. Essential oil therapy offers the individual tremendous power when used properly. There are essential oils for just about everything, including lymph movement, sweating, proliferaters (healers) and diuretics.

Some essential oils include, Rosewood, Lavender, Eucalyptus, Lemon, Rose, and Clary Sage.

Flavones

Also known as flavonoids, flavonals, flavonones, isoflavones and xanthones. Many flavones such as flavonoid glycosides are vital to calcium and vitamin C utilization. Bioflavonoids are cofactors in strengthening tissue, especially cardio- and vascular tissue. They include rutin, hesperidin and vitamin P. Fruits and vegetables have abundant flavones. Many antioxidants such as anthocyanidins and anthocyanins are related to flavonoids. These factors in foods strengthen the heart, brain, vascular walls and promote immune response. Also see: Phenols. Fruits and especially berries (Hawthorn, Saw Palmetto, blueberry, and others) are high in flavones.

Glycosides

Glycosides are bonded sugars, which can be broken down into one or more sugars (glycones). Even though glycosides are not considered a major classification of phytochemicals— as are alkaloids, phenols, terpenoids, carbohydrates, lipids, etc.—they bind with these major groups to form therapeutic actions. Some are anti-spasmodic, others act as diuretics, and still others affect circulation and heart action (cardiac glycosides).

Phenols

Phenols are also known as polyphenols, phenolic compounds and acids. They have an aromatic ring and have one or more hydroxyl groups. There are over eight thousand recognized phenols. They are generally broken down into flavonoids, phenylpropanoids, anthones, stilbenoids and quinones. Their actions within plants and human tissues vary greatly. They serve as: antioxidants, anti-viral compounds, anti-inflammatory compounds, anti-carcinogens, anti-spasmodics and diuretics, and have anti-microbial and tonic qualities.

Salts

Salts are the inorganic compounds of your body. They play a vital role in the function of cells and are vital for life to exist. The primary salts include chlorides, carbonates, bicarbonates, phosphates and sulfates. Plants are full of various mineral salts such as calcium phosphate, sodium chloride, and others. Their roles in the human body include:

- maintenance of proper water levels
- maintenance of osmotic pressure conditions for proper osmosis
- regulation of blood volume
- keeping the acid/alkaline (base) balanced
- the bases for essential components or constituents of various tissues, like bones and teeth
- proper coagulation of blood
- essential to the performance of nerve and muscle tissue
- acting as co-enzyme factors and activators
- effecting cellular transport and cell wall permeability
- essential to certain hormone functions

Saponins

These compounds have several actions in your body. They are considered anti-inflammatory and have expectorant actions. They are also part of the synthesis of adrenal gland steroids. Licorice Root and Devils Claw are herbs that have high amounts of saponins.

Tannins (Tannic acid)

Tannins are generally protective substances found in the outer and sometimes inner parts of a plant, tree, flower or fruit. Especially found in the leaves, bark, seeds and flowers.

Tannins act as astringents, having cleaning, shrinking and drawing effects upon tissue. They are considered a protective device for a plant against herbivores. Tannins are made up of simple and complex phenols, polyphenols and flavonoid compounds. These compounds are held together by carbohydrate structures and contain variations of gallic acid. Their main action is to bind and precipitate proteins. Tannins are common in fruits, various herbs (teas), grass and many plants. These types of foods are used to clean and strengthen various types of tissues within your body. However, moderate dosages of these aggressive substances are recommended because of their strong astringent effect. Tannins are used to clean and mature leather.

Terpenoids (Isoprenoids)

Terpenoids form the largest group of plant constituents and are particularly found in volatile oils. They are natural products and compounds consisting of oxygen, carbon and hydrogen. Terpenoids are derived from isoprene units and are subdivided according to the number of carbon atoms and their arrangements. Terpenoids are categorized into four basic groups:

1. Monoterpenoids/monoterpenoid lactones
2. Sesquiterpenoids/sesquiterpenoids lactones
3. Diterpenoids
4. Triterpenoids (largest group)

The above classes and related classes include camphor, carotens (beta-carotene), xanthophylls, carotenoids, terpenes, tetraterpenes, diterpenoids, iridoids, isoprenoids, prenols, retinoids, sesterterpenoids and steroids. If they contain nitrogen in their structure they become respective alkaloids. Terpenoids have a multitude of functions including functional oxidation, anti-inflammation, strengthening (tonic effects), hepatic stimulation, and catabolic and anabolic processes. They contribute to the aroma, bitter principles, antimicrobial (antifungal, antibacterial, etc.), antileukemic, carminative and adaptogenic properties of a plant. They also include properties to strengthen the heart and increase sex hormones. Terpenoids are vital in the formation of many vitamins.

☼ pH Factors of Foods

This section was written for those who want to have a greater understanding of why I recommend raw fruits and vegetables. This information becomes particularly vital if you're concerned about strokes or blood clotting. Knowing the meaning of alkaline and acid, and their effects upon tissue, will help you achieve vibrant health.

The **pH factor** is the measure of a chemical solution's acidity versus its alkalinity, on a scale of 0 (more acidic) to 14 (more alkaline). I recommend that you buy litmus (pH) papers, and use them to test your body's pH factor on a daily basis. This will help you observe firsthand the reactions that foods have on your body's chemistry, since the primary thesis of this book is that **alkalization is the key to tissue regeneration.**

To further understand the pH factors of foods and their relationship to health, let's back up a little and examine the very basics of life. This will involve a little chemistry and physics, but will help you to better understand the nature of things, including the processes of the body and the foods that you eat.

First, everything in this universe is made from building materials. The basic building materials of this universe are atoms, whereas the basic building blocks of cells are amino acids. At first, an atom appears as a simple structure—a nucleus (or center), made up of a proton, which is positively charged, and, orbiting magnetically around this nucleus, a negatively-charged electron. The number of electrons and protons that an element has will determine the type of element that it is. Oxygen, hydrogen, nitrogen, carbon, etc., are the basic elements and building materials of life. Water, for example, without which life could not exist, is simply two hydrogen atoms combined with one oxygen atom (H_2O).

Creation consists of opposites, and the movement of these opposites in relationship to each other creates electromagnetic energy. Magnetism is where opposites attract and likes repel. (If you have ever played with two or more magnets, you know what fun it can be to move magnets with magnets, and attract various materials to them.) Whether you know it or not, you too are like a magnet, attracted to the opposite of yourself. This "magnetism" helps you learn, and brings a balance to your experience in life.

Life in creation is controlled and expressed by two opposite forces, either positive or negative in nature. This type of polarization is essential for creation to exist. Without opposites like night and day, up and down, short or tall, everything would be the same—God undifferentiated. Creation depends upon these opposites to exist. You see this in your own life, as you have days that you call "good" or positive, and other days that you consider "bad" or negative. Yet, both of these aspects of life are essential to your experience of growth and awareness.

An element can start out negatively charged, which is called **alkaline**, creating a **cationic** reaction (cationic means to disperse or break apart). Through the process of ionization (chemical magnetism) the same element can become positively charged or anionic (**acidic**). **Anionic** means to compound, saturate, or come together. An example of such a change from negative (alkaline) to positive (acid) can occur with the element calcium. Plant calcium is alkaline, and works with magnesium, sodium and potassium to alkalize the fluids of the body. These elements are called **electrolytes**. However, once in the bloodstream, they can become ionized— or attracted to—other elements, magnetically, joining with these other elements and creating an anionic or acidic complex. This is seen where calcium joins with phosphorus to create calcium phosphate to form or rebuild bones, and is a positive effect. However, this process can happen with free radicals, like oxalates, which can then form calcium oxalate stones. This type of anionic reaction causes inflammation and tissue damage. It is very important to understand the meaning of acid and alkaline and their effect upon tissue, as this will give you an overview of disease.

ACIDS AND ALKALIES

Acids are chemical compounds that always have hydrogen as part of their make up. They have the ability to supply positively-charged hydrogen ions in a chemical reaction. The degree of acidity is determined by the number of hydrogen ions in the solution. Acids give protons to a substance creating a "bonding" effect, as in bone or stone formation.

Alkalies, or what we call "bases" in chemistry, are negatively charged and are attracted to protons. **Alkalies neutralize acids.** An example of this would be the toxic acids created from digestion (e.g., sulfuric acid and phosphoric acids), which are converted to non-toxic salts when combined with alkaline electrolytes. These non-toxic salts are then passed from the body through the kidneys. This neutralizing effect is vital because of the highly toxic and damaging effects these acids have upon the tissues of your body.

The pH balance—**the balance of alkalies to acids**—within the body is vital, and should be approximately 80 percent alkaline to 20 percent acidic. If we become too acidic from diet and lifestyle, we create too much of an anionic condition in the body, causing stone formation and inflammation. To reverse this is to alkalize, which is cationic and anti-inflammatory. This will break apart and liquefy calcium deposits, cellulite and lipid stones. These deposits can

> ## Acids and Alkalies
>
> - Acids burn and inflame tissues causing tissue failure.
> - Alkalies are cool and are anti-inflammatory to tissues.
> - Acids can destroy tissues (cells).
> - Alkalies can heal tissues.
> - In an acid medium, nutrients become anionic (coagulate).
> - In an alkaline medium, nutrients become cationic (disperse).
> - Acidosis creates bonding of fats, minerals, and other constituents creating stones of all types, including liver, gallbladder and kidney stones. It also creates the adhesion of blood cells and platelets. All this causes cellular starvation (through lack of nutrient utilization), strokes, and the like.
> - Acidosis and congestion (toxicity and mucus) is the root cause of 99.9% of all diseases.
> - Some foods (carbohydrates) require alkaline digestive juices to be broken down; others (protein) require gastric acid juices.

form or accumulate anywhere in the body, especially in the liver, gallbladder and kidneys. This alkalization and neutralization of acids requires the alkaline electrolytes. **If you're not eating a diet rich in raw fruits and vegetables, you're not getting enough of these vital electrolytes.** This compounds the over-acid condition within the body and creates dehydration.

ABOUT CATALYSTS

Nothing truly stands still. Creation is always in a state of flux. Atoms are always moving and changing. The question that should be asked is: "What makes things change?" First we could say our emotions, our desires, our likes and dislikes, even the primal need or desire of God to create. You could call this the original seed or desire of creation.

Secondly, you could say the mind, except the mind itself uses the past and present to create the future. One must think of something before he can experience or create it in this physical world. It is obvious that these two "bodies" (mind and emotions) of yours are the main creators of your experience. Without thought and emotions your physical body wouldn't know where to go or what to do.

But what about the physical body? What occurs at the physical level to move, react, respond, grow, expand or decay something? The term we use in chemistry is "catalyst." A catalyst is a vehicle, a transporter and an igniter. This is an element that changes elements, compounds or complexes into other elements, compounds or complexes. You could say that parasites are a catalyst as they take dying cells, putrid matter, and break these down into basic elements or compounds. Again, other elemental catalysts include enzymes (digestive, systemic, etc.), vitamins, minerals, oxygen and hydrogen, to name a few.

Let's look at hydrogen, which is simply one proton at the nucleus and one orbiting electron. If this hydrogen atom comes into contact with another atom that pulls its electron away, the result is a hydrogen atom without an electron, which is now called a **hydrogen ion**. This creates more magnetic potential (or activity), which creates an **acid**. An acid would give you a sour taste in your mouth. Compounds that combine with protons are called alkalies (or bases) and are, of course, **alkaline**. These atoms have an extra electron. An alkali is sweet tasting. One could say that protons influence acids, and electrons influence alkalies.

The result of this process of tearing down and coming together (oxidation and ionization)

should result in homeostasis—balance within the system. **Homeostasis is achieved when the body is more alkaline than acid.** When this balance (or homeostasis) is upset, from toxicity and predominately acid food eating (acidosis), tissues (organs, glands, etc.) fail to do their jobs properly. Thus, disease is the result.

OXIDATION AND IONIZATION

Knowing about oxidation and ionization will help you to further understand the alkaline (cationic) and acid (anionic) processes in the body. **Alkalization is the key to tissue regeneration**, so understanding these processes is essential for you in the achievement of vibrant health.

Oxidation and ionization are just two of the ways that encourage the breaking down and the building up, or changing, of matter from one form into another. Your bones are a great example of this as they are always being broken down and rebuilt to some degree. "Breakdown" and "buildup" keep life ever renewing itself, allowing for creation to eternally expand.

Oxidation is the process whereby elements combine with oxygen. In this combining, electrons get kicked out of the orbit of an atom's nucleus, and this increases the positive or proton valence. Oxidation can be either beneficial to the body, assisting alkalization, or it can create free radicals, causing destruction to cells. This is most evident in acidosis where inflammation is present. A superoxide radical is formed when oxygen compounds have not been completely broken down or utilized properly because of the inflammatory (acidosis) condition. This causes further cellular damage or destruction.

These oxygen compounds are less likely to be broken down properly when we are low on antioxidants or our immune system is underactive (hypoactive). When this breakdown and utilization of oxygen compounds is poorly functioning, free radicals are created, and without proper ionization or neutralization these free radicals join in creating more tissue damage. This is why there is so much current interest in antioxidants—like vitamin E, vitamin C, beta-carotene, pycnogenol, COQ10—and why they are such a hot commodity in the health market today. Antioxidants are attracted to free radicals —bond with them and neutralize their damaging effects.

Oxidation leads to ionization, or the transmutation of elements or compounds into simple ions. Water is one of the greatest catalysts for oxidation. You see this in action when water combines with metals to create rust. In our blood serum this oxidation creates electrolytes, which are conductors of energy.

Ionization creates both positive and negative ions. **Ions are your catalysts**, like enzymes, which create action and reaction, or building and destroying. Positive ions are sodium, potassium, magnesium and calcium, which are called **cations**. Negative ions include chloride, sulfates, phosphates and carbonates, and are called **anions**. It can become confusing, understanding how calcium, as we discussed earlier, can be alkaline at first, then charged or ionized and become acidic. However, nature must take an element and dispense it through the body, then make it useable. Calcium must first be dispersible in blood serum. Then it has to combine with other elements and become a building material. Too much ionized calcium will cause stone formation, bone spurs, and the like. Excessive ionized calcium must be converted back by alkalization/oxidation to its original electrolyte form, or be converted into a salt for easy elimination.

ANABOLISM AND CATABOLISM

The body uses what you eat to create new tissue, or to break down (or change) existing tissue. You can begin to see through ingestion and

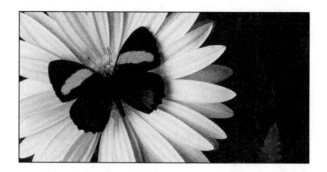

digestion that the body takes more complex compounds and elements, and breaks them down into their simplest forms. Cells have very small pores that only allow simple structures to enter. Simple constituents become the catalysts of life, creating action and reaction throughout your body and the universe. This is true biological transmutation, or God changing itself, creating the new and destroying the old.

Alkalies create **anabolism**—the building, rebuilding, growing and creating aspects of life. (This cannot take place without catabolism).

Acids create **catabolism**—the tearing down, breaking apart, and the destroying aspects of nature. (This cannot take place without anabolism).

Alkalinity disperses, moves and cleans the body; whereas acids coagulate, form masses and stagnate the body. As stated earlier, alkalization is the key to regeneration. The more anionic you become, the more acidic you become, causing acidosis. Acidosis causes malnutrition, inflammation, stone formation, pain, electrolyte depletion (dehydration), swelling, convulsions and death. On the other hand, most fruits, vegetables and herbs are alkaline-forming. **Nature seems to favor alkaline (cationic) solutions.** If your diet consists of 80 percent raw fruits and vegetables, and 20 percent nuts, seeds and cooked vegetables, you will experience tremendous health. If your diet consists of 100 percent raw fruits, vegetables, nuts and seeds you will experience incredible vitality and robust health.

☀ The Energy of Food

People today tend to focus a great deal of attention on the chemistry (or composition) of foods, especially vitamins and minerals, while mainly ignoring other properties, like astringent properties, antioxidants, tissue salts and the like. Even less do we think about the energy of a food, which is a reflection of the food's total chemistry.

Orthomolecular supplementation (vitamins and minerals) never cures. The power (or energy) of individual constituents can never match that of a whole food complex. In nature all things work together and with clockwork precision. **When you separate the nutrition in food, and only give back certain constituents, you miss the synergistic properties of the whole.** This causes a loss of proper utilization. Calcium, for example, needs phosphorus, magnesium, the flavinoid complexes, B complex, etc., to be properly utilized. If you take calcium tablets alone, you can't get this synergistic action. If you get calcium from nature, from raw foods, you get the whole deal—constituents and all. We just can't compete with nature.

Separated constituents, like vitamins and minerals, can increase your energy levels somewhat and in some cases make your symptoms disappear, only to return when you stop using them. An example of this, again, is calcium. Many people experience weak, brittle and/or ridged fingernails. They start taking a calcium supplement or gelatin and their nails will become hard again. However, as soon as they stop taking the calcium, their nails return to the weakened state. Your fingernails will give you clues about the condition of your bones or skeletal structure. You did not fix the "cause" of the problem, which is, in nine out of ten cases, a **calcium utilization problem**, not a deficiency problem. Calcium is very abundant even in our S.A.D. (Standard American Diet). However, we are destroying its utilization potential through cooking and processing. You must fix the utilization problem, and the bottom line of food utilization is energy and proper endocrine gland function.

"Are the foods you are eating full of energy, or have you destroyed the energy and nutrition in your food by cooking or altering it in some way?" This is the number one question to ask yourself. The higher the energy a food has, the greater healing ability it has. This is why fructose and glucose are essential. These simple sugars are one of the most important factors in encouraging cells to regenerate.

If I am consulting with a cancer patient, do I want to take away their energy, or give them energy? If I take more of their energy away they will die. Chemotherapy or radiation spreads (metastasizes) cancer as it destroys cells and weakens the body. This greatly lowers one's energy level, making one vulnerable to parasites and death.

The brain and nervous system cells are the highest energy centers in your body. Neurons require more energy than a typical cell. Understanding which foods have the highest energy is vital to your regeneration. The success I have witnessed with neurological weaknesses and injuries at our clinic is well known. We have seen spinal cord severations, even years after the injury, reconnect neurologically.

CONSCIOUSNESS AND FOOD

Energy is another word that can be used to describe awareness or consciousness. All life has an awareness or consciousness to it, at one level or another. Just because you cannot talk to plants or animals does not mean they do not have awareness. Some individuals have developed the ability to communicate with other forms of life. Foods also have an awareness or consciousness to them. Each type of food has its own unique individuality and reason for existing. God does not create something for no reason. In healing and regeneration we find this helpful to understand.

We noted that the brain and nervous centers of the body contain the highest energetic or electrical tissues we have. We find that fruits have the highest electrical energy of all the foods. Volt-ohm meters and electromagnetic meters can measure this energy. My own clinical studies have shown that fruits will regenerate brain and nerve tissue, whereas vegetables will not. I have found that, as a rule, **fruits are brain and nerve foods** as well as the **cleaners of** tissue. **Vegetables are the builders, which are** suited **for muscle and skeletal tissue. Nuts and seeds** are **structural foods** and are **strengthening to the body as a whole.**

Let's examine the electromagnetic energy of foods to further understand which foods are key to your regeneration and your vitality. Electromagnetic energy is rated in units called **angstroms.** The higher the quantity of angstroms a food gives off, the higher the energy of the food. When you eat foods picked fresh from nature, and eat them without cooking or processing them, the high electromagnetic energy of that food is transferred to your body and its cells.

This is true with chemistry as well. Chemical compounds and structures are broken down by digestion, and the individual components or elements are then absorbed through the intestinal wall into the bloodstream. From there they

Angstroms and Energy

ENERGY OF HEALTHY FOODS

Fresh raw fruits	8000 to 10,000 angstroms
Vegetables (fresh, raw)	8000 to 9000 angstroms
Milk (fresh, raw) for children under two years of age only.	8500 angstroms
Vegetables (cooked)	4000 to 6500 angstroms

ENERGY OF TOXIC FOODS

Milk (pasteurized)	2000 angstroms
Cheese	1800 angstroms
Refined white flour	1500 angstroms
Cooked meats	0 angstroms

BODY FREQUENCIES

Human (average)	6500 angstroms
Cancer Patients (generally)	4875 angstroms

are carried to the liver and to individual cells for energy or restructuring, and the remaining by-products are then excreted. There is a process called biological transmutation, where the body transforms one energy source into another. This process is not understood well in the health or medical fields. We are just beginning to see more of the picture from quantum physics. It is enough to say that through chemical (oxidation), parasitic, and enzyme action, life is constantly being transformed. According to physics, energy is always being changed—never created or destroyed. The previous chart will give you some idea of the electrical output of various foods.

The importance of the information in this previous chart will become clear when you understand that as homosapiens we need at least 6000 to 7000 angstroms of systemic energy at all times to even begin to smile, no less to be happy and healthy. According to Christopher Bird in his book *The Secret Life of Plants* (see bibliography), at approximately 4500 to 5200 angstroms, you are more susceptible to cancer or other seriously degenerative issues.

Fruits and vegetables that are frozen when fresh will resume the same level of radiation (electromagnetic energy) when defrosted. Refrigerated foods will slowly deteriorate. Bananas are one of the few, if only, fruits that increase in nutrition and sugars, and consequently in electromagnetic energy, after they have been picked unripe.

One of the laws of physics in this universe is the law of balance—homeostasis. The lower the energy of the food you eat, the lower your systemic energy becomes. This creates hypoactive or underactive tissues. **The more energetic the foods are that you eat, the more vibrant and healthy you become.** As we increase the energy of the physical body, we lift ourselves up out of despair and disease. This opens the senses to a whole new world of understanding and health. The vitality you can achieve is indescribable; it can only be experienced.

The body is a tremendous machine; fully aware of itself, with self-healing and cleaning mechanisms already built in. The body can get so healthy that you don't even realize that you are using it. No aches, no pains, no weaknesses, only pure energy. **If you wish to experience this pure energy you must consume pure energy.** It's that simple. Have vitality, have dynamic energy, have fun . . . go raw!

If you're green on the inside, you're clean on the inside.
— Dr. Bernard Jensen

☀ Whole, Living Foods

What you eat, drink, breathe, or put on your skin becomes your food or your poison. Our physical bodies were ideally designed to consume raw foods. Everything else, from toxic chemicals, minerals, metals, and the like, are considered foreign pathogens that inflame, stimulate, irritate or kill cells.

It's your body and you have to use it while you stay on this planet. If you feed and clean it correctly, it will give you great service, beyond your wildest dreams. Destroy it, and it will chain and bind you to this world in ways that you can't imagine. Remember, if no animal cooks its food before eating it, then why do we?

Tradition is killing us. Just because something becomes "tradition" doesn't mean it's true and the right thing to do. Cooked foods are dead foods—their chemistry has been changed (sometimes radically) and their energy destroyed. Many of the alkaline-forming foods now become acid-forming. Their enzymes are destroyed, leaving the burden of digestion entirely up to the body itself. This stresses the GI tract, pancreas and liver. It robs vital systemic energy from the body just to digest and eliminate these foods. Health is energy, which brings vitality and robustness. **This can only be achieved through raw, ripe, fresh fruits, vegetables, nuts and seeds.**

I personally recommend a 100 percent raw food diet. However, since this type of diet will detoxify you very quickly, highly toxic individuals who presently use a lot of chemical medications are advised to go about this transition more slowly. Even so, everyone with cancer, or spinal and neurological issues, should rapidly move toward consuming a diet of 100 percent raw foods. Fruits are the best regenerators of brain and nerve tissue, and for removing cancer from the body.

A diet of 80 percent raw and 20 percent cooked food will still rebuild you and clean you out, to a certain level. However, you will eventually reach a point where you might need to detoxify even more deeply. This is especially true in regenerating genetic weaknesses. The most important thing to remember is to keep yourself **alkalized**. The more acid-forming foods you consume, the more acidic you become. Consequently, your success in healing and regeneration will be very low, causing you to keep searching—reading book after book, going to doctor after doctor, and spending lots of your hard-earned money seeking the Fountain of Youth. But you will never find it. Ponce DeLeon never found it, *and* he missed the fact that his horse was feeding on it the whole time.

Cooking, heating, frying, and processing your foods causes radical changes in their chemistry and electromagnetic energy. These changes render food into poison or toxin that your body must fight against instead of using for energy and rebuilding.

ATTITUDE IS CRUCIAL

Health should be fun and challenging, not a chore. You are rebuilding yourself to become new again. As you build self-discipline, it will be much easier for you to become whole and alive. Don't settle for less than robust health. Change yourself. Expand yourself. Keep it simple. And don't allow anyone to stop you. Become free of all disease.

Today, health must be earned. There is no magical pill, and there never will be. What chemical could clean, alkalize and rebuild tissue? Your body doesn't even like to have a wood splinter in it, let alone toxic chemicals.

Sometimes we need to change our attitudes about things. Our attitudes are our roadblocks in life. They are similar to belief systems; both can limit your ability to experience truth. If you want to be healthy you must eat healthy, live healthy, breathe healthy, think healthy and **know yourself as healthy**. (You may want to think about that one.) "Knowing" is far more powerful than thinking. To know is simply to see truth for what it is. Knowing does not require thought. Thought is a process of interaction that leaves room for limitation and failure. When one is critically ill, a knowing of wellness is the most powerful force he or she can grab to start healing.

Have fun on your journey into health and spirituality. These are the greatest adventures you can pursue.

Summary

I spent the first three years in my naturopathic clinic using science via chemistry to seek a homeostasis, or chemical and biochemical balance, for the human body. I used tissue (cell) salts, vitamins, minerals and glandulars to try to achieve this. It wasn't until I studied the work of Dr. Royal Lee, of Standard Process Laboratories, that I realized the importance of synergistic elements and molecules. I realized that nature works together and in harmony with itself. It doesn't oppose itself.

I understood that the tremendous vitality I felt from my years of eating raw food was due to the *totality* of a food and its electromagnetic energies, not its separated chemistry. This is when I switched to botanicals (herbs). I have been using them now for over twenty-five years. I use them as detoxifiers, not for "treatment." Together with an organic, live food diet, herbs are the simple answers to robust health and vitality.

We explored in Chapter One the difference between detoxification and treatment, explaining that treatment deals with symptom-alleviation but not necessarily with the underlying cause of disease. It is time for us to break out of our treatment mentality and open up to the world of detoxification. Detoxification does not "treat" the symptoms (of the problem), nor does it treat from "deficiency" concepts; if it treats or addresses anything, it treats the root cause of the symptom(s). Detoxification takes into consideration alkalization, homeostasis, enhancement, revitalization, regeneration and cleansing. Eating your foods whole, fresh and raw, whereby the chemistry and energy is unchanged by human intervention, is the golden key that unlocks the door to health and vitality.

When you heat your foods you radically change their chemistry, creating acrylamides and other carcinogenic substances. This is especially true when using higher temperatures (frying, pasteurizing, canning, processing). The energy and nature of the foods you eat can make you vital or sick. The nature or vibration of a particular food creates reflex energy waves throughout your body. This can have a positive or negative effect upon your body's system and cells. The healthier you become, you will experience this. Simply by putting a food in your mouth, or even just touching or smelling a food, you can feel your body's response. I've seen the lymph system produce excessive mucus (or go into shock), just from smelling a harmful food or substance. Rather than choosing foods that you *think* your body needs, your body itself will *indicate* what it needs by what it is attracted to eat from among the many fresh raw foods that are available.

Detoxification is a system, not a treatment. It is a science that encompasses chemistry and how chemistry interacts with itself. It also encompasses physics and the energies of the universe and how your body is a part of the whole. It also encompasses God and how your spirituality, your mind and your emotions play an instrumental role in the functioning of your physical body.

Detoxification is the simple answer to curing disease and unhappiness. It cleans you out, and uplifts and reconnects you to God and nature. It rids your body of acidosis, toxins, chemicals, mucus and harmful parasites. It rids the mind of unwanted thoughts and cleans the angers and emotions from your being.

With all our scientific sophistication we have not even come close to making a supplement that replaces food. Chemistry, physics and physiology prove over and over again that fruits, vegetables, nuts and seeds are perfect foods for humans. They carry and support life in every way. Ninety-nine percent of the vertebrate species require and feed on these food sources. Why should we be any different? You can see in reviewing this chapter that there are literally hundreds of different constituents found in your foods. They have an incredibly broad range of effects that are most essential to life and the function of cells within your body.

If you wish to supplement your diet because your food is devitalized, then take a superfood complex. (The food industry has literally ruined many foods by picking them before they are ripe; and has compromised the soil, and thus the nutritional value of the food grown in that soil, in order to raise animals for slaughter.) A superfood complex is a supplement that is made from the whole food itself—generally the best that nature offers, nutritionally speaking. This means that you are getting the complete list of constituents needed for life to grow and maintain itself. Supplementing with manufactured supplements can throw your body's chemistry out of balance and affect proper utilization and ionization factors needed for proper metabolism.

Keep your life simple. If you relax and truly investigate and experiment on yourself, you will discover the truth. Detoxification is the golden key. Use it to open the door to the kingdom of true vitality and God, and to experience a disease-free life.

The doctor of the future will give us no medicine, but will interest his patients in the care of the human frame, in diet and in the cause and prevention of disease.

— Thomas Edison

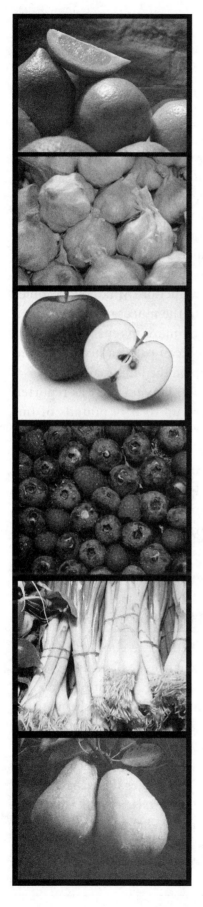

CHAPTER FOUR

Toxic Habits

Many concepts related to health and well being are erroneous. They have been passed down through our families and taught in our schools out of ignorance, or programmed into us deliberately via television and other media to sell products. The "Drink Milk for Calcium" myth is one of the biggest. The Protein Myth is equally huge. We have become a society of high-protein eaters mainly through the efforts of the industries that sell animal and grain products.

It is natural for anyone in business to develop slogans about their products to help sell them. However, when these industries cross the line and start advertising half-truths or untruths, then we have fraud and misrepresentation. These "untruths" damage the health of millions of people every year. This misleading advertising is abundantly true of pharmaceutical companies as well. Over-the-counter and prescription drugs kill hundreds of thousands of people each year according to *The Washington Post*, and many other sources.

This chapter will examine several deadly myths that relate to food, the myth of vaccinations against disease, and the myth of reliance on chemical poisons. It will conclude with information that will help you to protect yourself from some of the negative influences in your environment, including a reference list of Poison Control Centers in the United States.

When we make choices based on habit rather than from our alignment with the forces of nature, these habits can create toxic conditions within our bodies that result in serious illness or death. When we choose a level of imagined health or hygiene over environmental balance, we create farther-reaching toxic habits—patterns that can affect the health of our planet and all its inhabitants.

☼ The Problem with Milk and Other Dairy Food

Cow's Milk is for Cows. There is nothing bad about drinking milk from the time you first open your eyes at birth until you are two years of age. That is, provided the milk is from your mother, and is therefore fresh, raw and natural. Ideally, mother would be on a high-energy and highly-nutritional, raw food diet, before and during pregnancy. However, in our culture we tend not to breast-feed our children. Most of us were weaned on cow's milk or synthetic formulas, which are almost twenty times more concentrated than cow's milk.

Cow's milk tends to be high in proteins, minerals and fats—a necessity for baby cows that will grow to 300-500 pounds in one year. Needless to say, human babies do not grow that fast. Cow's milk has at least four times as much protein and over six times as much mineral content as human milk. Such heavily concentrated milk is extremely hard for infants to digest. Human enzyme production for handling milk products is much less than a cow's enzyme production. Without proper enzymes in the right quantity, human babies suffer digestive problems and mucus congestion in the sinus cavities, lungs, brain and ears. Many types of allergies are also created from the excessive congestion that started with cow-milk consumption.

Adults cannot digest milk at all and develop deeper congestive problems as they get older. Cow's milk is also low in essential fatty acids, which are vital to humans in the production of systemic cholesterol, steroids, brain and nerve tissue, etc. Raw cow's milk is more for skeletal/muscular growth, where human milk feeds brain and nerve growth. This is one of the main differences between frugivores and herbivores.

Roughly between ages three and four most children lose the enzymes that digest milk, especially lactase, which breaks down lactose—the main sugar in milk. This is because, biologically, we are supposed to be weaned after three or four years. Since we lack the proper digestive enzymes to break down milk, we get an increased mucus production. Milk now becomes highly irritating to the mucosa of the GI tract, which causes even more mucus. This mucus mixed with starch can cause a heavy mucoid plaque to build up on the intestinal walls.

Remember John Wayne? He was reported to have died with up to fifty pounds of impacted fecal matter in his bowels. Such impactions cause inflammation, pocketing (diverticulum), and tissue weakness of the intestinal wall. This leads to bowel restrictions, ulcerations, lesions and cancers. Several years ago, the now former U. S. Surgeon General, C. Everett Koop, M.D., told the world: "Dairy products are bad for you."

FROM ALKALINE TO ACID

Now, on top of all this, we cook (pasteurize) cow's milk. Heat changes the chemistry of the milk, as well as changing its nature from alkaline-forming to acid-forming. In chemistry, if we want to change a chemical compound, we add heat. Heating or cooking also destroys any water-soluble vitamins, especially the vitamin C and B-complexes. It saturates the fats and binds certain proteins to minerals, as well as binding minerals to minerals. What happens to a baby calf if you feed it pasteurized milk instead of its fresh, raw mother's milk? It dies.

CONGESTION DECREASES UTILIZATION

Colds, flu, mumps or any lymphatic or respiratory condition can be largely attributed to congestion from dairy products. Dairy products are highly mucus-forming and constipating. When you have a cold or respiratory problem, where do you think that clear, yellow, green, brown or black mucus originally comes from? Where do tumors come from? Or lymph node swelling, especially swelling of the tonsils?

The thyroid and parathyroid glands are located in the throat. They also get congested with the mucus formed from dairy products, creating hyper- or especially hypo-conditions of these tissues. The thyroid/parathyroid gland is responsible for calcium utilization by the body. When these glands begin to fail from the mucus congestion, toxins and inflammation that dairy products create, your calcium utilization begins to fail—which is the opposite result for why you consume these products in the first place. When a lack of calcium utilization at the cellular level begins, a host of conditions including depression, bone and tissue weaknesses, nerve and muscular weakness, and connective tissue weakness can also begin. All are side effects from mucus congestion that has built up in our tissues from the use of dairy products.

Calcium is an abundant mineral. The highest concentration of usable calcium is found in sesame seeds and sea vegetables like kelp. Calcium needs magnesium to be properly utilized. In fruits, and especially in vegetables, calcium and magnesium are compatible. Dark green leafy vegetables are full of calcium, magnesium and flavonoids, all of which need each other for proper utilization. In cow's milk, however, you have a lot more calcium than magnesium. This adds to the lack of utilization of calcium in milk. It has been estimated that less than 20 percent of calcium in milk is utilized. We utilize more calcium from fruit juice than we do from milk.

When milk is cooked, the minerals become ionized, changing its effect from alkaline to acidic. This can create stone formation, muscular weakness, GI tract inflammation, and other conditions. The truth of this can be seen in that many people who drink milk and take extra doses of calcium through supplementation are still getting osteoporosis. We must begin to think of **utilization** within the body **rather than supplementation**. High doses of calcium are not the answer, proper utilization is.

The thyroid/parathyroid and the adrenal glands are mostly responsible for calcium utilization within the body. I have found that when these glands are healthy, the body is strong where calcium issues are concerned. If you clean and regenerate these glands, your calcium utilization will be greatly enhanced. Use the Basal Temperature Test (found in Chapter 10) to study and check your thyroid function. Check your blood pressure to determine your adrenal weaknesses. Remember, if your systolic is under 118 you always have adrenal weakness.

PARASITES

Parasites are another result of milk drinking. Estimates are that 60 percent or more of American dairy cows have one or more of the following: the leukemia virus, salmonella and the tuberculosis virus. Furthermore, as milk and dairy products are the most mucus-forming of all the foods we consume, and refined sugar is the second most, both of these foods will cause excessive congestion to build up all through our tissues. Yeast, fungi and worms love to feed and thrive in this congestion. This causes Candida albicans and other infectious conditions. After observing thousands of cancer clients, I am convinced that milk and dairy products (even colostrum) cause and increase tumor growth and lymphatic congestion. Many congestive (tumor) type cancers, in my opinion, are initially started through the consumption of these types of foods.

DIABETES

Many studies have linked pasteurized milk consumption to diabetes. The antibodies produced to fight these altered, harmful, milk proteins also attack the beta cells in the pancreas. The beta cells are in the islets of Langerhans in the pancreas and their job is to secrete insulin.

BOVINE GROWTH HORMONE

Another major problem we see in milk is the effects from rBGH—or recombinant bovine growth hormone. The Monsanto Corporation created this bovine growth hormone from the E-coli bacteria. This growth hormone was initially created to increase milk production. Some studies have shown this growth hormone (rBGH) to be a carcinogen. In many studies it has been shown to proliferate (increase) the growth of cancer. I personally feel it stimulates the endocrine gland system, especially the thyroid and adrenal glands. This affects our growth, other developmental factors, and hormone balance. As a society we are faced with these massive hormonal imbalances that are destroying our health and our economy.

Learn the truth about the foods you consume. Don't be dissuaded by the media and other influences within our capitalistic society where money has become more important than human welfare. It is vital that you detoxify your body of all the built-up congestion from the many years of eating mucus-forming foods.

INTESTINAL FLORA

Many health-conscious people today take acidophilus with lactobacillus, and the like. Why? If you do not consume dairy products, why would you need to supplement with these products? These are bacteria that are involved in the breakdown of milk proteins and milk sugars. They can also be found in the body where toxemia (toxins) from dairy products are formed, e.g., in saliva, in the lymphatic system, in the vagina, etc. It is more important to your health to clean these toxins and the bacteria that feeds upon them out of your body entirely. It is also questionable whether these bacterial supplements survive the gastric acids, as it is.

It is not difficult to establish intestinal flora. You can't keep bacteria out of your body. This is pure nature. Bacteria are feeders, cleaning and feeding upon your wastes, the by-products of digestion and metabolism. Remember, your intestinal flora changes with your diet.

Success is nothing more than a refined study of the obvious.
— Jim Rohn, success philosopher

☼ Proteins—The Whole Truth

Look back to Module 3. 3 in the previous chapter for an introduction to the subject of protein and how it is metabolized. As you may recall, "protein" is a word meaning a "structure." Like a house, it's already built. It has form to it, like muscle tissue. However, like a house, it is built *from* various types of building materials. Protein structures are built from building materials called **amino acids**. Amino acids therefore are the building materials that your body requires and uses for building (growth), maintaining, and repairing itself. It also uses proteins (amino acids) for immune factors, transporters, and catabolic factors. A protein is also a general word for the total nitrogenous substances of animal or vegetable matter, exclusive of the so-called nitrogenous fats.

Proteins, or the total nitrogenous (nitrogen-based) substance of a food, consist of a variety of chemical compounds of two main types: **proteids** and **non-proteids**. Examples of proteids, both simple and complex, are albuminoids, globulins, proteases, peptones, glutinoids, etc. Examples of non-proteids, or simple compounds, would include creatine, creatinine, xanthine, hypoxanthine, amides and amino acids.

The human body requires numerous amino acids, and these are divided into two groups. First, are the **essential amino acids**, of which there are **eleven**. These are said to be mandatory for proper growth and repair. (Personally I do not agree with this conclusion as I have seen people with extreme cases of neurological weakness, repair and rebuild themselves solely on fruits.) Secondly, there are many **nonessential amino acids** the body also uses. The list at the right will show you both groups.

Protein structures also include carbon, hydrogen, oxygen, phosphorus, sulfur and iron.

As you can see, then, the word "protein" is actually an arbitrary word giving a "structure" to building materials. Protein is actually an arbitrary word that is assigned to any building material that the body needs. However, its factual definition is that of a completed structure, like tissue itself.

Amino Acids

ESSENTIAL AMINO ACIDS
(PROVIDED BY FOOD)
Cysteine
Histidine
Isoleucine
Leucine
Lysine
Methionine
Phenylalanine
Threonine
Tryptophan
Tyrosine
Valine

NON-ESSENTIAL AMINO ACIDS
(PROVIDED BY THE BODY)
Alanine
Arginine
Aspartic acid
Citrulline
Glutamic acid
Glycine
Hydroxproline
Hydroxyglutamic acid
Norleucine
Proline
Serine

CAN WE USE THE PROTEIN?

Digestion is necessary because the body can only use simple amino acids—the kinds that are found abundantly in vegetables and nuts. The liver can also produce its own amino acids and can synthesize even smaller nitrogen-containing compounds. The proteins found in meat must be broken down (hydrolyzed) into simple amino acids before the body can truly use them. I call meat "second-hand protein" because of the extensive digestion process needed to break down the "building" into simple "building blocks" or amino acids. Fruits, vegetables and nuts are much simpler for the body to break down, as these are basic amino-acid structures. It has been proven that a vegetable diet supplies more available nitrogen than a meat diet.

It is important to understand that nutrients act differently in an anionic (acid) environment versus a cationic (alkaline) environment. Amino acids become free agents for growth, maintenance and repair in an alkaline or cationic environment. In an anionic (acidic) environment they tend to bind with minerals, metals and fats, causing further toxic conditions in the body. This creates a loss of available amino acids, starving your body for building materials. You can eat all the proteins you want; however, your body cannot rebuild itself properly without proper bioavailability of amino acids.

"Bulk" type muscles, put on by high protein diets, will be lost during detoxification, as these are "stacked" amino acids not necessary to normal body functions. When protein breaks down, it creates sulfuric and phosphoric acids, which are highly toxic and damaging to tissue. It burns up our electrolytes to convert these acids into salts (ionization), thus neutralizing their damaging effects. Carbohydrates and fats create lactic and acetic acids, which require the same process, but are not as damaging. This is why we must replenish our electrolytes daily. The ionization and alkalization process is vital if you wish

to save your kidneys, liver and other tissues in your body. Those who deplete their electrolytes without replenishing them fall into heavy acidosis, which can cause convulsions, coma and death. Cancer and other highly acidic conditions of the body use sodium and other alkalizing electrolytes at a very fast pace. This is just another reason to consume as many raw alkaline fruits and vegetables as possible.

Foreign proteins from meats, dairy products, grains, eggs, and the like, are abrasive to the mucosa of the body. This causes a lymphatic (mucous) response that can cause excessive mucus to build up within the tissues and cavities of the body. This mucus build-up, with the trapped proteins, fills interstitial areas as well as lymph nodes, sinus cavities, brain, lungs, etc. Pimples, boils and tumors are expressions of this congestion or toxic build-up. Some of the final digestive stages of protein-matter result in the production of uric acid. Uric acid is abrasive and irritating, which inflames and damages tissues. Uric acid deposits can create arthritis in the joints and muscle tissue. Uric acid causes gout. The more flesh protein you put into your body, the more you work your immune system, and the more you invite the parasitic "kingdom" to grow inside of you. Many parasites (including many viruses, bacteria, and some "big boys" such as worms and flukes) feed on wastes from flesh-protein digestion.

Eating meat causes body odor from the rotting (putrefying) flesh within us. Meat can become impacted on the intestinal walls causing our mucosa and intestinal lining to decay along with the meat. It is important to note that putrefaction changes proteins into toxic chemical by-products. Fruits and vegetables, on the other hand, do not cause body odor.

Proteins are acid-forming, which can create inflammation and can cause tissue breakdown —the opposite reason to why we are supposed to eat them. I'm not saying to avoid proteins— just to be warned about quantities and certain types. Diets rich in nuts, vegetables and fruits yield a very strong and healthy body, supplying plenty of amino acids.

The body cannot use "flesh-type proteins" (grouped amino acids) until it breaks them down into simple amino acids first. This process starts in the stomach where gastric juices of HCL (hydrochloric acid) convert pepsinogen into pepsin. Pepsin starts to break down these protein structures into peptones/polypeptides. This is an acidic process. After the stomach moves this "pre-digested" process into the duodenum (small bowel), the proteolytic enzymes in the pancreas (which are alkaline) start changing the polypeptides into peptides. Finally, as these peptides are moving along the small intestines, your intestinal wall secretes enzymes (peptidase), which finally convert these peptides/peptones into amino acids. This extensive process robs the body of vital energy, only to achieve "second-hand" building materials.

Plant proteins are simple structures of amino acids which are considerably less energy-robbing. Plants, being full of electromagnetic energy, counter-balance this energy need. Meat protein, on the other hand, is much more structured and electrically dead. This requires a much more radical digestive process, which robs the body of vital energy. Because of the high acidic content, too much meat protein has also been linked to colon cancer, the second largest type of cancer in America today. Thousands of people die each year from the accumulated effects of eating high protein diets. The liver, pancreas, kidneys and intestines are destroyed when protein consumption is too high. Twenty to forty grams of protein a day is plenty, but most people eat 150-200 grams a day.

THE ENERGY OF MEAT

It has been said that meat gives you energy. Since this energy is mostly from the adrenaline found in its tissues, this is only a stimulated energy, not a dynamic energy. If you've ever visited a slaughterhouse you will see and sense the fear that these poor creatures experience just before they are killed. Physiologically, this fear pumps the medulla of their adrenal glands, producing epinephrine or what's commonly called "adrenaline." Epinephrine is a neurotransmitter, stimulating energy through the nervous system into the tissues of the body. This is mostly what gives protein-eaters a heightened sense of energy. However, after years of eating meat full of adrenaline, your adrenal glands become weakened and lazy at producing their own neurotransmitters. This begins to lower your blood pressure. (A systolic blood pressure of less than 118 is low.) As we begin to pass our adrenal weaknesses down genetically, future generations may see multiple sclerosis, Parkinson's, Addison's Disease, and other neurological weaknesses develop from a chronic lack of neurotransmitters.

High blood pressure can also be a result of adrenal gland weakness. When the adrenal glands become weak, we also begin to fail at producing adequate steroids (our anti-inflammatories), because meat is highly acid-forming (which creates inflammation). The body will use cholesterol in place of steroids where this inflammation is present. This becomes a serious problem because lipids, in the presence of acidosis, stick together and plaque themselves "in" and "onto" tissues.

Energy from eating meat can also come from growth hormones fed to the cattle (or other animals) for rapid growth. Energy should be dynamic or cellular, not created by stimulants. Dynamic energy comes from raw-food eating where alkalization, proper electrolytes, electricity, amino acids, proper synergistic compounds and complexes (vitamins, minerals, flavons, etc.) are found.

A CALL TO ACTION

It is time for humans to stop the toxic consumption of animal products, which today are so laden with toxic hormones, antibiotics, chemicals and the like, that they have become time bombs just ticking away inside of us. We *can* lift ourselves up from decay and toxicity and enjoy the vitality and internal cleanliness that a raw fruit-and-vegetable diet will bring. Such a diet breaks the chains of anger and despair, freeing us into the light of vibrancy and health.

Try a six-week diet free of animal products and see the difference for yourself. It's one thing to read and form opinions from conditioned thought. However, it's quite another to experience it directly for yourself.

All life transmutes compounds and elements into other compounds or elements, although this process is not well understood by the scientific community, as of yet. Your body can and does create amino acids from carbohydrates and fats. Your body uses the constituents in your foods, especially those biologically suited for you, to maintain and repair itself.

Nature will always have mysteries for us to seek. The mind, which is forever over-reacting, can keep the soul's attention here in the physical world indefinitely. The mind is like the seeker after God, forever looking for truth when it is always right in front of him. The mind (intellectualism) always likes to tear things apart to try to understand how they are made. Soul already *knows* how things are made. Break free from intellectualism and enjoy the simplicity of nature and God. It will free you from a lot of wasted energy. Become a raw-food, living-food eater and enjoy vitality and robust health. You will be much happier for it.

HIGH PROTEIN DIETS CAN CAUSE DEATH

Research studies done by some of the world's top educational institutions (including Simmons College and Harvard University, as reported in *The New England Journal of Medicine* and *The Archives of Internal Medicine*) have proven, over and over again, that meat protein is toxic to us when it is absorbed through our intestinal walls. This creates acidosis, affects an immune response and invites parasites. The following list will summarize what we have considered in the previous sections about the basic reasons to avoid meat and high protein diets.

- A protein structure is not useable by the body, as such, and must be broken down into its simplest compounds, called amino acids before the body can use it at all. This process *requires* energy instead of yielding energy.
- Many acids are created during the digestion and metabolizing of proteins, including uric acid (which causes gout), phosphoric acid, and sulfuric acid. These acids are irritating and inflammatory to tissues. They also stimulate nerve responses leading to hyperactivity of tissues.
- Protein is a nitrogen compound, high in phosphorous, which when consumed in large amounts, will deplete calcium and other electrolytes from the body.
- Proteins are highly acid-forming, lowering the pH balance of the body. This causes inflammation and tissue weakness, leading to tissue death.
- Proteins are not used as fuel by the body; they are building blocks and carriers. When proteins are broken down by digestion into amino acids, their main function becomes growth and repair of tissue. Simple sugars are the main fuels for the body besides oxygen. When we try to lose weight by burning proteins for fuel, this causes fat breakdown. However, it also causes tissue breakdown. You can destroy liver, pancreatic and kidney tissues by burning your building blocks instead of using proper fuels.
- In people who have adrenal weakness, a high protein diet causes the liver to create large amounts of cholesterol, which then begins to plaque throughout the body, especially through the vascular system, liver and kidneys. Stone formation also begins to take place in the liver and gallbladder.

- Animal proteins putrefy in the body causing body odor. This putrefaction causes a cesspool of toxins to build up in the intestines and the tissues of the body, both interstitially and intracellularly. This not only creates a base for parasites to grow, but the acidity creates inflammation, which blocks cellular respiration, eventually causing cellular death.
- High protein consumption does not fit our species, nor is it physiologically sound.
- Animal farming, as a food source, has devastated us economically, environmentally and spiritually. We are destroying our forests and green land to create pastures. This is destroying our planet in many ways. It affects the production of vital oxygen, diminishes heat protection, destroys beauty, limits erosion protection, limits our fruit and vegetable farming, increases toxic by-products of animals, robs topsoil and oxygen levels from grain farming, and destroys wild animal habitats. We waste thousands of acres in raising tons of grain needed to feed cattle and other animals.
- High protein diets contain excessive amounts of epinephrine (adrenaline) and thereby create aggression, anger and adrenal failure in humans who consume these foods.
- Meat has been proven to cause intestinal cancer. It is suspected in liver and pancreatic cancers, as well. The cesspool of putrefaction that builds up in the lymphatic system is possibly the starting cause of lymphomas.
- Meat-eating societies have a much shorter life span. An example of this is the Intuits of Northern Canada and Alaska whose average life span is approximately fifty years.
- Meat is nothing more than dead or dying cells, living in their own cesspool of stagnant, putrefying blood. And humans call this good nutrition.
- Meat stimulates, irritates and inflames the sexual organs, especially the prostate gland, leading to prostatitis.

- Today's animal meat is full of growth hormones, antibiotics, pesticides, herbicides, nuclear wastes, high levels of adrenaline, and other toxic chemicals from air and ground pollution. All of these compounds are considered carcinogenic. We find more cancer in cows, pigs and chickens today than ever before. And humans eat this. Some meat producers (farmers and ranchers) have also lost their integrity and sense of decency, and are grinding up their sick and dying cows, pigs and chickens and mixing this "dead," often "diseased," meat into their regular animal feed. This leads to "Mad Cow" and "Hoof and Mouth" disease. We see this now, especially in Europe, where meat growers have been feeding dead sheep meat to living cows. Cows are vegetarians. Hogs are not true meat eaters, either. This eventually leads to acidosis and disease within these animals, just as it does within humans.
- High protein diets lower manganese levels resulting in spasms, convulsions, neurotransmitter issues (myasthenia, S.O.B., heart arrhythmias including atrial fibrillation, etc.), neuromuscular problems, Parkinson's and Lou Gehrig's disease.
- Meat is full of dead blood cells (hemoglobin), which are full of iron. However, iron is a mineral, which if consumed in abundance can become toxic, especially oxidized iron (not plant iron). Iron toxicity creates a multitude of reactions within the body, including:
  - Decrease in chromium (needed in insulin transport issues)
  - Decrease in zinc (needed in insulin and energy production)
  - Damage to liver, pancreatic and kidney tissue
  - Lowering of calcium and calcium absorption and utilization
  - Increase in sodium levels (hence creating edema)
  - Increase in nitrogen and phosphorous levels (thus increasing acidosis)

- Dizziness, equilibrium and spastic conditions by decreasing manganese levels
- Meat eating leads to high blood pressure from sodium retention and lipid coagulation.
- Meat eating with vitamin C supplementation enhances iron absorption, thereby magnifying iron toxicity.
- Red meat eating is linked to the increase of N-Nitroso compounds from intestinal bacteria, which can be cancer-causing to the intestinal walls.
- Meat eating is known to be one of the chief and most direct causes of tooth decay.
- These are just a few examples of why high animal-protein diets are destroying the human race. Wake up and enjoy life without animal products. Your body will love you for it, as it becomes odor-free and vibrant. Love your planet and its animals too.

COMPLETE PROTEIN OR COMPLETE MYTH?

There is a myth about the need for "complete" amino acids or "complete proteins" in the human diet. We have struggled with this misinformation for years. Basically, the misinformation says that unless you eat foods containing all the essential amino acids in one meal you will not have what you need to create a "complete protein" and therefore your body will be protein deficient. This is one of the primary arguments for the consumption of meat and dairy products, or the consumption of soy products, beans, and white flour. Consider, however:

- What is the diet of a wild horse, an elephant, or a cow? These are herbivores and their strength is well known. Their diet is 100 percent grass and vegetable matter. If they needed the "complete protein" that is claimed, they must be getting it from plants.
- 70 to 80 percent of a grizzly bear's diet is grass. Bears don't eat much meat. When they do, it's generally the fat (not the protein) structure that they're after. Bears are omnivores.
- We are the highest species in the frugivore category, which is not designed to eat meat.
- Raw foodists who eat a balanced variety of fruits, vegetables and nuts are never deficient in the amino acids necessary for health. Quite the opposite. Plant amino acids are more energetic and easy for your body to break down and use. Meat requires a more radical and energy-robbing digestive process to obtain the amino acids that comprise it. The other important factor here is that meat protein leaves an acid reaction in the body, creating more acidosis, whereas vegetables leave an alkaline reaction, thus cutting acidosis.

Your body requires live foods to make it alive. If the components are not in fresh, organic fruits, nuts and vegetables you don't need them! And besides, there's nothing healthy about eating old, rotten, dead tissue—dead cells in stagnant blood.

The constitution of man's body has not changed to meet the new conditions of his artificial environment that has replaced his natural one. The result is that of perpetual discord between man and his environment. The effect of this discord is a general deterioration of man's body, the symptoms of which are termed disease.
— Professor Hilton Hotema, *Man's Higher Consciousness*

☀ Irritants and Stimulants

Most people consume large amounts of irritants and stimulants in their diets, so called because these compounds *irritate* and *stimulate* tissue, causing excessive mucus production and hyper- or hypo-activity of these tissues (organs, glands, etc.). Eventually, because of this abuse, these tissues fail, leading to chronic and degenerative disorders. Some of the irritants that people consciously or unconsciously consume each day are black pepper, caffeine, salt, MSG, preservatives, chemical and refined sugars. The list can get very long.

These compounds irritate the mucosa of the GI tract, causing mucus discharge, which becomes congested and impacted. They also create inflammation in the body, as most of them are acidic, or heat-producing, thus initiating an immune response. In the health field, however, Capsicum (cayenne pepper) is used by many for both high blood pressure and for increasing circulation. Cayenne pepper is not as irritating as black pepper. However, red pepper does stimulate the mucosa of the GI tract, which can cause excessive mucus production. Mucus congestion is at the heart of congestive conditions, including sinus congestion, bronchitis, pneumonia and earaches.

When an individual changes his or her lifestyle and begins to eat a raw, living-food diet, the body changes. The more raw food you consume, the more your body becomes pure and healthy. You will reach a point where you will not be able to eat pungent foods anymore. Cayenne pepper, onions and even garlic will become irritating to you.

Stimulants are one of man's passions. We intake hundreds of pounds and/or gallons of these substances each year. Coffee, tea and soda are consumed like never before. These drinks (being high in tannins, alkaloids, sulfuric and phosphoric acids, and the like) not only stimulate tissues, but also damage them. Do you know what happens to concrete if you pour soda pop on it? It breaks it down. If you put a piece of meat into a glass of soda, what happens to the meat? The same thing—it deteriorates. Soda pop inflames and destroys the lining of your GI tract, not to mention the liver and kidneys.

Coffee and commercial teas are also highly consumed today. These drinks irritate and stimulate the liver, GI tract, heart, endocrine gland system, (thyroid, adrenals, pituitary, thymus, etc.), and the kidneys. Among health-enthusiasts, coffee enemas are also very popular. I do not recommend these, however, because they are too stimulating to your intestines and liver. They only serve to stimulate these tissues, eventually causing extreme enervation and severe constipation. Use "good" herbal bowel regenerators that are non-addicting, and will clean and restore good bowel function. (See Resource Guide at the back of this book for recommendations of herb companies that make good formulas.)

Chocolate is another stimulant that men, women and children love to consume. Chocolate is highly acidic and has a high oxalic acid content. When your body is acidic and you consume foods that are high in oxalates, these oxalates bind with ionic calcium causing calcium oxalate stones, such as kidney stones.

Alcohol and refined sugars are other stimulants that are highly consumed by people today. These are highly acidic and mucus-forming. Beer adds to the yeast overgrowth in people, which creates the desire for more refined sugars, keeping this wheel ever-turning. In diabetes, alcohol keeps the blood sugar elevated and stimulates the adrenal glands, causing further weaknesses.

Of course, fermentation of food sugars in the stomach also causes alcohol. Organic wine would be the only alcohol I would recommend, and very little of that.

Refined sugars are acid-forming and cause a great deal of mucus production by the body. As previously stated, mucus becomes congestive leading to allergies, bronchitis, pneumonia, colds, flu, mumps, sinusitis, and all the "congestive" type conditions. Refined sugars, being acid-forming, also add to the inflammation of tissue.

Meat is also a well-known stimulant that is irritating and inflammatory to our tissues. As we noted in the last section, meat is full of antibiotics, hormones, nuclear wastes, steroids, adrenaline, pesticides, herbicides, and several other toxic chemicals. These substances are all stimulants, irritants and suppressors, all mixed together and found in the tissue of the meat. These chemicals (and adrenaline) can give you a temporary feeling of energy, only to make you more fatigued afterwards. Meat, being high in nitrogen, also pushes out calcium. Calcium and phosphorus need to be kept in balance. In meat, one finds a high phosphorus-to-calcium ratio, whereas vegetables have a balanced ratio between these two essential minerals.

The human intestinal tract is four times as long as that of a carnivore (cats, etc.) with a thousand times more absorption ability. Since meat (flesh) protein putrefies very quickly, and since our intestinal tract is so long, meat putrefies inside the body before we have a chance to eliminate it. Putrefaction causes acidosis, which also inflames and eventually destroys cells. This, of course, invites different types of our "parasitic" friends. These types of parasites are very destructive to weakened cells, tissues, organs and glands. Meat also yields sulfuric and phosphoric acids, which are highly stimulating, inflammatory and destructive to tissue.

Energy should always be dynamic or cellular, never stimulated externally. If you must consume stimulants for energy, this only goes to prove tissue weaknesses exist within you. In the long run, irritants and stimulants only weaken and destroy tissue (organs, glands). The nervous system (sympathetic, parasympathetic and autonomic) and the heart are especially hard hit with these. These substances cause palpitations and heart arrhythmias as well as neurological imbalances.

Free yourself and your body from stimulants and irritants and experience a world of dynamic energy—the cellular energy that explodes from healthy cells. Irritants and stimulants only serve as temporary energy, which in the long run, weakens and destroys your body. Stop consuming acidic irritants and stimulating foods that only serve to imprison you by making you a slave to the constant need for stimulation. These types of foods also make you weaker and more toxic. Animals do not ingest irritants or stimulants. Why should we?

Living is actually a struggle for fresh air. Keep the vast lung surface of the organism supplied with fresh, unpolluted air, and also observe all the other health rules, and there is no reason known to science why you should ever die.

— Prof. J. S. Haldane, English Astronomer

MODULE 4.4

☀ Vaccinations: The Poison Needles

"Like treats like" is a concept used by the allopathic (medical) and homeopathic (more natural) modalities to treat diseases. Along this line, one of the most toxic and oftentimes fatal concepts and practices that science has created is that of inoculation or "vaccinations," whereby live parasites are injected into the body, hoping the body will develop an immunity to them. The reason for this is that parasites (germs) are considered to be the cause of most diseases. Today, science is slowly moving away from this idea, replacing it with the concept of genetics or genes being the "bad boys."

An excellent example of the "like treats like" fallacy is the polio vaccine. The theory is: To build your immunity to this virus, simply take in more of the same virus, but in smaller dosages. The thought is that the body will develop immunity to the virus by building up antibodies, and that this will create a faster or ignored immune response to this pathogen (virus). Hopefully then, an immune cell will either destroy the viral cell before it becomes uncontrollable by the body, or simply ignore the pathogen all together. It can still be there, but inactive.

This is stupid thinking, to me, and the facts prove it. When the polio vaccine was introduced, polio went up 680 percent, as uncovered and reported by Dr. Leonard Horowitz in his book, *The Emerging Viruses*. An article in the *Tampa Tribune* several years ago told of an infant who contracted polio from the vaccination itself. The same thing happens with the flu vaccine. How many people do you know who took the flu shot and still contracted the flu? This is another example of the stupidity of this toxic practice, and one that has happened thousands of times.

No one should deny the dangers of vaccines. The measles, mumps, rubella (German measles) and polio vaccines all contain live but weakened viruses. Although health officials say that polio has been wiped out in the U.S. since 1979, they often fail to mention that all recorded cases of polio since that time are actually *caused* by the polio vaccine, or that we now simply call polio by another name—spinal meningitis. When are we going to lift our heads out of the sand and into the heavens?

A clean and vital body does not get sick. Its immune system is strong and its ability to protect itself is unbelievable. Natural immunity lasts a lifetime, whereas vaccinated immunity is short-lived—estimated at only approximately seven years. We forget that nature (God), through the botanical kingdom, supplies all that we need. It is far better to use herbal anti-parasitics, astringents and proliferants to clean and strengthen your body than it is to pollute it with toxic chemicals, active parasites and foreign proteins.

Many vaccines have been collaborative experiments. One such experiment was reported between Kaiser Permanente of Southern California and the U.S. Center for Disease Control (CDC) with the blessing of WHO (the World Health Organization). Between 1989 and 1991, this joint project used the virus from the Edmonston-Zagreb (E-Z) Measles on 1500 "poor, Black and Latino inner city children, primarily in Los Angeles. This experimentation had previously been attempted in Africa, Haiti and Mexico, with devastating results. Large numbers of children died directly from the vaccine and many more from the effects of its immuno-suppression, leading to the failure of these children to fight other pathogens." (*Cancer Cover-Up {Genocide}* by Kathleen Deoul. *See* Bibliography.)

Vaccinations have led to immuno-suppression and mutation, causing untold conditions many now suffer from. Human beings and their use of science have created much unnecessary pain, suffering and death, based in stupidity and in the desire to control nature and others. Diseases from the Gulf War Syndrome, AIDS, cancer, mutation of the body, and countless other conditions can be directly related to vaccinations. Since most vaccines are alive and manufactured from human and animal tissues like monkey kidneys, cattle and human embryos, chicken hearts and human placentas, contamination and mutation of these viruses /vaccines exist. While nature always keeps itself in balance and harmony, the human ego has brought about a dangerous level of mutation and imbalance in nature, causing a frenzy of devastating and soon to be horrendous effects.

Barbara Loe Fisher, president of the National Vaccine Information Center (NVIC), a consumer's group based in Virginia (USA), claims that vaccines are responsible for the increasing numbers of children and adults who suffer from immune system and neurological disorders, hyperactivity, learning disabilities, asthma, chronic fatigue syndrome, lupus, rheumatoid arthritis, multiple sclerosis and seizure disorders. She calls for studies to monitor the long-term effects of mass vaccinations, and wants physicians to be absolutely sure that these vaccines are safe and not harming people. (Good luck on that one.)

There is overwhelming evidence now from research and reported cases from the United States, Great Britain, Africa, New Zealand and throughout the world, that vaccinations are a toxic and deadly practice. Ask yourself: Why does your government and other agencies that were created to "protect" the American public i.e., Center for Disease Control (CDC), Food and Drug Administration (FDA), Vaccines and

Related Biological Products Advisory Committee (VRBPAC), Advisory Committee on Immunization Practices (ACIP), Human Resource Services (HRS), knowingly allow such atrocities to exist? What is the difference between what is happening now and what occurred in Nazi Germany, where hundreds of thousands of Jews were destroyed? The difference is that it is legal and has spread worldwide. It now involves millions of people. The bottom line to this is simple: money. These same people probably go to church and think they won't have to pay for such atrocities. If you think this world is heaven, think again.

Many medical journals (including the prestigious British *Lancet*) have reported some of the side effects of these "killer" vaccinations; including side effects of the measles vaccine, which has been linked to asthma and allergy-type conditions. The DPT (diphtheria–pertussis-tetanus) inoculation, which was first used in the 1940s, had widespread and disastrous results, including a multitude of deaths. Yet, states still legalized it. Japan outlawed it. The DPT vaccine has especially been linked to brain damage and neurological injuries (MS, Parkinson's, Lou Gehrig's disease, etc.).

The hepatitis B vaccine also stands out for many reasons. First, hepatitis B is not a difficult condition to overcome. Over 90 percent of hepatitis B cases are cured, and I've never seen a case *not cured* by natural means. Yet a vaccine was created for it, and this vaccine was administered to millions. It has now been linked to arthritis, diabetes, vascular conditions, Bell's palsy, MS and other neurological conditions. In New Zealand, it was reported that diabetes increased by 60 percent following the introduction of the hepatitis B vaccine. *The British Medical Journal* reported a link between the hepatitis B vaccine and both autism and inflammatory bowel syndrome.

One of the worst cases I've seen involved a sixteen-month-old female baby from Texas. She had a hepatitis B vaccination at three months of age, and shortly thereafter she went into constant convulsions. She became temporarily blind, and her left eye twisted to the left. She developed hepatitis and brain damage, and also had severe scoliosis of the spine. It took me two months to eliminate most of her convulsions. Her sight improved and the inflammation of her liver was diminishing. This was truly a sad case, but representative of what's going on in the medical community.

To add insult to injury, research has shown that the HIV virus was introduced in the Hepatitis B vaccine in four of the largest cities in the United States. Initially designed as a biological weapon, the HIV virus was introduced into the poor, ethnic groups and the gay communities. Dr. Horowitz, author of *The Emerging Viruses*, has done extensive investigative research into this matter and has collected a paper trail of who's who, as well as the times and places of this whole experiment. What evil thoughts created and initiated this process are way beyond me. Whatever happened to the medical oath: "First, do no harm"?

Vaccine investigator Neil Z. Miller questions whether we still need the polio vaccine when it *causes* every new case of polio in the country. Miller insists that before mass vaccination programs began fifty years ago, we didn't have cancer in epidemic numbers; that autoimmune ailments were barely known; and that childhood autism did not exist. Our children are now given twenty to thirty different vaccinations in their lifetime, each having its own devastating effects. Is it any wonder that the incidence of juvenile diabetes has soared to 600,000 new cases per year, and is rising? This example is representative of most of the diseases out there.

Those of us who work with cancer are appalled by the medical and scientific arrogance that has created this monster called "vaccines." Doctors and researchers who do not understand health and how nature works still continue their endless efforts to destroy us through the guise of "modern" medical practices, saying that, "It's the only way."

The problem of contamination has always plagued vaccine makers. During World War II a yellow fever vaccine manufactured with human blood serum was unknowingly contaminated with hepatitis viruses and given to the military. This resulted in more than 50,000 cases of serum hepatitis among our American troops who were injected with the vaccine.

I also want to mention the simian virus, number 40—also known as Sim-40 or the SV-40 virus. This virus was created in the early to mid-1950s when polio vaccines manufactured in monkey kidney tissue became contaminated. I have focused on this virus for many years now, and as research has shown, it causes cancer in animals and is probably linked to some lung cancers (mesothelioma) and bone marrow cancer (multiple myeloma).

Humans today are more toxic and weakened than at any other time in history. The immune system, through genetics, is now at an all time low. Since people have chosen the paths they have, particularly through inoculation with poisons, we are seeing chronic and degenerative weaknesses or conditions, even in infants. Remember, you cannot put parasites into a toxic body without severe consequences. Since we know so little about viruses it is extremely dangerous to be playing with them like it were some game. It is now thought that these viral proteins become a part of our cells' DNA structures in some way and are passed down through genetics. Again, it is important to understand God and the word "consciousness." As what we have experienced in life becomes a part of our memory patterns, so it is with all life, including the tiniest cells within the body. All life has memory and emotions, right down to the smallest created substances and elements. This has been proven over and over again with plants and animals, as well as with cells.

Men and women must awaken out of this "sleep state," and ascend in their awareness toward God. This will broaden their perspectives and their understanding of how simple and how beautiful health and life really is. It is time to fill yourself (your consciousness) with love, energy, health and vitality, and to rise above the lower levels of disease.

"Detoxification and Regeneration" is the only answer to our current dilemma. The consciousness of treatment has taken us down a devastating road. Cleaning your body out of all these toxins and strengthening your cells is logical, and proven to overcome the many conditions mentioned above.

It's your body. Think about it. Trust in yourself and God (nature). Learn all you can about true health and vitality through nature and the tools (food and herbs) that nature supplies for your health and vitality.

Wake up! It's almost too late *now*.

Resources

There have been many books written on the toxic practice of vaccinations. Check the Bibliography at the back of this book. Read, learn, and educate yourself. No one else will. If possible, check out these websites:

National Vaccine Information Center—
    www.909shot.com
www.hhi.org
www.newdawnmagazine.com
www.lightparty.com
www.cancer-coverup.com

I am much more interested in a question on which the "salvation of humanity" depends far more than on any theologians' curio: the question of nutrition.

— Friedrich Nietzsche, *Ecce Homo*

MODULE 4.5

☼ Chemical Toxicity: *Environmental, Hygiene, Household and Drug*

If you know anyone with chemical or environmental toxicity, you know firsthand the amount of suffering involved. I helped an individual who was so chemically toxic that the very smell of gasoline fumes made her faint. We have destroyed our home (Earth) with chemicals, and now it's too late. We can only stand by while the Earth detoxifies itself through many atmospheric and land changes. This is one of the biggest disgraces in human history.

Similarly, our physical bodies are ravaged with disease, as cancer is now climbing to one in every two males and one in every three females. That means that half the population has cancer and most of these will probably die from it. At the same time, the other half of the population is developing it.

The Natural Resources Defense Council relates that over 85,000 synthetic chemicals are in commercial use today, many now known to cause cancer, as well as damage to the brain, nervous system and reproductive systems. It is estimated that human technology releases over 6,000,000,000 pounds of chemicals into the environment every year. Whales and porpoises are beaching themselves in ever greater numbers. Fish are dying everywhere, and animals in the wild are developing cancer and birth deformities as never seen before. What is it going to take for humans to awaken to this? Every single individual, I don't care how wealthy or intellectual, is ingesting over 120 pounds of chemicals each year, including over ten different pesticides each day. Our immune systems cannot handle this level of insult to the body.

CHEMICAL AWARENESS

The list below consists mostly of carcinogens—or cancer-causing agents or chemicals. These chemicals are ingested through the air we breathe, the foods we eat, the water we drink, and the lotions, cosmetics, hair dyes, etc., that we put on our skin.

SOLVENTS
These are compounds that dissolve things.
- Propyl Alcohol
- Benzene Wood Alcohol
- Xylene
- Toluene
- Methyl ethyl Ketone (MEK)
- Methyl butyl Ketone (MBK)
- Methylene Chloride
- TCE

INORGANIC METAL POLLUTION
These can be found in dental wear, cosmetics, food, drinking cans, water supplies and cooking pots.
- Copper
- Mercury
- Thallium
- Lead
- Cadmium
- Nickel
- Chromium
- Aluminum

CHEMICAL TOXINS
- Chlorofluorocarbons (CFCS)—Freon can be found in air conditioners and refrigerators.
- Arsenic—can be found in pesticides.

- Polychlorinated biphenyls (PCBs)—can be found in transformers, commercial soap and detergents.
- Formaldehyde—can be found in furniture, pillows, mattresses, clothing, Formica cabinets, and carpets.
- Chemical medications
- Psychotropic drugs
- Chlorine in water supplies and pools
- Fluorine (a known carcinogen) added to water supplies.
- Inorganic Iodine
- Sulfa drugs
- Phosphates

EVERYDAY CHEMICALS

These are chemicals that you may be breathing, using, touching, etc.
- Aluminum cookware
- Household cleaners
- Automobile fluids
- Pesticides (neuro-toxins)—these are an excitotoxin (brain and nerve poison).
- Herbicides (neuro and liver toxins—these are an excitotoxin (brain and nerve poison).
- Fertilizers
- Paint
- Varnish
- Wax
- Glues
- Lubricants
- Bleach
- Gasoline
- Underarm deodorants (aluminum chlorohydrates and neomycin)
- Toothpaste
- Soaps

MYCOTOXINS

These are molds that can produce some of the most toxic substances.
- Alflatoxin—can be found in commercial fruit juices, rice, pasta, bread and vinegar.
- Zearalenone—can be found in commercial cereal grains, processed foods and feeds.

Top 20 Hazardous Substances

There are 275 substances on the current list from the ASTDR/EPA.

1. Arsenic
2. Lead
3. Mercury
4. Vinyl Chloride
5. Polychlorinated Biphenyls (PCBs)
6. Benzene
7. Cadmium
8. Benzo(a)pyrene
9. Polycyclic Aromatic Hydrocarbons
10. Benzo(b)fluoranthene
11. Chloroform
12. DDT, P' P'
13. Aroclor 1254
14. Aroclor 1260
15. Trichloroethylene
16. Dibenz (a.h.) anthracene
17. Dieldrin
18. Chromium, Hexavalent
19. Chlordane
20. Hexachlorobutadiene

- Sterigmatocystin—pasta
- Ergot
- Cytochalasin B
- Kojic Acid
- T-2 Toxin
- Sorghum molds
- Patulin

PHYSICAL TOXINS
- Fiberglass
- Asbestos
- Car and truck exhaust—carbon monoxide, lead, etc.
- By-products of chemical manufacturing
- Lead pipes
- Nuclear wastes

Common Water and Food Contaminants

PESTICIDES	POSSIBLE HEALTH EFFECTS
Chlordane	Known carcinogen.
Atrazine	Damages kidney, liver, heart, lung, tissue; a known carcinogen.
Alachlor	Probably carcinogen.
DDT and derivatives	Liver, kidneys, nerve, and endocrine damage.
Diazinon	Excitotoxin. Suspected carcinogen, liver and kidney damage.
EPN	Excitotoxin. Suspected carcinogen, liver and kidney damage.
Lindane	Excitotoxin. Suspected carcinogen, liver and kidney damage.
PCB's (polychlorinated biphenyls)	Excitotoxin. Suspected carcinogen, liver and kidney damage.
Phosphamidon	Excitotoxin. Suspected carcinogen, liver and kidney damage.
Chlorpyrifos	Excitotoxin. Suspected carcinogen, liver and kidney damage.
Dicloran	Excitotoxin. Suspected carcinogen, liver and kidney damage.
Endosulfan	Excitotoxin. Suspected carcinogen, liver and kidney damage.
2, 4D	Kidney, Liver and Lung damage.

TOXIC METALS	POSSIBLE HEALTH EFFECTS
Arsenic	Kidney, liver, endocrine and nerve damage.
Mercury	Brain and nerve damage.
Lead	Liver, kidney, muscle and nerve damage.
Sulfur	Accumulative, allergies, lymphomas, kidney and intestinal impairment, and inflammation.
Cadmium	Brain, nerve, liver, pancreas damage.

PETROCHEMICALS	POSSIBLE HEALTH EFFECTS
Benzene	Carcinogen.
Xylenes	Liver, kidney, endocrine and nervous system damage.
Carbon Tetrachloride	Suspected carcinogen.
Ethylene dibromide	Suspected carcinogen.
Permethrin	An excitotoxin (neuro-toxins) Suspected carcinogens, liver and kidney damage.
Toluene	Kidney, liver, nervous system, endocrine, circulatory damage.

FOOD ADDITIVES
- BHT
- Nitrates
- Nitrites
- MSG
- Artificial sugars (aspartame, saccharin, etc.)
- Tobacco for smoking or chewing

As you can see from the lists above there are high amounts of chemical toxins, mostly man-made, that have been introduced into our air, water and food supplies. Remember, for every cause there is an effect. All toxins are irritating, damaging and inflammatory (causing an immune response) to some degree or another.

TOXIC PESTICIDES

The U.S. Agriculture Department and independent research companies and organizations have reported that there are high amounts of pesticides and other pollutants on and in our foods. Tomatoes, strawberries, peaches, spinach, turnips, squash and many other foods can have as much as 80 to 100 different pollutants, especially pesticides, on or in them. Peanuts have over 180 pollutants, and raisins can have over 110.

As you read the potential and known side effects of pesticides, ask yourself if you're really in favor of Bio-Tech Engineering—whereby pesticides are genetically placed into the seeds of our foods. This means, of course, that pesticide residues will be in the foods themselves, and that we will have no way to remove them. Pesticides are like sulfur drugs, they have a cumulative effect. Once reaching toxic and deadly proportions they cause allergy reactions, inflammation, excessive immune responses and neurological failure.

TOXIC CHEMICALS

The following contains examples of everyday toxins that you "consume" through your foods, water, cosmetics, toothpaste, underarm deodorants, and other products. These are just a few of the extremely toxic chemicals that have been manufactured and released into our environment and food supply.

Aluminum (chlorohydrates, etc.)

Found in: Underarm deodorants, canned foods, industry, cooking utensils, etc.

Properties: Suspected brain and nerve damage, suspected in Alzheimer's and other brain and nerve syndromes. May affect the endocrine gland system, especially the pituitary.

Aspartame (NutraSweet®, Equal®)

Found in: Diet drinks (soda, etc.), candies desserts, many prepackaged foods, etc.

Toxic Chemicals

Educate Yourself About Toxic Chemicals

- EPA's Drinking Water Hotline
  1-800-426-4791

- Green Peace
  1-800-326-1959
  www.greenpeaceusa.org

- Agency for Toxic Substances and Disease Registry
  www.atsdr.cdc.gov

- Institute of Agricultural and Natural Resources, University of Nebraska
  www.ianr.unl.edu

- National Resources Defense Council
  www.nrdc.org

Properties: Artificial (low calorie) sweeteners. Known carcinogen excitotoxin (neurotoxin) affects brain and nervous system as well as the glandular system. U.S. consumes 7000 tons per year. (CNN)

Benzoic or Benzyl

Found in: Cosmetics, nail polish, shampoos, bath and shower products.

Properties: Suspected carcinogen, affects endocrine gland function, also suspected in birth defects.

BHA/BHT (butylated hydroxyanisole)

Found in: Breads, dry cereals, cake mixes, frozen pizzas, pork, potato chips, many oils, crackers, puddings, prepared donuts, gelatin desserts.

Properties: A preservative. Suspected carcinogen. Affects liver and pancreatic tissues. Forbidden in many countries.

Caffeine

Found in: Colas and other soft drinks, naturally occurring in cocoa, coffees, teas.

Properties: A stimulant. Suspected in birth defects. Affects endocrine system and nervous system. Over stimulates the GI tract.

Caramel

Found in: Colas and other soft drinks, bread, pudding, frozen pizzas, candies, snacks, etc.

Properties: A coloring. Suspected carcinogen, causes genetic defects.

Carrageenan

Found in: Cottage cheese, ice cream, sour cream, puddings, baby formulas.

Properties: A thickening agent. Suspected and indicated in ulcerative conditions of the GI tract. Affects blood clotting and proper nutrient dispersion.

Chlorine

Found in: Tap water, showers, pool, laundry products, cleaning agents, food processing, sewage systems, etc.

Properties: Anti-bacterial and parasitic. Contributes to asthma, hay fever, anemia, bronchitis, circulatory collapse, confusion, delirium, diabetes, dizziness, irritation of the eyes, mouth, nose, throat, lung, skin and stomach, heart disease, high blood pressure and nausea. Probably cancer causing.

DEA (Diethanolamine)
MEA (Momoethanolamine)
TEA (Triethanolamine)

Found in: Bubble baths, shampoos, soaps, skin washes and cleansers.

Properties: Foaming agents. Suspected carcinogen. May bind with nitrates and nitrites to form nitrosamines (tumor growers).

EDTA (Ethylendiaminetetraacetic Acid)

Found in: Shellac, solvents, and personal care products that foam (bubble baths, body washes, shampoos, soaps and facial cleansers).

Properties: Preservative. Hormone disrupters. Suspected in at least two types of cancer—kidney and liver cancer. Known to cause kidney, intestinal and skin disorders. Causes cramping and the like.

Gums (Arabic, Karaya, Xanthin, Cellulose, Ghatti, Tragacanth, etc.)

Found in: Ice cream, colas, candy, gum, beer, salad dressings, Isopropyl alcohol.

Properties: Thickening agent. May be linked to allergies and bowel disorders. Affects proper nutrient bioavailability.

Isopropyl Alcohol

Found in: Hair color rinses, body rubs, hand lotions, after-shave lotions, fragrances, and many other cosmetics. A petroleum-derived substance, it is also used in antifreeze and as a solvent in shellac.

Properties: A solvent and denaturant. (A denaturant is a poisonous substance that changes another substance's natural qualities). Inhalation or ingestion of the vapor may cause headaches, flushing, dizziness, mental depression, nausea, vomiting, narcosis and coma.

Lactic Acid

Found in: Printing industry, dyes, frozen pizzas, gelatin, cheeses, frozen desserts, olives, beer, carbonated drinks.

Properties: A preservative. Acidosis and inflammation.

Maltol Dextrin

Found in: Wood tars, many desserts and soft drinks, processed foods, ice cream.

Properties: Aroma and flavor enhancer. Suspected carcinogen.

Mineral Oil

Found in: Commonly used petroleum ingredient. Baby Oil is 100% mineral oil.

Properties: Disrupts the skin's natural immune barrier, inhibiting its ability to breathe and to absorb moisture and nutrition. Impedes the skin's ability to release toxins, promoting acne and other disorders. Ultimately causes premature aging.

Modified Food Starch

Found in: Baked beans, creamed canned foods, beets (processed), dry-roasted nuts, ravioli, drink powders, frozen pizzas, pie fillings, baby foods, baking powder, frozen fish (packaged), soups, gravies.

Properties: Thickening and filling agent. Alkali in sodium hydroxide. Suspected in causing lung damage. GI tract irritation, vomiting. Possible cramping and spasms.

Mono- and Diglycerides

Found in: Pies, butter, dry roasted nuts, cakes, cookies, some processed foods.

Properties: Binding and smoothing agent, softener. Suspected carcinogenic, possibly causing genetic and birth defects.

MSG (Monosodium Glutamate)

Found in: Many Chinese foods, sauces, canned and processed foods, frozen pizzas, beer, salad dressings, canned meats, tomato sauces, broths, gelatins, bouillon, soy sauce, etc. May be disguised by other names, e.g. glutamate, glutamic acid, autolyzed yeast, hydrolyzed proteins, natural flavors, caseinate, seasonings, carrageenan, maltol dextrin, yeast extract.

Properties: A common flavor enhancer. Excitotoxin (neurotoxin) affects the nervous system and glandular system. Spasms, headaches (including migraines), sweating, chest pain, diarrhea. Possibly linked to genetic conditions, brain damage, heart conditions, tumors, Alzheimer's and Parkinson's disease, asthma attacks, ALS, ADD, ADHD, GI tract conditions.

Nitrites, Nitrates (Sodium)

Found in: Processed meats, frozen pizzas, baby foods, etc.

Properties: Preservative, used in "curing." Known carcinogens. Extremely toxic. Overdoses cause death. Binds to form nitrosamines, especially in the presence of alcohol.

PEG (Polyethylene glycol)

Found in: Toothpastes, bath and shower products. Used to make degreasers and cleansers (oven, car, etc.)

Properties: Thickening agent. Affects endocrine function; has estrogenic effects; a suspected carcinogen.

Propylene Glycol

Found in: Antifreeze, make-up, lotions, deodorants, mouthwashes, toothpaste, hair products (shampoos, etc.) shaving cream, etc. Used in food processing. Used as solvents.

Properties: A surfactant or wetting agent. Skin irritant, causing inflammation and possible damage to skin. May cause kidney, liver, brain and pancreatic damage and abnormalities. Used to break down proteins and cellular structures.

Propylgallate

Found in: Gum, pickles, oils and shortenings, processed foods and meat products.

Properties: A preservative. Suspected in liver and pancreatic damage. Possible link to birth defects.

Red Dye #40 (Allura Red AC)

Found in: Red pistachio nuts, meats (hot dogs, etc.), gelatin, gum, cereals, baked goods, many candies, red sodas. Note: #40 is not used as much today. However, there are many artificial colorings that are very questionable.

Properties: A coloring. Suspected carcinogen and possibly linked to birth defects. Liver and kidney damage. Nerve toxin.

Saccharin

Found in: Many desserts, drinks and prepackaged foods.

Properties: An artificial sweetener. Suspected in some cancers (bladder, etc.) and possible tumor formation. Can affect heart rhythms, GI tract conditions and skin irritation.

Sodium Erythorbate

Found in: Meat products, baked goods, many beverages, etc.

Properties: Preservative. Banned in many countries. Suspected in birth defects and genetic conditions. Highly toxic.

Sodium Laureth and/or Lauryl Sulfate (SLES/SLS)

Found in: Mouthwashes, shampoos, bubble bath, shaving gels/creams, toothpastes, shower bars/gels, detergents, car wash soaps, engine degreasers, floor cleaner, cosmetics.

Properties: Said to contain nitrosamines and dioxane, which are both considered carcinogens. Suspected effects include: liver, kidney, lung and pancreatic damage. May affect calcium utilization causing teeth, bone and connective tissue weaknesses. May affect nerve and brain function. Suspected in hair loss, cataracts and poor eyesight, eye damage/development, shortness of breath, skin irritation/damage, and death.

Sodium Fluoride

Found in: Toothpastes

Properties: Known carcinogen. Affects brain and nerve function; weakens kidney tissue.

Talc

Found in: Deodorants, shaving products and skin products.

Properties: A known carcinogen that causes ovarian cancer in mammals.

Synthetic (Artificial) Flavorings or Fragrances

Found in: Packaged foods, mouthwashes, deodorants, cosmetics, perfumes, etc.

Properties: Many are neurotoxins affecting your brain, nerve, and endocrine function; many suspected as carcinogens.

Tannin (Tannic Acid)

Found in: Teas, coffee, beer, wine, soda. Found in many artificial flavorings, etc.

Properties: Flavoring. Suspected in liver, pancreatic and GI tract irritation. Occurs naturally in nature, in low doses and buffered.

Toluene

Found in: Nail polish, feminine products, as well as some cosmetics.

Properties: Suspected carcinogen, reportedly affects endocrine function. Research shows possible birth defects as one side effect. Can affect brain and nerve function.

Conclusion

Many of the toxins listed above have been detected in municipal water supplies, both above and below ground, including large city water supplies. Most of these toxins and pollutants come from manufacturing, industrial solvents, ammunition wastes, pesticides, herbicides, grain fumigants, and petrochemical use (gasoline, solvents, oils, cleansers) dumped into the ground. Boating is also a source of contamination of water supplies.

Reports indicate that over 125 cosmetic ingredients, and hundreds of others—commonly found in cigarettes, foods, lotions, salves, synthetic vitamins and many other daily used or consumed substances—are carcinogenic substances. Hundreds more accumulate in the liver, brain, kidney, pancreatic, bowel and heart tissue, obstructing proper cellular respiration and causing inflammation and damage to these tissues.

Many contaminants oxidize and become airborne thus causing liver and lung damage and cancer. Many more bond with each other to form radical substances like nitrosamines, which highly accelerate tumor formation and growth.

A large number of the above-cited pesticides, herbicides, fungicides, petrochemicals, etc., are hormone disrupters. They inhibit or stimulate the production of hormones or steroids, like estrogen and testosterone.

Benzene levels in air, water and food have skyrocketed. Benzene is a known carcinogen, which is used in solvents and food additives, and emitted from oil refineries, gas stations, rubber (tire) manufacturing plants and diesel powered vehicles. An astronomical amount of carcinogenic substances are released into our air and our water from tobacco smoke, gas and especially diesel emissions, body shops, airports, highways, railways, subways, most industries, boating, petro-production plants, etc.

Radiation is another high source of our cancers. Harmful radiation is found in dental offices and hospitals (with use of x-rays, nuclear medicine, and other processes), around high power wires, TV sets, microwave ovens, cathode-ray computer monitors and most medical diagnostic equipment—including Cat Scans, MRIs, mammogram and x-ray equipment.

Cancer has now reached epidemic proportions, estimated to be in every other person in the U.S.. According to Kathleen Deoul in her book *Cancer Cover-Up {Genocide}*: "One American dies of cancer every minute—the equivalent of crashing three fully loaded 747s every day! But it doesn't have to happen."

We live in a world of excitotoxins, also called "neurotoxins," which are affecting our relationship with the outside world and with ourselves. We have literally surrounded ourselves with cancer-causing agents—we live in them and around them, we drink, eat and inject them, and we are constantly putting them on our skin. Our houses are full of formaldehyde and other potentially toxic and carcinogenic substances released from carpets, Formica-type (laminate) cabinets, plywood, glue, curtains, synthetic garments, etc. Your clothes can be full of toxins, especially if they are dry cleaned. Perchloroethylene or "perc" —the chemical used in dry cleaning—is extremely toxic. Spills at dry cleaners can necessitate the removal of the building and the dirt beneath it.

Plastics are another server of toxins and potential carcinogens. Vinyls (phthalates) are found in PVC pipes, toys, baby teething objects, baby bottles and building materials. Never buy distilled water in plastic containers. As distilled water is void of substances, it therefore creates diffusion, pulling other substances (like minerals and chemicals) into it.

Even if we stopped using all chemicals today, it would still be too late. The human species remains steeped in ignorance as it continues to destroy its own home. No other species does this. Big industry and automobiles are some of the worst polluting offenders. Many factories that pour millions of toxic particles daily into the air do not want to use pollution control devices because of the expense. Although a lot of good research is going on by many honest individuals, this information seems to get suppressed or buried by a monetary-based society. But life has no price tag. Everyone must pitch in and help clean up this world of ours.

Become as free of toxic chemicals as possible.

☀ Protecting Yourself From Carcinogens

We are surrounded by and consume hundreds of carcinogenic substances each day. These substances act as igniters and accelerators. They damage tissue and inspire immune responses like gasoline enrages a fire. Many of these are neurotoxins, which attach themselves to your nervous system and endocrine gland system. This creates hypoactivity, or lowering of the function of these systems, which can create a multitude of symptoms including difficulty in breathing, heart arrhythmia, MS and Lou Gehrig's disease.

You must take full responsibility for your own health. Even our government has little concern about the levels of environmental toxicity. Politicians don't seem to realize that they are affected just as everyone else is. Why do you think cancer is soaring? The truth has been well hidden by those who wish to gain from all this. However, they will eventually succumb to these toxins, just as everyone else is.

PROTECT YOURSELF!

1. Live closer to nature, away from factories, power lines and heavy traffic.

2. Fill your house with live plants. Philodendrons (philodendron spp.) are known to absorb formaldehyde, ammonia, benzene, trichloroethylene and hydrates, as well as xylene. The following plants are great indoor plants and will help clean indoor air:

   - Philodendron (Philodendron spp.)
   - Spider Plants (Chlorophytum comosum)
   - Bamboo plant (Rhapis excelsea)
   - Corn Plant (Dracaena fragrans)
   - English Ivy (Hedera helix)
   - Bromeliads (Cryptanthus spp.)
   - Chrysanthemum (Chrysanthemum spp.)
   - House-type Palms
   - Ficus Tree
   - Golden Pothos (Epipremnum aureum)

3. Always wash your fruits and vegetables before you eat them. Use a vegetable wash or fresh lemon juice with hydrogen peroxide.

4. Eat an 80 to 100 percent raw food diet. Eat fruits even more so than vegetables. Fruits are full of antioxidant and astringent properties. They will keep your lymphatic (immune) system clean and moving. They also enhance the strength of a cell, especially brain and nerve cells.

5. In traffic, keep your car's outside air vent closed. Make sure your car's exhaust system is not leaking and in good order.

6. Use 100 percent natural hygiene products (soaps, shampoos, etc.). Read the labels. If they have chemicals in them, don't use them. (If you can't pronounce it—you probably don't want it.) What you put on your skin absorbs into your blood stream and circulates throughout your body. This can damage your brain, heart, kidneys and especially your liver.

7. Avoid dry cleaning, as the chemicals used are extremely toxic.

8. Use common sense with everything you do and use. It's your body and it carries you around this world, as any vehicle would. If it fails—you're stuck. Chemicals can be extremely dangerous.

9. Avoid cooking. If you must cook, steam your food in stainless steel. Always use stainless steel cookware.

10. Use and clean your air conditioners and air filters. Use the natural, high-filtration-type that removes 1-micron to 3-micron size particles.

11. Use R/O (reverse-osmosis) or steam-distilled water. Note: Avoid storing distilled water in plastic containers. Distilled water will leach some of the chemicals from the plastic into itself.

12. Drink from and use glass as much as possible. Plastic can be toxic to you.

13. Avoid walking for exercise near high traffic areas. Walk in a safe park or wooded area instead.

14. Avoid florescent lighting as much as possible. Be aware of what you eat, drink, breathe and what you put on your skin, as this is how you bring the outside world in.

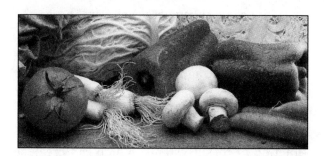

MODULE 4.7

☼ Poison Control Centers

Here are the telephone numbers for local Poison Control Centers in the United States. You may want to program the numbers for your area into your automatic dialing feature, if you have one. Please note that all phone numbers are subject to change. Check your state's Poison Control Center number for accuracy.

UNITED STATES

ALABAMA
205-939-9201
205-933-4050
800-292-6678 (AL only)

ALASKA
907-261-3193

ARIZONA
Statewide
800-362-0101 (AZ only)

Phoenix Area
602-253-3334
Tucson Area
602-626-6016

ARKANSAS
501-686-6161

CALIFORNIA
Davis Area
916-734-3692
800-342-9293 (Northern CA only)
Fresno Area
209-445-1222
800-346-5922 (CA only)
Orange County Area
714-634-5988
800-544-4404 (Southern CA only)
San Diego Area
619-543-6000
800-876-4766 (619 area code)

San Francisco/Bay Area
415-476-6600
San Jose/Santa Clara Valley
408-299-5112
800-662-9886 (CA only)

COLORADO
303-629-1123

CONNECTICUT
203-679-1000
800-343-277 (CT only)

DELAWARE
302-655-3389

DISTRICT OF COLUMBIA
202-625-3333
202-784-4660 (TTY)*

FLORIDA
813-253-4444
800-282-3171 (FL only)

GEORGIA
404-589-4400
800-282-5846 (GA only)

HAWAII
808-941-4411

IDAHO
208-378-2707
800-632-8000

ILLINOIS
217-753-3330
800-543-2022 (IL only)
800-942-5969

INDIANA
317-929-2323
800-382-9097(IN only)

IOWA
800-272-6477 (IA only)
800-362-2327 (IA only)

KANSAS
Topeka/Northern KS
913-354-6100
Wichita/Southern KS
316-263-9999

KENTUCKY
502-629-7275
800-722-5725 (KY only)

LOUISIANA
800-256-9822 (LA only)

MAINE
800-442-6305 (ME only)

MARYLAND
Statewide
410-528-7701
800-492-2414 (MD only)
D.C. Suburbs
202-625-3333
202-784-4660 (TTY)*

MASSACHUSETTS
617-232-2120
800-682-9211

MICHIGAN
Statewide
800-632-2727 (MI only)
800-356-3232 (TTY)*
Detroit Area
313-745-5711

MINNESOTA
Statewide
800-222-1222
Duluth/Northern MN
218-726-5466
Minneapolis/St. Paul Area
612-347-3141
612-337-7474 (TDD)
612-221-2113

MISSISSIPPI
601-354-7660

MISSOURI
314-772-5200
800-366-8888

MONTANA
303-629-1123

NEBRASKA

Statewide

800-955-9119 (NE only)

Omaha Area

402-390-5555

NEVADA

702-732-4989

NEW HAMPSHIRE

603-650-5000

800-562-8236 (NH only)

NEW JERSEY

800-962-1253

MARYLAND

NEW MEXICO

505-843-2551

800-432-6866 (NM only)

NEW YORK

Albany Area

800-336-6997

Binghamton/Southern Tier

800-252-5655

Buffalo/Western NY

716-878-7654

800-888-7655

Long Island

516-542-2323

516-542-2324

516-542-2325

Nyack/Hudson Valley

914-353-1000

New York City

212-340-4494

212-POISONS

212-689-9014 (TDD)**

Syracuse/Central NY

315-476-4766

NORTH CAROLINA

Statewide

800-672-1697

Charlotte Area

704-355-4000

NORTH DAKOTA

800-732-2200 (ND only)

OHIO

Statewide

800-682-7625

Columbus/Central OH

614-228-1323

614-461-2012

614-228-2272 (TTY)*

Cincinnati Area

513-558-5111

800-872-5111 (OH only)

OKLAHOMA

800-522-4611 (OK only)

OREGON

503-494-8968

800-452-7165 (OR only)

PENNSYLVANIA

Philadelphia/Eastern PA

215-386-2100

Pittsburgh/Western PA

412-681-6669

Hershey/Central PA

800-521-6110

PUERTO RICO

809-754-8535

RHODE ISLAND

401-277-5727

SOUTH CAROLINA

800-777-1117

SOUTH DAKOTA

803-952-0123 (SD only)

TENNESSEE

Memphis/Western TN

901-528-6048

Nashville/Eastern TN

615-322-6435

TEXAS

214-590-5000

800-441-0040 (TX only)

UTAH
801-581-2151
800-456-7707 (UT only)

VERMONT
800-562-8236 (VT only)

VIRGINIA
Statewide
800-451-1428
Charlottesville/Blue Ridge
804-925-5543
D.C. Suburbs
202-625-3333
202-784-4660 (TTY)*

WASHINGTON
800-732-6985 (WA only)

WEST VIRGINIA
304-348-4211
800-642-3625 (WV only)

WISCONSIN
Madison/Southwestern and Northern WI
608-262-3702
Milwaukee/Southeastern WI
414-255-2222

WYOMING
800-955-9119 (WY only)

CANADA

ALBERTA
403-670-1414

BRITISH COLUMBIA
604-682-5050

MANITOBA
204-787-2591

NEW BRUNSWICK
Fredericton
506-452-5400
St. John
506-648-6222

NEWFOUNDLAND
709-722-1110

NOVA SCOTIA
902-428-8161

ONTARIO
Province wide
800-267-1373 (ON only)
Eastern Ontario
613-737-1100

PRINCE EDWARD ISLAND
902-428-8161

QUEBEC
800-463-5060 (QB only)

SASKATCHEWAN
306-359-4545

*TTY—Teletype for the hearing impaired
**TDD—Telecommunications device for the deaf

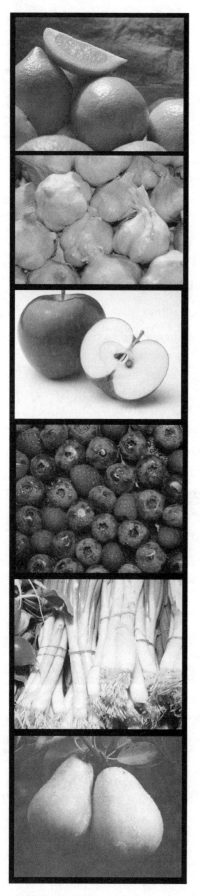

CHAPTER FIVE

The Nature of Disease

To understand how to get healthy it is first important to change your concepts about disease. Most people fear disease because they do not understand its causes. Medical doctors make diseases appear so complicated that the average person thinks only a trained specialist can help him. This is not true. To understand disease symptoms is simply to understand acidity and toxicity, and how the body responds to these conditions. In understanding this, you will see that disease is a natural process—the outcome of imbalanced decisions and actions.

In looking at disease it is also important to understand the original state of health (strength or weakness) that your cells received through genetics. In my experience, **the root causes of ninety-nine percent of all disease symptoms are genetic weaknesses, toxicity and overacidity.** This chapter will focus on these three areas, and discuss how these result in such common diseases as cancer, diabetes, male and female disorders, and such difficulties as weight gain or loss.

In the concluding module, called Body Language, you will find a listing of the many symptoms that point to a weakness or failure in one or more of the body's glands, organs or systems. You can learn to "read" the important information that your body is always giving you.

MODULE 5.1

☼ The Three Root Causes of Disease

FIRST ROOT: INHERENT (GENETIC) WEAKNESSES

Inherent weaknesses are cellular codes (cellular memories) that set the condition of tissue and how it responds to life. Your physical body is a genetic imprint of your family tree, and your cellular strengths and weaknesses come from your genetic history. This is true throughout your body. Cells were originally created by God, but the memory of how well a cell functions is what constitutes our genetics. As we mature, we either make our inherent weaknesses weaker or stronger depending upon our lifestyles. This is extremely important to understand because currently each generation is becoming weaker instead of stronger. Today, more than ever, people are consuming and injecting huge amounts of toxins into their bodies. We are now seeing cancer (a form of degeneration and chronic toxicity) in the early teens; chronic and degenerative issues in infants; and birth deformities as never before. When organs and glands are underactive from genetics, inflammation or toxicity, a host of imbalances and disease conditions can result.

It is easy to understand the concept of genetics. Our physical bodies came from Mom and Dad, which means we will have many of their characteristics, physically, mentally and emotionally. There is also a little of grandmother and grandfather in us too, as their characteristics, encoded in their genes, have been passed down through our parents. Geneticists say that we carry in our bodies and psyches the legacy of four previous generations. However, in my practice I have seen genetic patterns that have clearly been passed along for many more than four generations. Every cell in your body is a genetic cell—each a blueprint of its parent's cell.

Cells become strong or weak depending upon what genetics has dictated to them as well as from the effects of one's lifestyle—that is, by what you eat, drink, breathe, what is absorbed through your skin, and by what you think and feel (emotions).

Cells live and function from their memories of their experiences, just as we do. Certain experiences leave us weak and vulnerable, and the same is true of cells. Physical acids and toxins can weaken and injure cells. Genetic memories add to or subtract from the cell's overall state of health. The impact of all this together determines the strength or weakness of cells, organs and glands, and whether or not they will provide the necessary functions they were originally designed to perform. If you inherited a weakened thyroid, weak adrenal glands or liver, for example, the duties of these tissues will be compromised and their ability to produce hormones, digestive enzymes, steroids, or whatever, can be greatly diminished. This then affects your whole body and how it functions. Disease of one sort or another is the result. For another look at this issue see "About Consciousness and Disease" later in this section.

As a society we must begin to repair our weaknesses and rebuild our cells so that future generations can live. Remember, nature never procreates the weak. The weak are always consumed—this keeps nature healthy for all species and the same can be said of each cell in your body.

Let's look now at the two other primary causes of all disease, and the reasons that tissues fail in the first place: toxicity and overacidity (acidosis). Both create obstructions within your body.

SECOND ROOT: TOXICITY

Toxicity (which means poison) is a broad-range term that includes many things, from mucus accumulation from dairy foods, irritants and complex sugars, to chemical, toxic metal and mineral deposits. This toxicity (which is mostly acidic, and accumulates in the body) comes from foods, air, body-hygiene products, household products, building materials . . . the list goes on and on. Today, most of the foods people eat and the liquids they drink are acidic, mucus-forming, energy-robbing and protein-toxic. The refined starches we eat act like glue in the tissues of our body, causing plaque to build up, as we discussed earlier. This toxicity, being acidic, can inflame and congest tissue to the point of causing tissue death.

This toxicity and mucus is stored in all tissues, but noticed more in your sinuses, throat, thyroid, lungs, muscles, liver, kidneys and skin. This is why all these areas are affected when you have cold and flu-like symptoms. The body tries to "purge" itself of these toxins, or as many of them as it can, through natural processes called "disease." Many "diseases" are nothing more than elimination efforts by the body to purge itself of toxins, and/or dying or dead cells.

As previously stated, toxicity builds up intracellularly and interstitially (around cells) in the vascular system, in the organs and glands, in the bowels, and in the cavities of our body. Combine this toxicity with an over-acid diet and you get inflammation, ulceration, tumors and eventually cellular death (degeneration). These toxins and mucus create obstruction, blocking blood and lymph flow to and from cells. This greatly reduces a cell's ability to function and stay healthy.

Colds, flu, lymphatic conditions, lung conditions, gastrointestinal problems, infections, to name a few of many conditions, are all symptoms of this accumulation of toxicity in the body. Your immune system and/or parasites will naturally act upon this toxicity. Yet this natural response by your immune system to this toxicity and, of course, to the parasites who feed upon this toxicity, is oftentimes mistakenly called an autoimmune disorder. Parasites and immune responses are always secondary to the cause; they are side effects of the symptom.

THIRD ROOT: OVERACIDITY—ACIDOSIS

The body digests, absorbs, utilizes, reproduces, and eliminates in the presence of fluids. These fluids include digestive juices, blood, extra- and intra-cellular fluids, lymphatic fluids and urine. To fully understand the effects that food and toxins have within your body, however, you first have to understand opposites.

Creation exists because of the dynamic interplay of opposites, without which everything would be the same. (Of course, because God is One, the closer to God you get, the more the opposites merge.) The interplay between opposites creates movement, activity, shapes, sizes, colors, temperatures. As complicated as chemistry is, it rests upon two pillars or opposites: hot and cold, or yin and yang, the names for the two opposing dynamics within Chinese philosophy and medicine. Hot is called acid and cold is alkaline. Acids initiate change and alkalis balance. This is the basis of all matter.

The elements which comprise matter are either acid or alkaline in nature. Acid-forming elements include nitrogen, phosphorus and sulfur. Oxygen, calcium, magnesium, sodium and potassium are alkaline elements. Many of the alkaline elements are known as **electrolytes** because of their ability to carry and deliver electrical charges. Alkaline elements have oxygen and carbon dominating the hydrogen, whereas acids have nitrogen and hydrogen dominating.

To maintain health and vitality, all of your body's fluids should be alkaline, except for the stomach's gastric juices, hydrochloric acid and pepsin, which are acidic for initial protein breakdown. The acid or alkaline measurement in your body is classified in what is called **pH factors**. The pH means "potential of hydrogen." The pH scale is 0 through 14—with 0 being the most acidic, 7 being neutral, and 14 the most alkaline. Since each number on the scale represents a logarithm, there is a 10-fold difference between each number. This can be very significant when you understand that the pH of the blood should be 7.4, or slightly alkaline. Coma and death can take place when the hydrogen atoms in the blood lower (by adding hydrogen atoms) the pH to 6.95. The opposite can also be true. Convulsions and spasms can occur when the pH becomes too alkaline (less hydrogen atoms), which is rare. It is important to note that most convulsions and spasms are caused by mineral utilization problems.

All the food that humans eat can be divided into the above two categories: they are either acid-forming or alkaline-forming. This depends upon the ash left after their digestion, and upon the food's dominating inorganic minerals, which affect the pH of our body's fluids. Acid foods leave more phosphorus, iron and sulfur compounds, which push out alkaline minerals like calcium, magnesium, sodium and potassium. Acids crystallize, thus irritating and inflaming tissues. These crystals are deposited throughout the body causing inflammation, irritation and stimulation or agitation. Uric acid, for example, is a by-product of meat metabolism and/or fungal growth in the body. Uric acid buildup causes gout and other inflammatory conditions throughout the body.

There are many other acids formed during food digestion. These include sulfuric acid, phosphoric acid, butyric acid, lactic acid, acetic acid and pyroracemic acid, to name a few. These acids, if not converted to salts by electrolytes, will cause damage to tissue. The more acidic your body becomes, the more damage you create within it.

Men and women today eat mainly acid-forming foods, e.g., meats, grains, pasteurized dairy products, eggs and cooked tomatoes. As acidity is hot, these acids and compounds cause inflammation in tissues. Inflammation causes cellular weakness and an inability of the cell to transport nutrients across its membrane wall via cellular respiration, eventually leading to cellular death.

As previously stated, the only acid chamber in homo sapiens is the stomach, where protein digestion begins. Note: Immediately after the stomach contents move into the small intestines, bile and sodium bicarbonate are secreted to alkalize this mixture now called chyme. The rest of digestion is alkaline.

The accumulation of acids and toxic foreign proteins in tissues causes an immune response called inflammation. This inflammation is then diagnosed as an "itis" of some sort, e.g., gastritis, colitis, cystitis, nephritis, bursitis, and arthritis. These are not diseases, but inflammatory responses to acidosis. This is why the treatment of these conditions with more acid-forming drugs or steroids is ludicrous and will eventually lead to further degeneration of your tissues. It makes much better sense to alkalize and detoxify, that is, remove the acids and foreign proteins that are causing the problem in the first place. CNN recently reported that researchers at various universities have proven that the genetic pattern of cells (DNA and chromosomes) can and is being altered by acidosis, which weakens a cell, causing many changes in its DNA and chromosome structure.

ABOUT CONSCIOUSNESS AND DISEASE

Cells respond to states of consciousness just as we do. In other words, if someone walks up to you angry, you can get angry; if you hang around sick people, you can get sick. Everything *is* energy and everything *gives off* energy.

There are unlimited levels to energy. From a spiritual perspective, anger is a lower level of energy whereas love is a high level of energy. In spiritual circles we call energy "consciousness" or "awareness." God, or "total awareness," has been compared to a large mirror, while creation is thought of as that mirror divided up into unlimited pieces, or various states of awareness or consciousness. As I understand it, all life forms are merely pieces of this mirror expressing themselves in various individual states of consciousness or awareness. With birth into creation, we start out basically unconscious or unaware, and become gradually more conscious in response to life around us. As a computer that is being set up with more software, or programmed with more data, is therefore able to perform more functions, so each individual piece of the "mirror of creation" will expand its ability to express itself the more it awakens to its true nature. Since we humans are pieces of this mirror, we act in the same way—that is, the more we experience, the more we awaken or grow in consciousness.

While it is very difficult to express these things in words, if you look within yourself and at nature you can appreciate that all things are reflections of the same essence; that is, all are a reflection in some way of God and all of God's creation. Your cells are no different. They possess consciousness. They are subject to the laws of cause and effect, just like you are. What you put in, you get out. Your cells' DNA and chromosomes carry memory patterns far beyond those of simple genetics. They also include the traces of the day-to-day "experiences" that the cell goes through, much as your memory records your daily experience.

Viruses are proteins that affect the consciousness or life of a cell. They weaken a cell, setting it up for an immune response. As stated earlier, nature never procreates the weak, it eliminates it. Many proteins (like viruses, etc.) are the stimulus for this mechanism that allows the body to eliminate these weaknesses, so that it can replace the weak cells with the strong.

The problem for the cells is that the typical fuels and building materials—the foods that most people are consuming—can no longer support a refined level of consciousness or awareness. Most of the food we eat today is very low in energy and vibration or consciousness, which lowers the cell's energy and thus the body's overall energy, thereby creating disease and death. This low-energy lifestyle also lowers human awareness in general, which is why we have so much hate, gossip and deceit instead of love.

The role of parasites in disease processes should also be mentioned here. (See *Parasites Good or Bad?* Module 5.2.) Even though parasites are secondary causes of disease, they are contributing factors to the consciousness and vibration of a cell, thus affecting its DNA memory. Human stupidity in introducing live or even dead pathogens (parasites) into toxic bodies via the "vaccination" has led to a landslide of genetically weakened and mutated cells. (For a more complete discussion of vaccinations see Chapter Four, *Toxic Habits*.) Many "diseases" are created or inspired by vaccinations, including ADD, AIDS, and most importantly, cancer. We have allowed science to hurt, maim, or kill us, and then we have become conditioned by false propaganda that indicates that we are to blame, not science. Scientists play Russian roulette with human lives, all in the name of "progress" and under the guise of protecting us. We must move past these dark medical and chemical times where so much destruction of the species has taken place.

THE SIMPLE SOLUTION

It is time to awaken and get back to simplicity and the ways of God and nature. Nature has supplied us with all the herbs and the foods we need to clean, rebuild, and revitalize our physical and spiritual bodies.

Health is very simple: eat within the scope of your species; eat your foods fresh, ripe, raw and unprocessed, as all other animals do; rest and get plenty of sunshine; clean your body out of all the toxins, including chemicals, heavy metals, antibiotics, excessive hormones, excessive proteins, unnecessary mucus, destructive parasites, pesticides and the like. Basically, alkalize yourself with your diet. We humans have the highest neurological development of any species, and fruits are the highest electrically-alkaline foods on the planet. I have seen fruits regenerate the nervous system where vegetables did not.

Use herbs to rebuild tissue and promote tissue function. Use freshly-made fruit and vegetable juices as "power" supplements to your diet. Add a super-food complex or blend to your diet to enhance deficient foods. A super-food, as its name implies, is one that contains some of nature's most nutritious and energetic foods, like royal jelly, wheat grass powder, and alfalfa powder, in a capsule, pill or powdered form.

If you do all of the above, you will see your body kick into action. It will clean itself out and rebuild itself, regardless of the disease you may have. As a health professional, I've never seen a case of any disease that did not respond to this program. Every person I have worked with has greatly improved, and in most cases their diseased conditions have been entirely eliminated.

Always try. I don't care how advanced or immobile you are. I've seen complete spinal cord severations repair themselves after years in which the patient was almost completely immobilized. I have seen the body realign and reshape itself from various deformities. If you follow nature's laws, you will find that the power of God and nature is unlimited.

Remember, there is a reason for everything, including health and disease. It's all about the law of cause and effect: your decisions and actions set the cause in motion and you eventually experience the effect. Don't get lost in an endless scientific barrage of "treatment" concepts. Always try to understand what is causing something. Ask yourself what the side effects might be of whatever you do, eat, drink, breathe, feel or think. All these things *become* your experience—physically, emotionally, mentally and spiritually.

"Disease" is only a word used by the medical community and associated with a set of symptoms that the body displays. When an allopathic doctor refers to a disease, he/she does not understand the true nature of the body and its response to genetics, toxicity and acidosis. They do not understand the chemistry and physics of nature and the need for human beings to live and consume in harmony with it.

Forget diseases. Clean and strengthen your body (cells) and there is nothing you can't overcome (cure). Life begets life, death begets death. The strong survive and the weak are consumed. This is especially true at the cellular level. Make your body (and the cells that run it) strong again and you will experience vitality and robust health and live a disease-free life.

Summary

Almost all tissue failure begins with acidosis and toxicity. As tissue fails, or becomes congested, disease symptoms begin, both local and reflexed. By "reflexed" we mean that many times we feel pain in one area, but the problem or weakness originates in another part of the body. An example of this is when the gallbladder is inflamed you may experience right knee pain or weakness. You would never correlate the two because of the distance between them.

We commonly and mistakenly call the symptoms of acidosis and toxicity "disease," and attempt to treat these symptoms with suppressive drugs. This is not only foolish, but also deadly, as this eventually causes tissue failure leading to tissue death. Never treat the symptoms; cure the cause. If you treat the symptom, you never cure what created the symptom in the first place. This means that in the future the root cause of the symptom of your disease will take its toll on you, and could end your life.

Treatment never *cures*. Don't treat—regenerate. It's our only hope of survival. Simply remove the inflammation throughout your body by detoxification. Detoxify yourself of all the chemicals, unnecessary mucus, toxic heavy metals, unnecessary parasites and acids. A clean and alkaline body is a healthy and strong body.

Nothing is mysterious when you understand the truth behind it. Disease is simply a natural process, an effect that the body experiences when its cells begin to fail from toxicity in the form of excess mucus, vaccinations, metals, chemicals and other pollutants, and from acidosis, that is, inflammation. Cleaning out the body and strengthening the cells are the only ways to bring about genuine healing.

☀ Parasites, Good or Bad?

For the last 200 years or so scientists have spent a lot of time and money in researching the ominous parasite. We have poured antibiotics into our bodies until we have developed severe allergies, excessive fungal growth, lymphatic suppression, tissue damage and new diseases, including strains like MRSA—methicillin-resistant staphylococcus aureus. And in many cases, the use of antibiotics has resulted in death. The pharmaceutical cartel, the U.S. Government, and various scientific communities have experimented with the oftentimes deadly "vaccination," as we discussed in Chapter 4. Vaccinations have proven to be one of the greatest killers ever invented. From this methodology we have started a genetic landslide that we cannot stop, which is why we are seeing chronic and degenerative conditions in infants and young children. We have created so many mutations in bacteria from the use of antibiotics; we have created so many mutant and deadly viruses that these pathogens are rapidly destroying the human species.

People oftentimes become so intellectually obsessed that they cannot see the forest for the trees. Let's take a simple look at why nature (God) created parasites. Webster's Dictionary defines a parasite as "an organism that feeds off of another." For our purposes I would change this definition to "an organism that feeds upon the toxicity and weaknesses of others."

To understand the parasite's function better, let's look at what happens if we shoot and kill a deer. (This is an example only.) Flies are the first creatures attracted. Their work is to lay eggs, which become maggots. What is the job of a maggot? The same as other proteus (protein-splitting) types of parasites—to eliminate the dead carcass of the deer. This is the way nature cleans itself. Otherwise, the bodies of all dead animals would still be here. Nature is constantly changing from one form into another.

Did you know that maggots are currently used in hospitals to debride (clean) wounds? In World War I, when medical attention was slow and so many of the wounded men developed maggots in their wounds, the maggots kept their wounds partially clean so that many were able to survive.

Certainly God did not design parasites to attack healthy tissue or we would all be dead.

Parasites are everywhere, and you can see their vital role on this planet in helping nature eliminate the weak so that the strong survive. This keeps the cycle of nature going. The atoms in this world are never destroyed, just changed by different actions, including oxidation, ionization, and parasitic action, just to name a few.

An example of how we can accumulate parasites within our physical body was seen in a case involving a nineteen-year-old female. She came to me undernourished and thin from malabsorption of her foods. She was tired all the time, and was never feeling as good as she should. She had muscle aches and digestive problems. As I started her on my detoxification program she began to eliminate a lot of mucus, which is standard. She also began to notice "weird-looking creatures" in her stools. She drew me pictures of what she saw; pictures which even astounded *me*. Two were tapeworms—one a beef tapeworm, and the other a common tapeworm. She saw roundworms and pinworms, flukes ("jellyfish-looking" creatures), and other unidentifiable parasites. She panicked and went to the Emergency Room of her local hospital where the ER doctor told her that "there is no such thing as parasites in Americans." The young lady insisted that the ER doctor have her stools tested, which he did after much apprehension and discussion. The report came back from the lab that this sample was full of parasites.

We are a host to many parasites, mostly microbial. However, I would guess that about 40 to 75 percent of homo sapiens have the larger ones that you can see if you look for them. There are many different types of parasites including yeasts, fungi, warts, viruses, bacteria, worms of all types, and flukes. Most people have many of each of these types in their bodies. All people have yeast (Candida) or fungus in them. Over thirty different strains of fungus can be found in most people. The yeast-type fungus is mostly located in the mouth to aid sugar and starch digestion. Those with overgrowths of a fungus type called Candida albicans which grows through-

out the body suffer from fatigue, listlessness, itching, skin irritation and infections, just to name a few of the symptoms.

Candida creates a craving for sugars and starches, and patients are typically and incorrectly told not to eat fruits because of the sugars. As we've learned in a previous chapter, fructose and glucose are two of the principal energies or fuels for a cell. These sugars are simple sugars and are essential to the body as its main source of fuel. Fruits are vital in helping the body eliminate Candida because they are high in antioxidant and astringent properties. These properties clean the lymphatic congestion out of the tissues, which is essential since congestion is the "home" of these little critters. Complex sugars, however, are another story. They are super fuels (or food) for Candida, but are unusable as fuel by the body until they are broken down into simple sugars. Using an herbal parasite-and-lymphatic-cleansing program to make a more effective "kill," will immensely help anyone suffering from disorders linked with Candida.

VIRUSES

I have included the term "virus" under parasites. However, we still do not know for sure what a virus is. Some scientists think that they are components of decomposed cells. Others think they are microorganisms. We do know that they are some sort of protein structure, and that they have no known "life" to them, like bacteria or protozoa. I believe that **viruses are a protein catalyst for immune response**. When a cell becomes weakened, it can release its own "virus" (protein) causing an immune response against itself for elimination. The weak are always consumed in this world. This is just the order of things so that life will continue to perpetuate itself. The strong always survive, one way or another, and this is true cellularly as well. It is vital that the body eliminates its weaknesses to increase its strength.

Many types of viruses, including the herpes virus (which appears to be a proteus-type), are "protein splitters." They appear in overacid conditions, especially when high protein is consumed. In cases of herpes simplex or genital herpes, the elimination of protein in the diet will make these viruses inactive or dormant.

Science has been so ignorant of the true role of parasites that it has created the devastating concept of vaccinations, introducing deadly and DNA-altering viruses, in the name of immunity. Because most viruses are cultivated in animal tissue and blood, contamination of these cultures is common, and has created such monsters as the Sim-40 virus, which has been implicated in causing many cancers. The HIV and E-boli viruses are other examples of man-made viruses which were knowingly released into unsuspecting human guinea pigs, creating a horrible nightmare of pain and suffering, which has included the deaths of thousands of people.

The U.S. Government has inoculated thousands of military personnel in the name of "immunity." The Gulf War Syndrome is just one devastating example of the horrible side effects of this ignorant type of thinking. The people who initiated these programs should be held accountable for more suffering and death than even Hitler perpetrated. Hundreds, if not thousands, of people, have contracted polio from the polio vaccine itself. Thousands of others have developed cancer and other disease conditions because of the introduction of live bacteria and viruses into already toxic human beings. Such devastation created within the human organism will take us many generations to overcome . . . if we wake up fairly soon.

BACTERIA

We are all familiar with the word "bacteria" meaning those single-celled organisms without a true nucleus. There are several different types of bacteria. First, the rounded or spherical-type,

---

A Spiritual Perspective

We do not need to live in fear of nature's laws and the creatures that uphold them. We must simply learn how nature works. Parasites do not create or cause disease, they are only feeders. We often forget who created everything, and that this Creator knew just what to do and how to make things work. A look into the wonders of the physical body should make a believer out of anyone.

Just stop a minute and consider: "What gives you your awareness?" Not the thought processes of learning, comparing or deciding, but the awareness behind the thought—the *you* that is *you* whether you're in your car, at the beach, or at home; the you that you can't escape from no matter where you go.

You are always present, for time is nothing more than a succession of Nows. You, as awareness, always live in the present moment. The mind, however, lives in time—past and future.

Take time to observe yourself. Learn to relax. Control your thinking processes. Stop desiring so much, and learn to live each moment fully. Enjoy and experience each moment for what that moment brings; then enjoy the next moment for what that moment brings. Living in the past or future is living a "dead" life. Life truly exists only in the eternal now.

---

which occur as single cell units called *micrococci*, or as pairs called *diplococci*. In this category we have the cluster-type called *staphylococci*, which is well known, as is the chain-type called *streptococci*. Cubical groupings of this chain-type are called *sarcinae*.

The second type of bacteria is the rod-shaped or *bacilli*. If they are oval-shaped they are called *coccobacilli*. Those forming chains are called *streptobacilli*.

Third, we have the spiral-type, of which the rigid ones are called *spirilla*. The more flexible spirals are the well-known *spirochetes*. The curved spirals are called *vibrios*.

Bacteria are microscopic, and they live and thrive in lymph congestion. Lymph tissue, remember, is your septic system, which moves cellular wastes and by-products of metabolism out of the body. These wastes and by-products can appear as mucus on the skin, in the gastrointestinal tract and throughout the body where toxins are present. Bacteria love complex sugars, milk and starch by-products. This is why, when you "catch" a cold, the body starts purging the lymphatic system, causing a discharge of this mucus and the parasites feeding within it. One notices this purging especially from the sinuses, lungs, kidneys and bowels. However, the body also starts purging itself throughout the entire system, causing that "achy-all-over" feeling.

There are bacteria (also called flora) all along the GI tract helping the body to break down foods. Many vitamins are created by the actions of bacteria. A good example of this would be the various bacteria that live in your GI tract that create B-vitamins from the breakdown of the foods you eat.

PROTEUS

Another type of parasite is the proteus or proteolytic type, which are the protein-splitters. Like the herpes virus, this parasite attaches to or enters weakened cells. These are acid type parasites, which thrive in the body when it becomes overly acidic. Their job is to decompose proteins or weakened cells. When a healthy cell is living in an alkaline environment, you will never see this type of parasite. However, a diet high in protein is a calling card to the most destructive parasites. High protein diets over-acidify the body causing damage to the liver, pancreas, and especially the kidneys. This also creates body odor because of the excess of undigested proteins that are stored interstitially in tissues.

WORMS

We have been discussing the microorganisms. Now let's look at the larger "boys"—worms of all types, as well as flukes—which can become a major problem within us. There are many types of worms: pin, hook, round, spiral types, and many different varieties of tapeworms. They can grow and travel throughout the body, but especially love the liver, heart and GI tract, including the stomach. I have seen worms even in the lungs. Tapeworms, of course, can get very large and long. I have personally seen them twenty-six feet long.

In one case, a middle-aged female had her gallbladder removed when she was in her early twenties. At the time she had a lot of pain both in the gallbladder area and in her back. But when the removed gallbladder was examined there was nothing wrong with it. Over the next twenty years the pain grew intensely. She could not eat excessive fats or dairy products or she would vomit. Her stomach area became extremely sensitive to touch. She also began eating her meats very rare, almost raw. When I started her on my detox program she found three large tape worms in her stools. Now the pain and sensitivity in her abdomen are completely gone.

Another case that I worked with was a young butcher from Portugal. He had severe neurological weakness, very similar to multiple sclerosis. Based on his rate of nerve decline he was given two months to live. As soon as he started the detox program he started vomiting handfuls of worms. Within three months of detoxifying he was driving around Lisbon again.

Years ago, adults use to "de-worm"—that is, remove the parasites from their children every spring. Day-to-day activities and the ingestion of foods bring many parasites into the body. These parasites then become feeders on our own toxins and weak cells. Many times worms grow in the intestinal tract. After several years, they then become the problem causing a multitude of symptoms. We have forgotten some of the basic facts of life, especially when it comes to parasites and their role in nature.

Many people have flukes (which look like little jellyfish) and mainly grow and accumulate in the liver and pancreas. When they grow in the pancreas this can cause digestive problems and diabetes.

Summary

Keep the body pure and clear of mucus and impurities, and strengthen your cells. Remember that parasites are secondary to the cause. They only thrive in a base of toxicity and mucus, as this is their food source. Healthy cells are not food for parasites. Only the strong survive in this world. Become healthy and vital and your life will change in every way imaginable.

Watch your stools as you clean and detoxify yourself. Some of the larger parasites you may actually be able to see in your stools during your detoxification program. For those who are curious, a textbook on parasitology will give you the pictures or illustrations you need. Smaller parasites can only be detected via a stool sample done by your healthcare practitioner or through a laboratory.

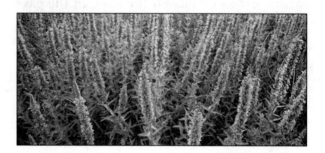

Most Common Parasites

Parasites range in order of size, from smallest to largest: Viruses, Bacteria, Yeasts, Protozoa and Worms (Nematodes).

NAME	WHERE FOUND
BACTERIA	
Streptococci (several)	Lungs, Lymph, Sinus, Small Intestines
Salmonella	GI Tract, Liver, Brain
Shigella Dysenteriae	Dysentery
Staphylococcus Aureus	Lungs, Lymph, Joints, Eyes
Clostridium Difficile	Colon
E-Coli	Kidneys, Bladder, GI Tract
Pseudomonas	Lungs, Lymph, Urinary Tract
Campylobacter JeJuni	GI Tract—Main Cause of Diarrhea
FUNGI (MUSHROOMS, YEAST, MOLDS)	
Candida Albicans (Moniliasis) (Yeasts)	Lymph System, GI Tract
Yeasts (Other)	Throughout the body
Molds	Skin
Fungus (general)	Lymph System, under Fingernails and Toenails, in GI Tract, etc.
PROTOZOA	
Trypanosoma Cruzi	Heart, Muscle
Giardia Lemblia Trophozolte	Small Intestines, Gallbladder
Neospora Caninum	Brain, Spinal Cord, All Tissues
Sarcocystis (Amoebas)	Muscle, CNS, Heart, Lungs, Glands, Liver, GI Tract
Isospora	Intestines
Pneumocystis	Lungs
Cryptosporidium	Intestines
Entamoeba's SPP	GI Tract
Plasmodium SPP. (Malaria)	Liver, Red blood cells
Toxoplasma Gondii	Brain, Spinal Cord, All Tissues
WORMS	
Tape worms, beef, pork, etc.	GI Tract, Liver, Brain, Bladder
Hook Worms	Skin, Blood, Lungs, Intestines
Round Worms (Trichinosos, etc.)	Intestines, Eyes, Brain, Ears
Pin Worms (oxyuris SPP)	Large Intestines, (mature in small intestine)
Flukes (Many Types) Liver, Lung, Pancreatic	Pancreas, Liver, Lungs
Whip Worms (Triehuris Trichiura)	Intestines
Frichina Worm (tichinella Spiralis)	Muscles, Intestines
Blood Flukes (Schistosomes)	Blood, Bladder, Small Intestines, Veins

☀ Why Do We "Plaque" Cholesterol and Other Lipids?

Your liver produces an abundant amount of cholesterol, which is an important lipid used by the body for many reasons. By definition, a lipid is any one of a group of fats or fat-like substances characterized by their insolubility in water and solubility in fat solvents such as alcohol, ether, and chloroform. The term is descriptive rather than a chemical name such as "protein" or "carbohydrate." Lipids include true fats (esters of fatty acids and glycerol); lipoids (phospholipids, cerebrosides, waves); and sterols (cholesterol, ergosterol). A large portion of a cell's membrane wall is cholesterol. The adrenal glands use cholesterol to make cortical-type steroids, which are, in part, the body's anti-inflammatories.

So why does cholesterol build up in the lining of the vascular system and throughout other tissues in the body? This build-up is known as plaque. To answer this question you must first understand inflammation, or acidosis, and the role of steroids in the body.

Inflammation simply means that the body is on fire. This inflammation or fire can exist at low levels or become a raging blaze. Cancer is an excellent example of a raging fire. As we discussed earlier, inflammation is caused by acidosis from what you eat, drink, breathe, what you put on your skin, what you think and what you feel.

Inflammation is diagnosed as an "itis." *Where* the inflammation is discovered will determine what type of "itis" it is. An example of this is arth*ritis*, which is inflammation of the joints. "Itis's" are treated by the allopathic medical community with a steroid shot—like cortisone, prednisone, or the like. Since we know that the adrenal glands use cholesterol to make cortical-steroids, the question to ask is: "Why don't my adrenal glands produce adequate amounts of their own cortisone?" The answer is that if the adrenal glands are weak or underactive in the tissue that produces these steroids, the body cannot adequately defend itself against this strong inflammation.

Lacking adequate steroids, the body then has no choice but to turn to water and electrolytes in an attempt to manage this "fire." But water and electrolytes also cause edema (swelling) in the area of the inflammation. The liver will also begin to increase its production of cholesterol, thus giving the body additional anti-inflammatory compounds. Cholesterol is one of the main ingredients of steroids.

All of these anti-inflammatory compounds are essential to the protection of a cell against the highly damaging effects of acids. The creation of plaque occurs naturally, chemically, in an acid environment. Alkalization is essential for the removal of this "protective shield" of plaque which itself can become a problem.

Most people consume 90-100 percent acid-forming foods. Eating this way keeps the body's pH factors acidic. The acid by-products after metabolism also add to this already over-acid condition,

---

Check for Acidity

Buy some litmus papers, also known as pH-testing papers, and keep checking your saliva and urine, approximately one to two hours after you eat. This will help you to see what is causing your over-acid condition.

---

causing inflammation (fire), which is a killer of cells. As stated earlier, the body, in its infinite wisdom, tries to compensate for this by several methods, including: steroid production, cholesterol (lipid) plaquing, calcium extraction, and electrolyte or fluid retention. This attempt by the body to alkalize itself is only self-preservation.

Alkalization is key to tissue regeneration, to the breaking up of stones, and to the removal of plaqued lipids. Lipid plaquing from inflammation/acidosis causes poor circulation leading to tissue death, heart attack and strokes. Acidosis also creates a coagulating of fats and nutrients, which also leads to strokes, heart attacks, memory loss, graying of hair, pain in tissues, stone formation and other conditions.

REMOVING THE FIREWALL, SAFELY — It is not difficult to remove this plaque and to break up lipid-type stones if you consume an 80-100 percent raw-food diet. Raw foods remove inflammation through alkalization and increased steroid production, thus dissolving stones and plaqued lipids. This will unclog the body, increasing blood flow to tissues, which in turn increases nutrition and energy to cells. This will restore or regenerate these weakened areas. Such restoration does not take very long if you are persistent with the diet.

MODULE 5.4

☀ Adrenal Gland Weakness = Female and Male Disorders

The adrenal glands greatly affect the quality of life that each individual wants to and *can* experience. This is why you should always seek to strengthen all the cells/glands in your body. Your body is your transportation while you are on this journey in the physical world. Disease and weakness locks you away from life, while health and vitality make you more a part of it. Enjoy your adventure into health. It's more rewarding than you can imagine.

Let's look at some other problems that can arise when the adrenal glands are weak and the diet is predominately acid forming.

FEMALE IMBALANCES

Women are especially hard hit in the area of adrenal weakness. One of the first indicators of this is low blood pressure. With underactive adrenal glands, blood pressure starts out below 118 systolic and eventually can swing the other way, creating high blood pressure, or it can keep getting lower.

Another indicator of adrenal weakness for women will be trouble with the menstruation cycle. In this situation a female is likely to begin her menstruation early in life, at anywhere from three- to twelve-years-old. (Yes, I have known of three-year-old females menstruating.) She often has excessive bleeding and her monthly cycle is not on time. The opposite can also happen: women having sparse and infrequent periods. However, this is not as common.

Adrenal weakness in women can also manifest as fertility problems, lack of sex drive, frigidity, and vaginal dryness. If the adrenal weakness continues, she can develop ovarian cysts, uterine fibroids, fibrocystic issues, a-typical cells, fibromyalgia, and breast, ovarian, cervical and/or uterine cancers.

The main issue, of course, is estrogen. Without proper progesterone and other anti-inflammatory steroids a woman becomes estrogen dominant. The estrogen levels in her body, especially ovarian estrogen, dominate without the counterbalance of progesterone. Most estrogens are acidic, especially ovarian estrogen, which breaks down the inner lining of the uterus each month. Of course progesterone stops this, and heals the inflamed tissue while repairing the damaged cells.

Because of estrogen's ability to break down the uterine lining, birth control pills are made from estrogen. Estrogen stimulates a woman's natural menstruation cycle. With all this in mind, ask yourself: "Why does a medical doctor give a woman *more* estrogen after removing the uterus?" Also, with the above information, would estrogen build up bones or tear bones down? Yes, tear down. This is why estrogen replacement programs usually make the problems much worse.

MALE IMBALANCES

Now let's take a look at the male issues, which spring from the same adrenal weaknesses. These imbalances would be prostatitis and prostate cancer. The same reasons apply: acid-type hormones like testosterone and androsterone dominate without proper steroids (like progesterone) counterbalancing the inflammation caused by these acidic compounds or hormones.

A lot of good romance is lost because of glandular weaknesses. This would include many other conditions that plague men, including erection problems, impotency, and premature ejaculation. Health brings it all back.

PROBLEMS COMMON TO BOTH

In both males and females with lower steroid production, from underactive adrenal glands, we also find lower back and pelvic weakness and deterioration. This also leads into sciatica and other lower extremity nerve pains, especially when the thyroid is involved. Since the thyroid/parathyroid affects calcium utilization, we begin to see bone loss, fingernail problems, and connective tissue issues, including varicose veins, hemorrhoids, macular degeneration, hernias, heart arrhythmias and aneurysms.

The adrenal glands also create neurotransmitters. When the adrenal glands are weak, the nervous system can also be involved, causing anxieties, shyness, feelings of inadequacy, panic attacks, asthma, multiple sclerosis, Parkinson's, or any other neurotransmitter weaknesses, including blood pressure irregularities. It is shocking to see the huge number of reflex conditions that result from just one pair of glands that become hypoactive. Add to this the fact that most people have thyroid and/or pituitary weaknesses as well, and the list of diseases that can result gets longer and longer. There is nothing mysterious about diseases when you begin to look at the overall picture.

You are the only one in control. Stop, explore yourself, and rid yourself of the thoughts, images, and feelings that bind you. Become free and healthy and your body will readjust itself to match. Become love.

☀ Cancer

Diseases are a natural process or effect born out of a cause. Learn to eliminate the cause and the effect will also be eliminated. In my opinion, after thirty years of experience in clinical work and observation with cancer clients, there are basically two types of cancer. First, the congestive or tumor types, which deal with the lymphatic system—the body's sewer. Second, the degenerative type, in which the tissue or cell itself is dying and the immune system is trying to eliminate these cells. This later type may *appear to be* an "auto immune" runaway, in which the immune cells start attacking themselves and the normal cells of the body. But, as I will discuss later, there is little understanding of the real purpose of this process within the allopathic medical community today.

Both of these types of cancer and their causes are intertwined. We can see this by looking at the congestive or tumor-type cancers. Congestion in the body, as stated earlier, can be caused by dairy products, refined sugars, chemicals, metals, foreign proteins, etc., all creating inflammation. In the presence of inflammation, mucus is discharged from the mucosa as an anti-inflammatory response. This mucus can accumulate if the lymphatic system is stagnant, or if too much mucus is produced and the system becomes overwhelmed. As this congestion develops, it blocks proper cellular respiration. This, in turn, causes cellular weaknesses and cellular death. This also causes further inflammation leading to additional cellular death. The cycle of congestion and inflammation now starts a cycle of cellular decay, opening the doorway to cancer.

As previously stated, this degeneration (or the killing of cells) results from prolonged inflammation (acidosis). This acidosis is caused mainly from what you eat, drink, breathe, and what you put on your skin. However, cancer can develop from acidosis by the dominance of acid-type (catabolic) hormones (steroids) such as estrogen or testosterone. These types of hormones or steroids, when unchecked by anabolic (anti-inflammatory) steroids, which are produced in both the adrenal glands and the gonads, cause additional inflammation. All this leads to tumor or fibrocystic formation and the destruction of cells. Estrogen is one of the primary examples of a very acidic/inflammatory-type hormone. When allowed to go unchecked by steroids, estrogen eventually causes degeneration of tissue through inflammation. Breast, uterine and ovarian cancers are the results of this.

Parasites and mutations are almost always involved with both types of cancer. Parasites do not feed on healthy tissue, only tissue that has become weakened or is dying. They definitely live and breed in "toxic waste dumps" in lymph and lymph nodes. I think cells also release their own virus (protein) when they become too weak to support life. These viruses and parasites cause cells to mutate in response to the invaders. Your immune system is designed to eliminate these types of cells. This is why we see an abnormal immune response in the presence of cancer or any degenerative condition. As a matter of fact, your immune system is designed to respond to *any* type of invasion—be it parasites, foreign proteins, which include your own weakened cells, and any other pathogen that doesn't belong or can cause harm to the body. This would include acids from metabolism or digestion that can damage cells and tissues.

Cancer doesn't just suddenly appear. It used to take years to form tumors or to degenerate tissue. However, with the pounds of chemicals and hormones that most people consume each week, tumors can grow within months or even days. This is also true of hormonally-fed cancers. **Hormone imbalances are mainly due to chronic endocrine gland weakness, especially weak adrenal glands.**

The word and condition known as "cancer" was virtually unknown until humans started playing with vaccines and toxic chemicals. Contaminated vaccines have been blamed for many conditions that people now suffer from. One such vaccine is the polio vaccine. As we've mentioned previously, in the early to mid-1950s it was determined that polio vaccines manufactured in monkey kidney tissue became contaminated with a monkey virus called simian virus number 40. This virus is known as Sim-40 or

---

Vaccination Facts

- The FDA estimates that most doctors report only 1 to 10% of the injuries, and/or deaths from vaccinations to VAERS (Vaccine Adverse Event Reporting System). This was set up as a central reporting agency to oversee the side effects of vaccinations.

- The health of hundreds of thousands of children and infants are compromised each year from the 20 to 30 vaccinations that are "required." Some children suffer serious injuries, and some die as a result.

- Vaccinations have been linked to many cancers, and the sharp rise in diabetes (especially juvenile), multiple sclerosis, Bell's Palsy, vascular disorders, arthritis, and other conditions.

- The American Academy of Pediatrics knows of the toxic and horrific side effects of vaccinations and *still* recommends their prolific use.

SV40 and has been proven to cause cancer in animals. It has also been linked to mesothelioma (lung cancer) and multiple myeloma (bone marrow cancer). This is just one vaccine. How many different vaccines have *you* had? And what are their side effects?

As you weaken the cells in your body via foods, chemicals, vaccinations and the like, your cells take on this weakness as their expression. This happens the same way that you, in every moment, express yourself according to the experiences you have and the memory of these experiences. Your cells are no different. With each minute, hour, day . . . the strength or weakness of each of your cells becomes a part of its memory patterns in DNA and chromosomes.

At the moment of conception the condition of each cell and its memories that are passed down to you become a part of your body, and thus determine how your body functions and the conditions that it can experience. Since we keep making our genetic condition weaker by continuing to wear down our bodies through diet and lifestyle we are seeing a landslide of chronic cellular and tissue weaknesses. We then pass them on to our children, who then pass them on to their children. And with each successive generation, the cellular patterns and functions become more chronic, causing disease symptoms to appear now in infants. Through this process of genetic transmission we have created frightening consequences.

Many allopathic doctors claim that cancer is an autoimmune disease. However, I find this conclusion to be misleading, and commonly used as a catch-all for the unawareness of the actual cause of disease processes. Your body's immune cells are especially designed to attack and consume weak, mutant, dying or parasitically involved cells. This is especially true of the natural killer cells (NK), including the T-cells (thymus) and B-cells (bone marrow). These natural killer cells are much larger than the smaller macrophages, neutrophils, basophils, etc., that do basic body cleanup. We have an army inside of us that is always active. This process is extremely necessary for internal survival. The weaker a cell or tissue becomes from inflammation, toxicity, or even genetics (and the parasitic response to these), the more immune response will be needed. The increased elevation of white blood cells is in response to all of the above, and especially to foreign pathogens.

DETOX FOR CANCER PREVENTION AND CURE

It is vital to clean, strengthen, and thus regenerate your cells and tissues. Detoxification is the process one must go through to accomplish this. Detoxification naturally begins as you alkalize yourself through a raw food diet. This process strengthens cells by removing the obstructions and acids that cause inflammation and block nutrition to your cells. Detoxification allows cells to gain nutritional energy and to properly eliminate their wastes via cellular respiration. This then begins the rebuilding process within the body.

It has been proven that diets high in animal protein are cancer causing. Animal protein is acidic (inflammatory), putrefactive and congestive. The congestive aspect is caused by the mucus, formed from its abrasive and putrefactive aspects. The toxic chemicals, vaccinations, and hormones eaten by or injected into these animals also create tissue toxicity within the body. This causes your immune system to respond, causing inflammation. Meat also causes a biochemical imbalance within your body. The high levels of iron and phosphorous push out your calcium, magnesium, and other vital electrolytes, which then weaken and dehydrate your body.

As you can see and imagine, one cannot treat cancer, which is created by the above, with chemotherapy that acts on the body like Draino® acts on your plumbing system, or burn it away with radiation (fire), either. Both of these choices cause more cancer, or cause cancer to move (metastasize) to areas where these therapies have destroyed or weakened the cells and tissues. Radiation destroys the oxygen-carrying and utilization factors of a cell. However, glucose can still enter through the cell membrane wall. This eventually causes fermentation within a cell, and that cell will die from auto-intoxication. This creates a delayed response.

At first these treatments seem to reduce the tumor or stop the cancer. But then watch out – cancer can explode throughout the entire body. Of course this will invoke additional immune responses, creating the appearance of "autoimmune problems."

The bottom line in all cancers is overacidity/inflammation and the build-up of cellular toxicity. Both lead to enervation or the loss of cellular energy and function, thus the loss of systemic energy and health. This results in the over-working of the immune system. Most of the tissues responsible for the production of immune cells in cancer patients, especially the thymus gland (where T-cells are produced) and the bone marrow (where B-cell production takes place), become hypoactive.

A HEALTHY LYMPH SYSTEM IS ESSENTIAL

With all of this in mind, it becomes vital that you understand your lymphatic system. I have discussed this "sewer system of the body" in some detail in Chapter 2. **Your lymphatic system is where ninety percent of all disease processes begin**. When this highway system is congested and cannot eliminate well, it backs up the whole "sewer system" of the body, causing a lack of or improper elimination of cellular/metabolic wastes (acids), as well as toxic chemicals and metals that have been ingested. These toxins must be eliminated or cellular death will result.

Your lymph system is a vital part of your immune system. To enhance your immune system, clean out your lymphatic system first. Remember, your kidneys, colon and skin are the exit doors of your lymphatic system. If your septic system is obstructed or full, you don't remove it, you clean it out. Most people have lost proper kidney filtration. Their intestinal bowel walls are impacted, and many don't sweat well. This means that their doors are partly closed in allowing their sewage or wastes to be properly eliminated. This then backs up the lymphatic system and enlarges the lymph nodes. When this goes on for many years, you will see all types of lymphomas, non-estrogen types of breast cancer, throat cancer (especially when the tonsils have been removed), and neck, colon, kidney, liver and many other cancers.

This is why **detoxification is essential in the elimination of cancer.** By alkalizing and cleansing your tissues and fluids, your cells will begin to strengthen, and the sludge of toxins that snuff the life out of your cells will be gone. This then brings a tremendous joy, energy, and vitality.

Out of 100 clients who came to our clinic and followed a detoxification regimen, 80 were able to eliminate their cancers. **I know of no better way to heal, clean and rebuild the body than through detoxification and regeneration of its cells, through diet and herbs.** If you take responsibility for your health and open your heart, it is unbelievable what you can accomplish. Don't allow anybody to tell you that there is nothing that can be done. We've had individuals who were given only one day or even hours to live who pulled themselves back. In the last thirty years I have seen some amazing results in regeneration. Never compromise your immune system or let anyone destroy it. And most importantly, do not have your lymph nodes removed. The consequences can be devastating. Don't treat, regenerate!

MODULE 5.6

☀ Neurological Disorders and Injuries

It saddens me to see so many quadriplegics and paraplegics in this world with supposedly no help. Nothing could be further from the truth. My first tough case was a thirty-four-year-old female who had a spinal injury at the C3-C4 level. At the time of the accident she had a complete spinal severation. This accident occurred when she was twelve years old, and left her with only movement of her head. She had immense spasms and was in extreme pain. It took me eleven months, but this young lady went from severe degeneration throughout her body (she could only move her wheelchair by a tongue-operated control) to the ability to shake your hand and lift either leg as many times as you wanted her to. She could "feel" from head to toe.

Another case involved a man in his early twenties who had a C4-C5 level injury. He had been paralyzed from his upper body down to his feet for two years. Within six months on our program his nerve response was helping him to move his feet and he could stool on his own. This was quite significant, as quadriplegics and most paraplegics lose their ability to have a bowel movement on their own. This greatly backs up the body's lymphatic system causing cell auto-intoxication.

In our arrogance and blindness we humans overlook the truth that is always right in front of our faces. If the body can miraculously repair itself in ways such as broken bones, deep cuts, re-growth of various gland and tissues, then why can't it repair nerves? Well it can, but not on cooked, dead foods, and foods that make the body's pH acidic.

Neurons are the highest energy centers in the body. Not only do they require an alkaline "soil" to regenerate in, they require the highest energy foods—fruits. Fructose is a high-energy, simple sugar, which lends its energy effortlessly to your cells. This holds true in all neurological issues including multiple sclerosis, Parkinson's, Bell's palsy and even asthma. Note that all of these neurological weaknesses have an adrenal weakness as a precursor.

In all neurological issues, including injuries, it is vital that the adrenal glands be enhanced along with the rest of the endocrine gland system. It is also vital to live on a 100 percent raw food diet. I had a forty-year-old female brought to me one time with advanced multiple sclerosis. They brought her lying on a stretcher, completely rigid. After three months on a fruit diet she could sit up, feed herself, and even mobilize her own wheelchair. Since she was so thin and small I needed to encourage her body to produce more muscle tissue, so I started her on vegetable juices and salads, as these foods are full of amino acids. Guess what? She lost her mobility temporarily. Why? The answer can be found in the difference between the electrical charge of a fruit versus that of a vegetable. When I put her on a diet of fruits alone she began to regain strength. The power that raw foods have to revitalize the physical body is almost unlimited. I've seen the body pull itself back from some pretty precarious edges. It took a while for this young lady to regenerate herself, but with such a degenerative condition it would naturally take a significant time to turn the body around. A predominately fruit diet was essential to maintain nerve response.

It is important to realize here that your body cannot regenerate itself with toxic chemicals. Toxic chemicals are seen as invading foreign proteins that will only serve to further acidify your tissues, creating further damage, and constant inflammatory immune responses that have to be treated with steroids—causing a vicious circle. Electrical stimulation is not the answer either. People dance around the truth refusing to embrace it. Money is generally the motivating factor. Because of greed, people would rather create moneymaking "treatment" systems (like illness-care institutions, drugs, surgeries) than learn the underlying truth about disease.

THE SAME ANSWER—ALKALIZE

Strengthen every cell in your body through diet and herbs. Remember Alkalize, Alkalize, Alkalize! It is the only way. I also recommend a high quality, herbal, brain and nerve formula to further strengthen the spinal column, nerve centers and brain tissue. Also it is essential to enhance the adrenal glands. This is where a great many of the body's neurotransmitters and steroids are created.

Another consideration in neurological disorders and injuries is the thyroid/parathyroid. The parathyroid hormone is necessary for proper

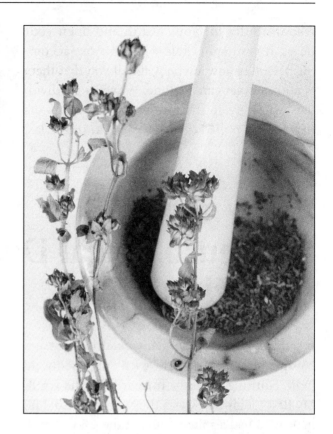

calcium utilization. You can find out how well your thyroid is working by taking the Basal Temperature Test (see Appendix A). With good calcium utilization and an **all raw-food diet** your success is almost guaranteed.

At the very least, the quality of life of those suffering from nerve damage are much improved with the elimination of urinary tract infections, over-spasticity, pain, cellulitis, obesity, and deterioration of tissue. At the very best they experience total recovery. The whole body can become healthy and vital again.

Don't ever give up or believe the body can't regenerate itself. Our bodies become very acidic and toxic from the foods that we have been taught are good for us. The body cannot regenerate when it is full of inflammation, mucus, parasites, toxic chemicals, metals and excessive hormones. Dead animal flesh, cooked mucus-forming dairy foods, acidic "fatty" grains and refined sugars only serve to destroy the body. Become alive again. Regenerate yourself and let the miracles begin.

☼ Diabetes: Types I and II

U.S. Government figures, January 2003, report 17 million Americans with diabetes. For a disease that is so devastating in its effects upon the body, diabetes is one of the easiest to overcome. I say this respectful of the fact that there are some difficult cases, especially in the more advanced "brittle" types, or what is called type I or juvenile diabetes.

There are basically two types of diabetes. Type I, which is usually called juvenile or brittle diabetes, fits in the category of insulin dependent. Type II, or what is referred to as late onset diabetes, is considered non-insulin dependent diabetes. It can, however, become insulin dependent.

In my opinion there is very little difference between these types except the associated tissue weaknesses in type I, which have become much weaker through genetic transmission. To better understand the disease called diabetes let's examine the tissues and cells involved and the cause behind their failure.

THE ROLE OF THE PANCREAS

One of the glands involved in diabetes is the pancreas, which is both an exocrine and an endocrine gland. The pancreas is located behind the stomach, in front of the first and second lumbar vertebrae, situated horizontally with its "head" attached to the first part of the small bowel (the duodenum). The "tail" of the pancreas extends to the spleen.

The pancreas has two vital jobs to perform, without which the body could not live. First, is the secretion of major digestive enzymes. Sodium of bicarbonate is also released at this time to alkalize the stomach contents so these digestive enzymes can work. Second, the most pertinent to diabetes, is the production of insulin by the beta cells for glucose utilization. When the cells in the pancreas become weak and fail to do their respective jobs, both aspects or functions can be affected. There are several other functions of the pancreas, which we'll discuss later.

Digestion is one of the first things we think about when we think of the pancreas. Even though not directly related to diabetes, proper digestion is a vital process whereby foods are broken down so that their nutrition and energy can be used for cellular fuel. Without this the entire body becomes weak, affecting all its functions.

The body secretes various digestive enzymes in basically four places: the mouth, stomach, pancreas and small intestines. The mouth, pancreatic and intestinal enzymes are similar to each other and are alkaline in nature, affecting carbohydrate, sugar and fat digestion. The stomach is the only acid chamber in your body and its role is to start breaking down protein structures. This is accomplished by HCL (hydrochloric acid) releasing pepsin. HCL and pepsin are acidic in nature. It is important to note here the importance of bile and sodium bicarbonate, the former released by the liver/gallbladder and the latter by the pancreas. These are alkalizing agents, which now alkalize the acid stomach contents (called chyme) so that the alkaline pancreatic and intestinal enzymes can finish up the job.

If there is inadequate bile flow and inadequate sodium bicarbonate, the acids from the chyme will neutralize the alkaline digestive enzymes from the pancreas, halting proper food digestion or breakdown. The HCL will then burn or inflame the walls of the intestines. This can eventually lead to ulcers and intestinal "itis's." Since acids neutralize alkalis, the alkaline digestive enzymes of your pancreas and intestinal tract are inhibited from properly digesting your foods. This causes fermentation and putrefaction, which now becomes the process that breaks down the remaining food particles, instead of the proper enzyme action. This, of course, releases much toxicity and alcohol, which further impedes the proper breakdown of your foods into building materials and fuels. This alcohol creates additional blood sugar problems and acidosis.

Letting Others Do It For You

I've seen case after case where a loved one drags their mate into my clinic and wants me to tell the other person what they have to do. They push their ailing friend or loved one into a detox program. They make the juices for them, they prepare their food for them and they prepare their herbal supplements for them. Nine times out of ten, this breeds failure. The sick person's heart and true desire to be well is not there.

You must be a part of your own healing. This is partly why you get sick. If you want to be well and healthy, *you* must create this with your own desires and actions, just as you would anything that you desire to experience or have in life.

It's great to have your loved ones on your side in this process, but not to the point of overshadowing your own desire and goals for yourself. If you want to be well, it must come from *you*. Become a shining example to the world of just how powerful God really is. But first you must show yourself.

The function of the pancreas that directly relates to diabetes is performed by the beta cells, which produce and release the insulin that assists in the utilization of glucose fuel by the body. Insulin, being a protein-type hormone, assists the transport of glucose through cell membrane walls. It is important to note here that fructose from fruit moves through cell walls by diffusion, not active transport, as in the case of glucose. This means that the need for insulin to assist fructose into a cell is highly questionable, yet diabetics are commonly told not to eat fruit because of its sugar. I have always put my diabetic patients on fruits with tremendously positive results.

The part of the pancreas called the Islets of Langerhans is where the beta cells are found. As previously stated, these cells produce and release insulin. When this part of the pancreas becomes hypoactive from inflammation or congestion, this can cause inadequate amounts of insulin to be produced.

The Islets of Langerhans consist of three types of cells: alpha cells, which secrete glucagon and raise blood glucose; beta cells, which secrete insulin, lowering blood glucose levels; and delta cells, which secrete somatostatin. Somatostatin inhibits the secretion of insulin, glucagon, a growth hormone from the anterior pituitary, and gastrin from the stomach. As previously stated, in diabetes mellitus it is the beta cells that are affected.

In both types of diabetes, but especially type I, this weakness in the pancreas is usually passed on genetically. However, through one's lifestyle, pancreatic weakness can be created in this lifetime. This would be especially true of type II or late onset diabetes. It might take several generations for a weakness from inflammation or toxicity to actually cause diabetes. You would probably experience hypoglycemia or gestational diabetes before this would manifest as any permanent type of diabetes. Of course there is a broad range of diabetes, as the degree of pancreatic weakness varies. Remember that someone had to start this weakness originally. The question remains: "How did they start it?"

Diabetes is considered another autoimmune problem, where lymphocytes attack the beta cells and destroy them. In my experience this is a misunderstanding of the body's protective mechanisms. Remember, your immune system is designed to eliminate the weak. It does not attack itself for no reason. The allopathic medical community cannot find a reason for this autoimmune response other than to say it is probably in the genes. However, the real reason for this response becomes obvious when you understand that in nature the strong survive while the weak perish. Nature never procreates the weak. Nature eliminates it.

I have seen diabetes created just from pancreatic flukes. Flukes are parasites that can infiltrate the liver and pancreas. Cleaning out most of the harmful parasites within the body is part of a good detoxification program. However, parasites do not originally create disease or tissue failure. They are secondary to toxicity and tissue weakness.

ADRENAL GLANDS

One of the most important relationships that is widely overlooked is that between the pancreas and the adrenal glands. The cortex of the adrenal glands produces andrenocortical hormones. Adrenal steroids called glucocorticoids (namely cortisol and corticosterone), act principally on carbohydrate metabolism. Cortisol and cortisone have many functions, including anti-inflammatory and carbohydrate digestion or metabolism. This action is catabolic in nature, meaning it's involved in the breaking down process.

The adrenal glands also produce neurotransmitters which affect pancreatic function. Therefore it would be important to work on both of these glands. It is always important to strengthen the adrenal glands as they have a vital relationship with every cell in the body.

Body Fuels

- Glucose and fructose are essential simple sugars required to "run" your body, just as your car needs fuel to run.

- Simple sugars require much less insulin than complex sugars.

- Complex sugars, like maltose, dextrose, and refined sucrose must be broken down into simple sugars before the body can use them. This creates heavy insulin requirements and also leads to excessive glucose, causing fat storage.

- Amino acids are your building materials, and sugars (glucose, fructose, etc.) are your fuels.

- Never use proteins for fuels. This creates tissue damage, cancer, and death. Proteins are building materials, not fuels.

THYROID/PARATHYROID

The thyroid/parathyroid gland must also be considered because of its control of metabolism and calcium utilization factors. Without proper calcium utilization all the cells in the body can become weakened. Calcium also plays a role in zinc, selenium and iron utilization, which affects glucose utilization and cellular functions.

HYPOTHALAMUS AND PITUITARY

Another area of weakness to consider in diabetes is the hypothalamus and pituitary gland. The posterior part of the pituitary gland, controlled by the hypothalamus (the master computer in the body), releases an anti-diuretic hormone which when underactive causes diabetes insipidus. It is also important to note that the transverse bowel is at the heart of eighty percent or more of the upper brain weaknesses, including and especially the pituitary and hypothalamus areas. With a greater understanding of the GI tract, especially the colon and its relationship to the organs and glands, you will appreciate why a healthy GI tract is necessary to assist the health of the rest of the body.

GI TRACT AND DIABETES

Your gastrointestinal tract has a relationship to all the organs and glands within your body. Just as the hub is the center of a wheel, the GI tract is considered the hub of your body. When the GI tract gets impacted with putrefying plaque from meat and flour products, the resulting inflammation and toxicity produced is echoed to the related areas. This is why cleaning and strengthening the GI tract is vital to your success in any disease condition, including diabetes.

THE TRUE CAUSES OF DIABETES

There are many theories regarding what causes diabetes, from plaqued cholesterol around the beta cells, to autoimmune problems, to genetics. Others say it's from stress and obesity.

Every cell in your body is a genetic cell. Some become weaker than others depending upon the above. These weaknesses are magnified and passed on through each new generation. Because of our unawareness of this fact, the human species is currently facing serious tissue weaknesses, resulting mainly in chronic and degenerative diseases.

Remember there are only **two causes of disease**, any disease. Number one is **toxicity** and number two is **acidosis**, in the form of inflammation. These two causes are the effects of what you eat, drink, breathe, what you put on your skin, as well as what you think and feel. These are the ways that you either strengthen your body or weaken it and the cells within it.

TREATING DIABETES

I have always put diabetics on a raw fruit and vegetable diet. This type of diet will clean and rebuild the pancreas and adrenal glands. Food combinations are also vital to follow (see instructions for food combining in Chapter 7, *Eating for Vitality*), as the fermentation and putrefaction of foods adversely affect the pancreas and blood sugar levels. I also use an herbal detox program and a pancreatic support formula with the diet (see Chapter 8 for herbs and herbal formulas that provide this support). In type II diabetes, if you follow a good detox program and use high quality herbs, you should be off insulin within three to eight weeks.

I would always advise the assistance of **a qualified healthcare practitioner** who can help guide you though this detoxification process. It is vital that you watch your blood sugar levels. They can drop very fast and you do not want to give yourself too much insulin when your blood sugars are more normalized. This could put you into a coma.

Use common sense. Take your time and be smart in what you do. If you are on insulin, and you're self-regulating or checking your sugars daily, you do not have to worry if your sugars temporarily go up. Some fruits may temporarily raise your blood sugars. If you notice a particular fruit doing this, just eliminate that fruit until you stabilize your sugars. Remember your goal is to **clean and regenerate the pancreas and adrenal glands**, not to treat diabetes.

Don't forget that complex sugars like sucrose, maltose and dextrose can overload your system with glucose. Trying to drive this excessive glucose into your cells with insulin is not the answer. Avoiding these complex-sugar foods is the answer.

You will also note that proteins, especially meat, will also raise your blood sugars. Meat is not a balanced food, as it consists of mostly protein. Therefore your body will break down fat and convert this to glucose for balance. The responding glucose will then raise your blood glucose levels.

There are so many contributing factors to diabetes. Keep it simple. Eat the food that was designed for your body—fruits, vegetables and nuts.

"There are no incurable diseases, only incurable people." This means that some people will not be cured because they don't want to be. Many use their disease for attention from family members or others. Many individuals become lost to themselves and seek love and attention from others as a support mechanism. Become strong in yourself; spend time alone with yourself.

Learn as much as you can about foods and their true effects upon tissue. Never fear God and nature. The devastating effects of diabetes are great, but its cure is simple. If it takes you six months to a year to cure yourself, that's better than a lifetime of misery. Be free of your diseases. Get healthy.

MODULE 5.8

☀ Obesity and Excessive Thinness

Understanding the "cause" of each of these common issues is essential in helping you to "fix" the "cause" behind them.

Always ask yourself: "Why am I experiencing a particular symptom?" "What am I doing to my physical body that is promoting these symptoms?" Remember: Cause and Effect.

The medical world is lost in self-described diseases, lost to the real cause behind all symptoms. Treating what they do not understand has killed a lot of people! The medical community is not educated about real causes, nor do they understand that your lifestyle (e.g., what you eat, drink, breathe, what you put on your skin, as well as your emotional and mental states) has everything to do with your health, vitality, or suffering.

To understand the cause—or the why behind obesity or thinness—you need to understand a little more of how your body works, the basic chemistry of life, and your genetic weaknesses.

Throughout this book I have provided enormous information about basic chemistry, the types of foods the human body is designed to eat, the physics (energetics) and the genetics surrounding this subject called "health and vitality." Here, under each of these topics of obesity and thinness, we will further explore the underlying causes. The causes may be the same for each of these conditions, and yet may be found in different locations in the body, and result in differing experiences within individuals.

THE DANGER OF HIGH PROTEIN DIETS

In trying to lose weight or put on weight we often use high protein diets. High protein diets are toxic to us, especially when this protein is from animal sources. Your body must spend a lot of time and energy to break down these protein structures (complex amino acids) into simple amino acids. This breaking down process is essential before your body can use these amino acids, as the body cannot use protein structures at all. Of course, the energy needed to do this will cause stored fat to be broken down as the body scrambles for energy to achieve protein conversion.

Proteins (amino acids) are on the nitrogen-dominant side of chemistry, which make them acid forming. Amino acids are your building blocks and carriers for tissue growth and repair. **They are** not designed or used for cellular fuel. If we try to burn amino acids for fuel, and not carbohydrates, this will cause excessive energy demands. On top of this, proteins are stimulants. Animal proteins contain neurotransmitters in them, which weaken our production in our adrenal glands. We also create acidosis, inflammation, and disease trying to burn amino acids for fuel. Excessive protein consumption (20 grams or more a day) results in damage to the gastrointestinal tract and kidneys. Our muscle tissue will also tear itself down; we then become weakened and in many cases die. Yes, die! There are tens of thousands of deaths from protein-related toxicity/acidosis each year. As said, protein is acidic and high in phosphorus (nitrogen) and iron, which burns your electrolytes out, especially calcium. Being acidic and abrasive, proteins cause inflammation and mucus build-up in the body. This all eventually leads to cellular death. It is important to understand the true biological needs of our bodies and the devastating effects of high protein diets. A high protein lifestyle with dairy products is by far the number one cause of the breakdown of the cells in your physical body and, of course, it is the number one cause of the allopathic concept of diseases.

OBESITY

The number one cause of obesity is, of course, the poor functioning of the adrenal glands. You have two adrenal glands, one sits on top of each kidney, and there are two basic functions of these glands.

Each adrenal gland has two zones, the inner portion and the outer portion. The **inner portion** (the adrenal medulla) produces the neurotransmitters for your autonomic nervous system (ANS). This nervous system is your "worker bee" nervous system, which controls your breathing, heart, bowels, muscles, etc. In my experience it is safe to say, genetically, that well over 95 percent of humans have adrenal and kidney weakness. In the younger generations, probably 100 percent have kidney and adrenal weakness. Understanding that these tissues (cells) control the body's Great Lymphatic System is beyond essential! The lymphatic system is the body's sewer system, which is responsible for removing all cellular wastes. Remember that cellular wastes are *acids*. We will return to consider this system later, especially when we discuss excessive thinness.

The **outer portion** of the adrenal glands (adrenal cortex) is where cortico-steroids are produced. Steroids control metabolism of minerals and sugars.

In obesity, these steroids are low. Cortisone controls sugar metabolism, so when cortisone is low, it in turn affects sugar metabolism, causing incomplete sugar metabolism and thus excessive glycogen (fat) to be stored. I have observed blood and saliva results for years with one major conclusion: you cannot refer to these statistics or readings alone, and ignore overall body symptomology.

It is important to understand that sugars (carbon) are essential to cell life, without which death is assured! Simply learn that fruits, berries, melons, and vegetables are your carbohydrates. They are made up of simple sugars essential for cellular energy (ATP/ADP/AMP). Combining simple sugars into complex sugars creates starch (e.g., *di-* = two, *poly-* = many). Complex sugars are difficult to metabolize, for anyone. Therefore, they are extremely fattening. Of course, this leads to fermentation, which causes excess fungal growth to deal with this excess fermentation. When your steroids are low (cortisol especially), you begin the journey to *hypo*glycemia (low blood sugar), then, over time, *hyper*glycemia (high blood sugar, diabetes). Consuming starches like grains and potatoes with an adrenal gland weakness is fattening.

Investigating the second cause of obesity will lead you to your thyroid glands. Your thyroid glands control the "rate" of metabolism—how fast or how slowly you digest your foods. In hypo (low) thyroidism, your digestion is slowed down. Therefore, your foods may not properly digest, especially if you are eating more than two meals a day. This poor digestion fosters fermenting in your system, and is fat producing. Add these two weaknesses (in the adrenal and the thyroid glands) together, and an individual can gain a lot of weight.

NOTE: One should never overlook the pituitary gland in these cases as well. Always remember to keep fatty and processed foods out of your diet!

EXCESSIVE THINNESS

Excessive thinness is also a major problem, possibly more so than obesity in that thinness results from a core problem of mal-absorption. Hyperthyroidism, of course, will cause this, as one's rate of metabolism is increased, "burning" energy at a much higher rate. However, by far the main cause of thinness is mal-absorption. It is vital to understand mal-absorption, the system it includes, and the other problems that can occur from being excessively thin.

Mal-absorption begins when your kidneys begin failing to filter your cellular wastes. Protein-rich diets are the main cause of kidney damage and, through the long genetic past of humanity's high protein diets, it has lead to many common health ailments experienced today.

As said earlier, your kidneys (and skin) are the eliminating organs of your lymphatic and glymphatic (glial lymph system in the brain) systems. The lymphatic system, because it deals predominantly with acids, is a lipid (mucous) based system, with cholesterol as one of the main lipids of this system. Remember, lipids are anti-inflammatories or antacids. When your kidneys fail to filter this system, mucous builds up around the cells in the interstitial spaces. This is because cellular metabolic wastes are backing up interstitially. When this mucous build-up occurs <u>in</u> the gastrointestinal tract walls, it <u>blocks</u> the absorption of nutrients from the villi (along the intestinal wall), into the blood; and for lipids, into the lymphatic capillaries. THIS CAUSES STARVATION.

Now, here is the kicker—your adrenal glands (remember, one on top of each kidney) are always involved in both issues, excess weight or thinness, one way or another. Therefore, your kidneys are always involved in excessive thinness as well.

So, with this understanding, what else is involved genetically? **Your lymphatic system!** As previously noted, this is the system linked to all the medically diagnosed diseases, especially cancers. The lymphatic system is your body's sewer system, where your body eliminates its acids, and it is your main immune system as well. By the way, it is also the fatty-acid carrier system to your liver. It is your body's lubrication system. Amazingly, it is six or more times bigger (at least) than your blood system! This is obviously vital for you to know. This system is where inflammation is born, fighting the stagnation of acids around your cells.

Excessive thinness obviously has the same cause as obesity. Being too thin can mean starvation from mal-absorption. To fix this problem one must detoxify the body. This means one must address the Great Lymphatic System, which includes the kidneys and adrenal glands. This in itself can cause more thinness, temporarily. However, it is an essential process to go through, as there simply is no other way to fix this issue.

EMOTIONAL COMPONENTS OF WEIGHT GAIN AND LOSS

As a society, we have become extremely emotional and codependent—that is, emotionally and mentally weakened. Humans are spiritually starved. This has a profound effect on obesity, as we have been taught to substitute sweets or refined foods—so called "comfort foods"—in times of emotional weakness and pain. Since we are frugivores, sweets fit our biological needs. However, these sugars should be simple sugars (which are mostly fruits, berries, melons and vegetables), not complex sugars.

Your adrenal glands also affect your emotional state (including anxiety, shyness, loneliness, feelings of isolation). They control your autonomic nervous system, including your breathing and heart rhythms. They also control sugar metabolism. Weak adrenal glands will lead to emotional weakness, neurological weakness, obesity from incomplete sugar metabolism, and the low neurotransmitter effect upon your autonomic nervous system.

Your thyroid gland also affects how you see yourself, or your self-image. Do you love yourself or not? It also brings about loneliness and isolation. Any symptom of depression is relative to the parathyroid.

Oftentimes, obesity and excessive thinness can follow the symptoms mentioned above. The largest individual I have had the pleasure of helping was a seven-hundred-pound male. He was struggling with the above symptoms, but as he learned about true healing he began to work himself out of these issues. The last time I saw him he had worked himself down to around four-hundred pounds.

LOW-FUNCTIONING ENDOCRINE GLANDS

Your endocrine glands control literally everything that goes on in your body. The pituitary is your main gland (like a CEO), since it controls all others. When your endocrine glands are "down," you may experience many different symptoms, as indicated in the list that follows.

Pituitary Gland: Short or above-average height, obesity, all other gland issues, irregular and excessive menses in females, bed-wetting, vitiligo (skin pigmentation issues), etc.

Parathyroid Glands (four sit on the Thyroid gland): Bones and connective tissue (spider or varicose veins, hernias, aneurysms, prolapsed colon or organs) weaknesses, weakened skin integrity, depression, low or high calcium levels, heart arrhythmias.

Thyroid Gland: Lethargy (tiredness), slow or fast digestion, obesity, calcium issues.

Thymus: Low T-Cell formation (immune system), stunted growth, reduced/compromised immune responses.

Pancreas: Poor digestion of carbohydrates and starches, blood sugar problems such as Type I diabetes (insulin production problems); even the breakdown of polypeptides and peptides into amino acids.

Adrenal Glands: Mineral utilization problems (low zinc, selenium, iron, etc.), sugar metabolism issues such as Type II diabetes, obesity, vaginal dryness, autonomic nerve issues like shortness of breath or asthma, heart arrhythmias, Multiple Sclerosis, Lou Gehrig's Disease (ALS), Parkinson's Disease, dizziness/equilibrium problems. NOTE: There are many more things the adrenal glands affect or control, like kidney filtration.

Ovaries (females): Produces ovarian estrogen and its base (alkaline) steroid progesterone. Controlled by the pituitary gland. Some issues are excessive bleeding during menstruation, inability to carry a fetus full term, premature births, inability to conceive, etc.

Prostate (males): Affects erections and sperm production in the testes. Aids in the production of testosterone. Some issues are premature ejaculation, inability to get or maintain an erection, frequent urination, slowed urination, etc.

SUMMARY—COMING HOME TO WELLVILLE

Getting healthy is a natural process and takes place all through your body as you learn to fix your lymphatic system, hydrating it interstitially, and therefore allowing your body to heal itself. Remember, acid can destroy, base can rebuild. This is in ALL conditions! It is all about the chemistry and magnetics (energy) of life. In this world at least!

I have always addressed both the physical and the emotional aspects of weight gain and loss. First and foremost, you **must** look at your diet and change what you eat and drink. And, you must change your thoughts from obsession with disease to preoccupation with getting healthy and feeling great again. For some, such a reorientation may be occurring for the first time.

If you are extremely obese, begin your program in balance. You may eat some cooked food, but start to eliminate the "fungal and fattening foods" called starches. Protein and dairy are an absolute *must* to get rid of. However, if protein is an issue, have some baked fish with a large salad, one to two times per week until you feel strong enough to let go of the fish.

The beautiful thing is that, with raw uncooked foods like fruits, berries, melons, and veggies, you can eat as much as you want and as often as you want. You cannot go hungry! However, your body can fool you into thinking you are hungry. One must push past this. If you can, you are coming home to **Wellville**. One day at a time. **Be here now in every moment.** Do not call yourself fat or thin. This is setting your mind up to accept these conditions.

Enjoy your journey into the incredible world of true health and vitality. Make a time for yourself to renew and expand your whole being. Great love to you and your newfound journey. Remember, it is one of regenerative detoxification.

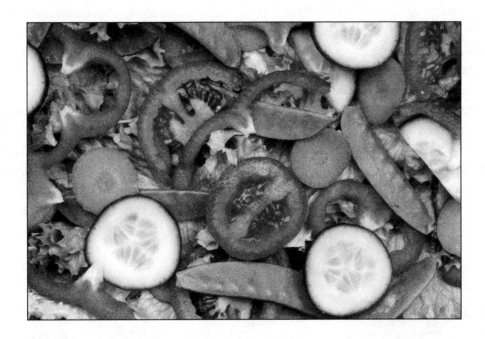

☀ The Skin and Its Disorders

Your skin is the largest vital organ you have. Its jobs range from temperature control and protection to elimination. Your skin is also the largest eliminative organ you have and is sometimes referred to as your "third kidney." Your skin is supposed to eliminate each day as much as your lungs, kidneys and bowels do. This elimination is in the form of mucus, toxins (acids) and gases.

The effects or by-products of many of the foods you consume will congest and inflame your system. Skin conditions are only signs of this process. As the body attempts to eliminate these by-products, you can experience anything from dandruff, pimples and rashes, to dermatitis, psoriasis and skin cancer. Psoriasis and skin cancer being the most toxic and parasitically involved of all the skin conditions.

Parasites are scavengers. They are found anywhere there is toxicity and dead or dying cells, including in the layers of the skin and on the top of the skin. You can call all these symptoms "diseases" if you want, however the cause is always the same. Only the degree of seriousness is different. Most allopathic medical doctors use cortisone or steroids like prednisone to treat these skin conditions, which only serve to drive the toxins and parasites deeper into the tissues, thus blocking proper elimination even further.

As the skin and eliminative organs become backed up with toxins, so does the liver. If you have any skin conditions—from ordinary pimples to dermatitis or psoriasis—you must detoxify yourself, especially the lymphatic system, liver, kidneys and bowels. Stop eating dairy products and refined sugars, all of which cause heavy congestion within the tissues of the body. Fungi love this type of congestion and toxicity as a food source. This creates a condition called Candida albicans, which is a yeast overgrowth. Yeast is part of the fungi family. You can kill most of these fungi (yeasts) with any good herbal parasite formula. However, if you do not remove the toxicity and congestion they feed on, they will be back.

Fevers are one of the greatest tools the body uses to help eliminate through the skin. Increasing the body's temperature increases perspiration, thus increasing the elimination of toxins, poisons and mucus. This is why the body will produce cold and flu-like symptoms as a result of parasitic attacks, stimulation, or detoxification (alkalization). **Never stop a cold or flu-like symptom or a fever.** These are not diseases, but a natural response by the body to increase the elimination that is vital to getting well.

If you do not sweat, your skin becomes congested, leading to dryness or inflammation. Many females have this problem so they use moisturizers to make the skin soft and oily again. This only adds to the problem, as these lotions add to the congestion in the subcutaneous layers

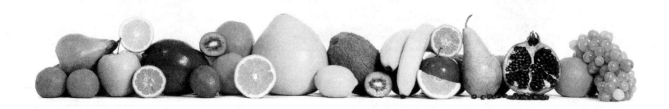

of the skin. Congestion and toxicity block the skin's oil ducts and exit pores, making the skin dry and scaly. The health of your skin is an internal issue not an external one. In other words, a healthy body inside means healthy skin outside. If you must feed the skin externally, use pure, raw, organic grape seed oil or olive oil. Or mixed tocopherol vitamin E, jojoba oil or pure essential oils would be advised.

If you have hypothyroidism, which 60 to 70 percent of the population does, you will have a difficult time perspiring. The thyroid gland affects one's ability to sweat, either making you sweat too much or not enough. Lack of exercise and low activity is another reason people do not sweat enough. Refer to Chapter 9, *Healthy Habits*, and read the sections on cold-sheet treatments and dry skin brushing. These are just two simple ways to increase skin elimination. A raw food diet is just as essential to great skin health as it is for the health of any cell. When your skin begins to prolapse (drop) or wrinkle, this is not old age. This is skin weakness.

You must care for your skin as you would any vital organ. Remember that the thyroid and liver are related to the skin, so detoxify the liver and keep your thyroid functioning properly. Use the Basal Temperature Test (see Appendix A) for a more accurate determination of your thyroid function.

Enjoy healthy skin. As you detoxify and regenerate, your whole body will thank you and pay you back with robust health. I have helped people of eighty and ninety years of age to regain vibrant, healthy, wrinkle-free, toned and tightened skin. The body is a most wondrous, intelligent machine. Take care of yours, as it is your vehicle during your earthly stay.

MODULE 5.10

☀ Mind, Emotions and the Cells

Up to this point we have been discussing the impact and effect that the various foods and toxins you consume have upon your body. Let's examine the more subtle processes that affect you and your body and also create disease.

The two most powerful tools you use to create your experience here in the physical world are your mind and your emotions. Your physical body is just a clay shell that carries your awareness around. You would not be able to create the events in your life if it were not for the thought processes that allow you to imagine the sequence of events you wish to experience. Without the emotions, however, there would be no desire to create. As the mind takes images of the past and present and puts them together to create the future, it is the emotions that drive you to manifest these images. The stronger your feelings are toward some idea or image, the more you're going to "experience the experience," no matter what it is. Added to these twin creative aspects is your ego, which is your sense of individuality. Put all these together and you have the play of life.

The mind and emotions can work for us in a positive manner, or against us in a negative manner by controlling and enslaving us. I suggest that you use your mind and emotions to enhance and revitalize you. Remember, the mind works from images. What you imagine becomes your reality on one level or another. So, turn this process to your benefit. Imagine yourself healthy and vital. This is where your emotions can come in. Get excited about a new life, full of vitality and vibrancy. Let your emotions be the drive to your success. Read and surround yourself with books and information on raw foods and detoxification. It is vital that we, as souls, understand our bodies, for they are our vehicles on this journey through creation. You must learn how to properly use the body for your highest good. What you create mentally and emotionally becomes your experience.

True health and vitality is found when we have these mental and emotional "bodies" in balance. Each of these bodies impact one another. Your emotions, especially the negative ones like anger, hate, and jealousy, can make your physical body sick and full of disease. These emotions are stored in the liver and kidneys. They block proper pancreatic function (digestion) and other glandular functions as well. Emotions can even shut down our mind, affecting our ability to comprehend, think and make rational decisions. They especially can close off the heart centers. Once the heart center is closed, your ability to get healthy drastically decreases, even to the point where death is the inevitable result.

Among the cancer clients whom I could not help were those who had their heart center closed, for one reason or another, and had a hard time opening to love. In some people this is a complex and deep-seated issue. This is where meditation, deep personal prayer, and spiritual counseling comes in. One should start enjoying life for what it is. Observe nature and surround yourself with flowers and plants, as these are very healing. Nature embraces with energies of love. If we can let go of the past, we can enjoy every moment for what it is. Let all hate, anger, and opinions go. Give them over to God. An old saying I use personally is, "Let go and let God."

Love, happiness, joy, health and mental control all keep the heart open. Unhappiness, depression, despair, anger, jealousy, rage, envy and negative states shut down or keep the heart center closed. The mind must also be kept in control. They say the mind is a great servant but a lousy, even destructive, master.

The thinking process keeps us from enjoying the present moment, the "eternal now" as it is called. Remember when you were a child and the present moment seemed to last forever? Those days were long and filled with play and excitement. As you grew up, these timeless moments were lost at the hands of thought and desire. The way teaching is done in most of our school systems promotes competition and limits free thinking, just as the materialistic world of possessions limits freedom and happiness. These circumstances have greatly reduced our overall awareness and our ability to experience God, the source of true vitality, happiness and bliss.

By detoxifying your physical body you can start a chain of events that will allow you to clean and bring under control your emotional and mental processes. You can help this process by allowing old thought patterns and the emotions that can surface during detoxification to finally be released and forgotten. There are several ways to do this.

Begin by watching your thoughts. Step away from them and become the observer. Become detached about the outcome of things and from other people's opinions and emotions. Let go. Give it all over to spirit, God, the wind . . . whatever you believe in. Let go of all of your negative emotions and mental chains. This allows the greatest healing power to flow through you and your mental, emotional and physical bodies, bringing a vibrancy and awareness that is indescribable and rare. Enjoy life moment by moment. Allow yourself the freedom to expand and experience. Break out of the old conditioned states of thinking and feeling and become vibrant and healthy. Do it now!

GLANDS, EMOTIONS AND HEALTH

It is important to note that when your glandular system is out of balance, so are you. This is especially true of the triad: the pituitary, thyroid and adrenal glands.

When the thyroid is hypoactive, calcium utilization drops. This can bring on all types of states of depression from mild to chronic. When the adrenal glands become hypoactive, anxieties can overwhelm you. Responses vary from mild shyness and introversion, to apprehension, to chronic worry and anxiety, to acute anxiety attacks, to paralyzing fear and reclusiveness. Bipolar disorder, schizophrenia and other similar conditions are all manifestations of the above, as they affect your calcium, serotonin, neurotransmitters, and the like. This is why the health of your physical body is so important to your mental and emotional bodies. They are all interconnected to the point that you experience all three as one expression.

Summary

Learn the secrets that lead to the health and vitality of your physical body, emotions and mind. Take charge of these tools or bodies. They are your instruments of expression while you are in this world. Detox and clean your body. Let all your emotions be carried away or replaced with love. Go beyond your mind into the world of the Now. Be "you"—not your mind. Only use thought to create what you need, not what you want.

MODULE 5.11

☀ Body Language: What is Your Body Trying to Tell You?

Nothing happens in life without a reason. All things exist and change from a cause. If you take a long walk down the road, it's because you decided by thought and emotion (the desire) to do so. Cells in your body are the same way. They act and respond via thought and emotions. However, the types of thoughts and emotions that act upon the cells are carried on in a subtle, almost subconscious way.

Cells already function automatically. However, hormones, steroids, neurotransmitters, serotonin, etc., influence them. These substances create a reaction in tissue (cells) that make them respond or react in a particular manner, depending upon the initial thought or emotion. A good example of this is fear. If you see something that terrifies you, your adrenal glands will produce adrenaline (epinephrine) to stimulate the heart and blood flow, and to encourage muscle movement. This gives you much added strength and energy to run or fight. The adrenal gland first got its message to release adrenaline from the brain, which received its message through your awareness.

Cells respond to stimuli. This can have positive results or negative results depending upon the source of the stimuli. As I have reinforced throughout this book, the foods you eat, what you drink, breathe, and what you put on your skin, can have a positive and enhancing effect or a negative effect upon cells, tissues, organs or glands. A negative effect can cause hypoactivity of cells and their respective tissues. These negative influences can even kill cells.

As your cells become weakened or die, they can change their morphology (function). They can be invaded by parasites to finish them off, and/or be consumed by an immune cell and thus eliminated.

As this process of cellular deterioration takes place, your body as a whole begins to suffer. This creates a domino effect causing a change in the way your body functions. These many changes are like signs. Linked together they become a body "language" for you or your healthcare practitioner to read. If you are observant and learn about your body's language or communication methods, you will be able to determine what organs and glands are failing you. This module should be used in conjunction with Module 5.12, Health Questionnaire, which concludes this chapter. That Questionnaire will allow you to reflect upon various bodily processes and systems, and to pinpoint their weaknesses.

For now, the lists that follow are some "body language" cues, or side effects, that I have learned in my thirty-plus years of experience as a healthcare practitioner. Some of these might sound like diseases to you, but they are merely the effects of organ or glandular weaknesses and failures.

THE LANGUAGE OF THE GLANDS, ORGANS AND SYSTEMS

Thyroid (Endocrine Gland System)

Weakness or failure of the thyroid will show up as:
- Obesity (if your pancreas is weak, you can be thin and still have a thyroid weakness)
- Low Metabolism (can give you poor digestion)
- Low Body Temperature (cold extremities and cold intolerance)
- Hair loss and balding
- Failure to sweat properly, affecting skin elimination (creates dry skin and other conditions)

Parathyroid (Endocrine Gland System)

Calcium requires a parathyroid hormone so it can be utilized properly by your body. Failure to utilize calcium results in:

- Bone loss (Osteoporosis, spinal deterioration or herniated disks)
- Bone (calcium) spurs
- Arthritis (adrenal gland weakness must also be present)
- Connective tissue weakness, causing prolapsed conditions (dropping) of skin, bladder, uterus, bowels, and other organs
- Varicose veins and spider veins
- Hemorrhoids
- Depression
- Nerve weakness
- Spasms, cramping of muscles, convulsions
- Dehydration
- Ridged, brittle or weakened fingernails
- Anemia (low calcium causes poor iron utilization)
- Scoliosis
- Ruptured Discs
- Hernias
- Aneurysms
- MVP (mitral valve prolapse—heart)

Adrenal Glands (Endocrine Gland System)

Linked to the nervous system, inflammation, carbohydrate utilization, healing and repair of tissues. Weakness or failure of these glands will be seen as:
- "itis's" (all inflammatory conditions)
- Fibrocystic conditions
- Fibromyalgia, scleroderma and sciatica
- Ovarian cysts
- Excessive bleeding
- Endometriosis and atypical cell formation
- Prostatitis
- Prostate cancer
- All female cancers
- M.S. and Parkinson's Disease
- Tremors
- Tinnitus (ringing in the ears)
- Shortness of breath
- Cholesterol plaquing
- Dehydration

- Anxieties, excessive shyness, emotional sensitivities, and other related conditions
- Sleep disorders
- Memory problems
- Early puberty, initial menstruation, and irregular menstruation
- Conception problems
- Sexual problems (including lack of or excessive sex drive, impotence, erection problems, frigidity in women, and fertility problems)
- Low Energy (Chronic Fatigue)
- Low endurance

Pancreas (Digestive and Endocrine Gland System)

Hypoactivity (underactivity) of the pancreas can cause the following:
- Gas and bloating during digestion
- Undigested foods in your stools
- Excessive thinness
- Loss of muscle tissue
- Moles growing on your skin
- Low blood sugar (Hypoglycemia)
- High blood sugar (Diabetes, etc.)
- Acid reflux
- Gastritis
- Enteritis
- Nausea

Liver and Gallbladder (Hepatic/Blood System—Your Chemical Factory)

When the liver or gallbladder becomes toxic, inflamed and full of stones, the following symptoms may appear:
- Bloating and Acid-Reflux conditions
- Enteritis
- Poor digestion
- Anemia
- Low amino acid utilization
- Low hemoglobin and albumin count
- Skin toxicity (resulting in dermatitis, eczema, psoriasis, and other conditions)
- White stools
- Liver spots (skin pigmentation changes)

- Starvation
- Low cholesterol production = low steroid production = more inflammation
- Lower resistance to inflammation
- Lowers cell wall protection
- Gastritis
- Nausea after eating
- Loss of muscle tissue (low protein utilization)
- Low cholesterol levels
- Sugar problems (high or low blood sugars)

Gastrointestinal Tract (Digestive and Eliminative Systems)

Your gastrointestinal tract (stomach to anus) is the "hub" of your body. When it fails to do its job because of impactions and inflammation, this can weaken and starve the body. When the GI tract fails, the rest of the body will soon follow. The following are just some of the side effects of its failure:
- Malabsorption and starvation
- Gastritis, enteritis and/or colitis
- Diverticulitis (when "pockets" are formed from impactions)
- Gas
- Diarrhea
- Constipation (also connected to adrenal medulla weakness)
- Parasites (worms, and others; the unfriendly type)
- Crohn's disease
- GI cancer (now second most prevalent type of cancer in the U.S.)
- When the GI Tract becomes toxic, it sends toxicity to all parts of the body
- Appendicitis
- Lymphatic congestion (blocks proper lymphatic elimination)
- Nausea upon eating

Lymphatic System (Immune and Eliminative "Septic" System)

The job of the lymphatic system is to clean and protect the body. This system is just as important as the blood system. The lymphatic system is the most neglected and needs the most attention. All diseases begin when this system becomes over-burdened and fails. The following are just some of the noticeable effects:

- Colds and flu-like symptoms
- Many childhood diseases (mumps, measles, etc.)
- Most respiratory congestive issues
- Sinus congestion
- Earaches
- Hearing loss (causing the need for tubes in the ears)
- Sore throats
- Cysts and tumors
- Boils, pimples and the like
- Lymphatic cancers
- Appendicitis
- Low immune response
- Low lymphocytes (when the lymph gland called the spleen is affected)
- Low platelets and a lack of blood cleansing can take place.
- Lymph edema from removed or degenerated lymph nodes
- Lymph node swelling
- Allergies
- Cellulitis
- Blurred vision
- Cataracts and glaucoma
- Snoring
- Sleep apnea
- Tonsillitis
- Stiff neck
- Cervical spine deterioration from stagnant lymph system in neck (especially when tonsils have been removed)
- Dandruff

Kidneys and Bladder (Eliminative/Urinary Tract System)

These organs are vital in your body's elimination process. Without proper elimination of metabolic wastes, both cellular and digestive, toxic by-products will cause auto-intoxication of cells. This causes cellular weakness and death. The following are side effects or warning signals that your body experiences when the kidneys and bladder become weak.

- Bags under your eyes
- Vision problems
- Lower back weakness and pain
- Kidney stones (contributing factor to parathyroid weakness)
- Urinary tract infections—UTI (burning upon urination)
- Loss of bladder control (incontinence)
- Difficulty urinating (can be urinary tract infections as well)
- Increased acidosis
- Dehydration
- Edema (contributing factor)
- Toxemia
- Headaches
- Can affect your breathing

Heart and Circulation (The Circulatory System)

Many conditions that affect the heart and circulation have already been covered under various glands and their effects upon the body. This is because many conditions within the body are reflex conditions that have an origination point other than the obvious symptoms. Examples of this are mitral valve prolapse and heart arrhythmia, which have their origins in the parathyroid, where connective tissue and the nervous system can be affected. The adrenal glands, of course, play a vital role in the nerve that feeds the heart. Cholesterol will plaque itself if the adrenal glands are weak and acidosis goes unchecked. All this can lead to strokes, heart attacks and blockages in the vascular system. One must think this out and take all this into consideration when dealing with the heart and circulatory issues. The following are some of the symptoms the body will manifest when these heart and circulation tissues are affected:

- Poor circulation leads to cellular death (which leads to a multitude of problems)
- Gray hair
- Memory loss
- Chest pain or angina
- Feeling of "heaviness" or "weight" on top of your chest
- Petechiae (bruising easily)
- Blood Regurgitation (back flow) from weak valves (causing chest pain)
- High or low systolic blood pressure (adrenal gland relationship)
- High diastolic (bottom number)
- Tired feeling (especially during exercise)
- S.O.B. (shortness of breath) from water buildup, congestive heart failure (CHF), and myocardial edema (fluids around the heart). Water build-up is an inflammatory issue from acidosis.
- Low endurance (also adrenal gland relationship)
- Cramping or spasms upon exercise
- Contributes to lymphatic blockages, causing sluggish lymphatic issues
- All types of heart arrhythmias (however, thyroid and adrenal gland weakness is mostly to blame.)

Skin (Integumentary and Eliminative System)

Your skin is the largest eliminative organ you have. It's supposed to eliminate as much waste each day as your kidneys and bowels. However, when the liver, bowels and lymphatic system is backed up, this overburdens the skin and it becomes sluggish and impacted. This causes many of the skin conditions that exist. On top of this, when the thyroid is weak it becomes more difficult to sweat. This inhibits proper elimination through the skin even more. A breakdown of the skin's normal functions will result in:

- Skin rashes
- Dry skin
- Eczema
- Boils, pimples, etc. (related to lymphatic system)
- Dermatitis
- Psoriasis
- Splitting of the skin

Lungs (Respiratory System)

Breathing and the lungs are how we bring the biggest factors of energy and oxidation into our body. Without oxygen, of course, you would die. Oxygen helps elements to transmute into other elements or compounds. Transmutation is the true process of nature. The following body language obviously indicates lung congestion, toxicity and acidosis:

- Bronchitis and pneumonia
- Asthma
- S.O.B. (shortness of breath)
- Chronic coughing
- Emphysema
- C.O.P.D. (chronic obstructive pulmonary disease)
- Pain in lung areas
- Fatigue (also thyroid and adrenal gland weakness)
- Low endurance (also caused from adrenal gland weakness)
- Sore throat (begins here)
- High carbon dioxide levels
- Toxemia

☀ The Health Questionnaire

Now that we have looked at body language in Module 5.11, this Health Questionnaire will enhance that understanding of your body by highlighting what organs, glands, or systems are failing to perform properly for you. After you discover your body's areas of weakness then you can use the diet recommended in this book, as well as herbal formulas designed for these specific areas. See Chapter 8, Module 8.3 for *Herbal Formulas* applied to each system, and see the Resource Guide for recommended companies that supply herbs and herbal formulas.

This Questionnaire would also be invaluable to share with your healthcare practitioner, as it details many things that are not always covered in simple medical history questionnaires, and may reveal topics that you haven't discussed. Use it as a way to work together to find the best possible approach to your program of detoxification and regeneration.

THYROID/PARATHYROID (GLANDULAR SYSTEM)

Are you overweight?	Yes _____	No _____
Do you get cold hands and feet?	Yes _____	No _____
Do you have hair loss or are you bald or going bald?	Yes _____	No _____
Is it easy to put on weight and hard to loose it?	Yes _____	No _____
Are your fingernails ridged, brittle or weak?	Yes _____	No _____
Do you have varicose or spider veins?	Yes _____	No _____
Do you have, or have you had, hemorrhoids?	Yes _____	No _____
Do you get cramping in your muscles?	Yes _____	No _____
Is your bladder strong or weak?	Strong _____	Weak _____
Do you have an irregular heartbeat?	Yes _____	No _____
Do you have mitral valve prolapse (heart murmur)?	Yes _____	No _____
Do you get headaches or migraines?	Yes _____	No _____
Do you now have, or have you ever had, a hernia?	Yes _____	No _____
Have you ever had an aneurysm?	Yes _____	No _____
Do you have osteoporosis?	Yes _____	No _____
Do you have scoliosis?	Yes _____	No _____
Do you get irritable easily?	Yes _____	No _____
Do you have low energy levels?	Yes _____	No _____
Do you suffer from symptoms of depression?	Yes _____	No _____
Did you score low on your bone density tests?	Yes _____	No _____
Do your tests come back showing low calcium levels?	Yes _____	No _____
Do you have, or have you ever had, a goiter?	Yes _____	No _____

Do you have spine deterioration or herniated discs?	Yes _____	No _____
Have you or any family member been diagnosed with Hashimoto or Reidel disease?	Yes _____	No _____
Do you sweat profusely or hardly at all?	A lot _____	Little _____

ADRENAL GLANDS (GLANDULAR SYSTEM)

Medulla (Adrenal)

Do you have MS, Parkinson's or palsy?	Yes _____	No _____
Do you have anxiety attacks, or feel overly anxious?	Yes _____	No _____
Do you feel excessive shyness, or inferior to others?	Yes _____	No _____
Do you have low blood pressure (below 118 systolic)?	Yes _____	No _____
Do you have tremors, nervous legs, etc.?	Yes _____	No _____
Do you have tinnitis (ringing in the ears)?	Yes _____	No _____
Do you have shortness of breath or is it hard to take a deep breath?	Yes _____	No _____
Do you have heart arrhythmias?	Yes _____	No _____
Do you have a hard time sleeping?	Yes _____	No _____
Do you have Chronic Fatigue Syndrome?	Yes _____	No _____
Do you get tired easily?	Yes _____	No _____
Have you ever been diagnosed with Addison's Disease or with congenital adrenal hyperplasia?	Yes _____	No _____

Cortex (Adrenal)

Do you have elevated blood cholesterol levels?	Yes _____	No _____
Do you have lower back weakness?	Yes _____	No _____
Do you have, or have you had, sciatica?	Yes _____	No _____
Do you have arthritis or bursitis?	Yes _____	No _____
Do you have any "itis's" (inflammatory conditions)?	Yes _____	No _____

Explain_____

_____

_____

FEMALE ONLY

Are your menstruations irregular?	Yes _____	No _____
Do you get excessive bleeding during menstruation?	Yes _____	No _____
Do you have or have you had ovarian cysts?	Yes _____	No _____
Do you have or did you have fibroids?	Yes _____	No _____
Do you have or did you have endometriosis or A-typical cells?	Yes _____	No _____

Are you fibrocystic?	Yes _____	No _____
Do you have fibromyalgia or scleroderma?	Yes _____	No _____
Do you get sore breasts, especially during menstruation?	Yes _____	No _____
Do you have a low or excessive sex drive?	Yes _____	No _____
Have you had a hysterectomy?	Yes _____	No _____

Partial _____ Complete _____ When _____

Did they take any other organs out at the same time? (c.a. gallbladder)	Yes _____	No _____
Have you had a D & C?	Yes _____	No _____
Have you had a miscarriage?	Yes _____	No _____
Have you had difficulty in conceiving children?	Yes _____	No _____

Other _____

MALE ONLY

Do you have prostatitis (frequent urination, especially at night)?	Yes _____	No _____

If yes, how often?

Do you have prostate cancer? PSA counts:	Yes _____	No _____
Do you have testicular hypertrophy (enlargement)?	Yes _____	No _____
Do you have a low or excessive sex drive?	Yes _____	No _____
Do you have erection problems?	Yes _____	No _____
Do you have premature ejaculation?	Yes _____	No _____

Other _____

PANCREAS

Do you get gas after you eat?	Yes _____	No _____
Do you feel your foods just sitting in your stomach?	Yes _____	No _____
Do you have acid reflux?	Yes _____	No _____
Do you see any undigested foods in your stools?	Yes _____	No _____
Do you have hypoglycemia (low blood sugar)?	Yes _____	No _____
Do you have diabetes (high blood sugar)?	Yes _____	No _____

Type I _____ Type II _____

Are you thin and have a hard time putting on weight?	Yes _____	No _____
Do you have gastritis or enteritis?	Yes _____	No _____
Do your foods pass right through you (diarrhea)?	Yes _____	No _____
Do you have moles on your body?	Yes _____	No _____

GASTROINTESTINAL TRACT

Is your tongue coated (white, yellow, green or brown),
especially in the morning?   Yes _____   No _____

Do you have a hiatal hernia?   Yes _____   No _____

Do you have gastritis?   Yes _____   No _____

Do you have enteritis?   Yes _____   No _____

Do you have colitis?   Yes _____   No _____

Do you have diverticulitis?   Yes _____   No _____

Do you get or have diarrhea?   Yes _____   No _____

Do you get or have constipation?   Yes _____   No _____

How often do you have a bowel movement?   _____

Have you ever had stomach or intestinal ulcers?   Yes _____   No _____

Do you have, or have you ever had, any type of gastrointestinal
cancers: stomach, colon, rectal, etc.   Yes _____   No _____

Explain _____

_____

_____

Do you have Crohn's Disease?   Yes _____   No _____

Do you have "gas" problems?   Yes _____   No _____

Other GI problems _____

_____

_____

LIVER/GALLBLADDER/BLOOD

Do you have a problem digesting fats?   Yes _____   No _____

Do fats or dairy foods cause bloating and/or pain
in the stomach area?   Yes _____   No _____

Are your stools white or very light brown in color?   Yes _____   No _____

Do you get pain in the middle of your back (especially
after eating)?   Yes _____   No _____

Do you get pain behind the right, lower rib area?   Yes _____   No _____

Do you have "liver" or brown spots on your skin?
(not freckles)   Yes _____   No _____

Do you have any skin pigmentation changes?   Yes _____   No _____

Do you have skin problems? If so, what type?   Yes _____   No _____

Are you anemic?   Yes _____   No _____

Do you have, or have you ever had, hepatitis?   Yes _____   No _____

A _____ B _____ C _____

HEART & CIRCULATION

Do you have any gray hair?   Yes _____   No _____

Do you have a hard time remembering things?   Yes _____   No _____

Do your legs get tired or cramp after you walk?   Yes _____   No _____

Do you bruise easily?   Yes _____   No _____

Do you get chest pains or angina?   Yes _____   No _____

Have you ever had a heart attack (Myocardial Infarction)?   Yes _____   No _____

Have you ever had open-heart surgery?   Yes _____   No _____

Do you have heart arrhythmias?   Yes _____   No _____

    What kind? _____

Do you have a heart murmur or mitral valve prolapse?   Yes _____   No _____

Do you ever feel pressure on your chest?   Yes _____   No _____

Do you get "prickly" pains anywhere, especially

    in the heart area?   Yes _____   No _____

    Where? _____

Do you have, or have you ever had high blood pressure?   Yes _____   No _____

Your average blood pressure is _____ over _____

SKIN

Do you get or have skin rashes?   Yes _____   No _____

Do you get skin blemishes?   Yes _____   No _____

Do you have eczema or dermatitis?   Yes _____   No _____

Do you have psoriasis?   Yes _____   No _____

Do you itch anywhere? Where?   Yes _____   No _____

Is your skin dry?   Yes _____   No _____

Is your skin excessively oily?   Yes _____   No _____

Do you get or have dandruff?   Yes _____   No _____

LYMPHATIC SYSTEM

Are you allergic to anything?   Yes _____   No _____   What? _____

Do you ever get colds or flu-like symptoms?   Yes _____   No _____

Do you have sinus problems?   Yes _____   No _____

Do you have or get sore throats?   Yes _____   No _____

Do you have swollen lymph nodes?   Yes _____   No _____

Do you have, or have you had, tumors?   Yes _____   No _____

    What type? fatty _____ benign _____ cancerous _____

    Where? _____

Do you have a low platelet count (blood)?   Yes _____   No _____

Is your immune system low or sluggish?	Yes _____	No _____
Have you had appendicitis or an appendectomy?	Yes _____	No _____
When? _____		
Do you get boils, pimples, and the like?	Yes _____	No _____
Do you have allergies?	Yes _____	No _____
Have you ever had abscesses?	Yes _____	No _____
Have you ever had toxemia?	Yes _____	No _____
Do you have, or have you had, cellulitis?	Yes _____	No _____
Have you ever had gout?	Yes _____	No _____
Do you get blurred vision?	Yes _____	No _____
Do you have mucus in your eyes when you wake up in the morning?	Yes _____	No _____
Do you snore?	Yes _____	No _____
Do you have sleep apnea?	Yes _____	No _____
Have you had your tonsils out?	Yes _____	No _____
What age? _____		

KIDNEYS & BLADDER

Have you ever had a urinary tract infection?	Yes _____	No _____
Have you ever had "burning" upon urination?	Yes _____	No _____
Do you have problems holding your bladder (parathyroid)?	Yes _____	No _____
Have you ever had kidney stones?	Yes _____	No _____
Do you have bags under your eyes (especially in the morning)?	Yes _____	No _____
Is your urine flow restricted?	Yes _____	No _____
Do you get cramping or pain on either side of your mid-to-lower back?	Yes _____	No _____
Do you have, or did you ever have, nephritis?	Yes _____	No _____
Do you have, or did you ever have, cystitis?	Yes _____	No _____

LUNGS

Do you get or have (or have you had) bronchitis?	Yes _____	No _____
Do you get or have (or have you had) emphysema?	Yes _____	No _____
Do you get or have (or have you had) asthma?	Yes _____	No _____
Do you get or have (or have you had) C.O.P.D?	Yes _____	No _____
Are you on inhalers or nebulizers?	Yes _____	No _____
How often? _____		
What type? _____		
What is your oxygen saturation? _____		

Do you get pain when you breathe?   Yes _____   No _____

Do you get pain when you take a deep breath?   Yes _____   No _____

Did you ever have, or do you now have, lung cancer?   Yes _____   No _____

Do you have a collapsed lung?   Yes _____   No _____

Are you a smoker? If yes, how often do you smoke?   Yes _____   No _____

Have you ever had pneumonia?   Yes _____   No _____

Have you ever worked around toxic chemicals,

    in coal mines or around asbestos?   Yes _____   No _____

Do you cough a lot?   Yes _____   No _____

Do you get any mucus when you cough?   Yes _____   No _____

    What color is the mucus? _____

OTHER (*What are your main health complaints or concerns?*)

Please list and elaborate on any conditions or symptoms that this questionnaire has not covered
or asked you. _____

_____

_____

_____

_____

_____

_____

_____

_____

_____

PAST SURGERIES

Please list any past surgeries you have had (e.g. tonsils removed, gall bladder removed,
hysterectomies, open heart surgery, etc.).

    Surgery _____ Year_____

        _____ _____

        _____ _____

CHEMICAL MEDICATIONS

Please list any chemical medications that you are presently taking.

    Medication _____ Reason _____

        _____ _____

        _____ _____

        _____ _____

NATURAL SUPPLEMENTS

Please list any natural supplements you are currently taking.

Supplements _____

_____

_____

_____

_____

Vitamins & Minerals _____

_____

_____

_____

_____

ALLERGIES

Please list anything that you are allergic to: _____

_____

_____

_____

_____

GENETIC HISTORY: List major diseases or conditions.

Mother _____

Father _____

(Maternal) Grandfather _____

(Maternal) Grandmother _____

(Fraternal) Grandfather _____

(Fraternal) Grandmother _____

Sister _____

Sister _____

Sister _____

Brother _____

Brother _____

Brother _____

Other _____

_____

_____

_____

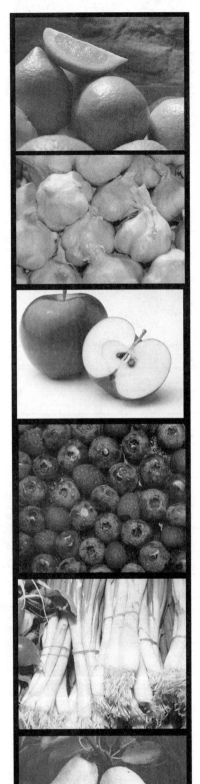

CHAPTER SIX

Eliminating Disease

Through Cleansing and Rebuilding Tissue

Most healthcare systems today, especially the allopathic, focus on treating symptoms. These include fevers, infections, sugar imbalances, neurological failure, and skin rashes, just to name a few. Statistics now tell us that cancer is in every other male and in every third female. With diseases just about to eliminate us as a race, it is obvious that this treatment concept isn't working. With the treatment method, symptoms are only controlled or temporarily eliminated, only to return when treatment is stopped. Oftentimes, the symptoms come back with a vengeance, as in cancer. You cannot "treat" chronic or degenerative conditions, as treatment just worsens the condition.

Regeneration and detoxification, on the other hand, mean the complete elimination of the cause of the symptoms. If you correct the cause of the problem, the symptoms will automatically go away. Regeneration means rebuilding tissue that is failing; and detoxification is the method used to remove the inflammation and toxins that have caused these tissues to fail in the first place. Always ask yourself what the cause of your symptoms may be, and focus on that. People are too busy chasing effects.

As we learned in detail in the previous chapter, there are only three basic causes of disease symptoms: 1. acidosis, which causes inflammation, leading to congestion, ulceration and atrophy (tissue failure); 2. toxicity, which causes congestion, inflammation and cellular damage, thus leading to tissue failure; and 3. tissue weakness or tissue failure itself caused by genetics, acidosis, and/or toxicity. Acidosis (over-acidity or inflammation) and toxicity are the main causes of tissue failure, which can cause innumerable effects or symptoms. This is true especially when this "tissue failure" affects the endocrine gland system. These three causes are behind 99.9 percent of all diseases.

In thirty years of clinical work I have never seen a condition that could not tremendously improve, or in most cases completely disappear, with these methods of regeneration and detoxification. These two concepts are interdependent, as you cannot regenerate the body without detoxification. They are the twin pillars of health and vitality.

I have seen bones and backs straighten and strengthen themselves—from curvatures (scoliosis), old fractures, and similar conditions. I have also seen complete spinal cord severations reconnect after more than ten years. I have seen glands and all types of tissue rebuild themselves.

Your body is a living, conscious machine. It can rebuild itself after surgeries, major cuts and wounds, so why not after nerve damage or atrophy? The truth is, it can! But not on a diet of dead animals and other cooked, dead foods.

Regeneration has three main components to it: **Alkalize**, **Detoxify** and **Energize**. All three work together and are inseparable. Alkalization is vital to tissue regeneration because it is anti-inflammatory. It builds electrolytes for proper ionization, oxidation and neutralization. It allows for proper cellular respiration and for disbursement of nutrients throughout the body.

Detoxifying, of course, cleans all the obstructions, irritants and stimulants, like mucus, heavy metals, chemicals and pesticides out of your body. This allows for proper digestion, absorption, utilization and elimination.

Energizing your cells with energy from living foods is also vital to robust health. Without the power of *live* foods, which are full of nutrition and electricity, you cannot accomplish alkalization and detoxification.

Detoxification is the only way to establish a true homeostasis within the body. This homeostasis can then be elevated to unlimited heights.

Vitality and vibrancy should always be one's goal. Life then becomes exciting, joyful, and bubbling with energy.

Take the time for yourself and don't settle for anything less than total health—free of disease. The road to regeneration is not the easy way. It can be filled with ups and downs depending upon your toxicity levels and weaknesses. However, regeneration is the only way to lasting health, vitality and longevity.

Up to this point we have covered a lot of information about you—the type of species your physical body belongs to, and the types of food that are best suited for your body. We've examined how your physical, emotional and mental bodies work. We've discussed foods and their chemical make-up, and we've covered those foods and chemicals that are toxic to you. We've also covered various disease symptoms, what they are, and what causes them.

Now let's get to the heart of the matter: **What do we do about our health issues?** How do we start this journey into health? This chapter will begin with *Naturopathy and the Science of Detoxification*, and then cover the detoxification process in detail. You may want to tag this chapter for ongoing reference, as it will supply you with step-by-step guidelines, warnings, and hints to take you through this vital process.

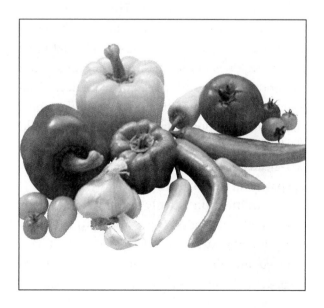

☀ Naturopathy and the Science of Detoxification

Naturopathy is one of the greatest sciences, for it is the study and practice of nature. Its basic foundation is health and vitality, and it encompasses all aspects of nature that influence regeneration.

In nature, all forms of life consume some sort of food to sustain health. Most of nature eats intuitively. Human beings have lost a great deal of this intuitiveness, and therefore they primarily consume what society teaches them to eat. Since money is one of the major motivating factors in today's world, many products and foods are sold for financial gain at the expense of personal health. As our species has become the sickest and most disease-ridden on this planet, Naturopathy was born out of a desire to regain this lost intuition for what truly are the appropriate foods to sustain human life.

As we've discussed previously, your body is like an engine that requires a fuel source, but it needs to be cleaned and rebuilt as time goes on. If you use bad fuels, your car won't run properly and will eventually stop running. The same is true of your body. Since men and women have chosen to fill their bodies with bad fuels—foods that leave a lot of residues in their tissues—they must clean the body out, or suffer the consequences. **Diseases are nothing more than signs and symptoms that reflect the body's need to clean and rebuild itself.** Fresh, uncooked foods, especially fruits, are self-cleansing. They not only feed the body, they keep it clean internally as well.

Detoxification is truly a science and an art unto itself; a necessary response to the consumption of toxic and congestive foods that have clogged and obstructed the human body. In nature, detoxification is a continual process that all of life goes through, at one level or another. The process of cleaning your body of toxins, mucus and acidosis can create symptoms that are seen as diseases by some doctors, and so we have been taught to fear this natural process.

All life in the physical world takes in energy, metabolizes it, and then excretes the remains and by-products. Most of the time this is done automatically. However, the human is the only species on this planet that *chooses* to eat foods that are not harmonious with its species. Humans also *choose* to alter the chemistry and energy of the foods they eat by processing and cooking them. This changes the nature of these foods and the way they are metabolized. Many of these foods then become irritating, mucus-forming, and inflammatory to the body. Some foods, like processed grains and dairy products, act like glue in your tissues; and others, like meat and processed foods, contain deadly chemicals and heavy metals. Added to this destructive situation is the chemicalized air we breathe and the products we use on our bodies and in our homes. The external environment also exerts its influence. "Acid rain" has resulted from so much acidic air pollution from factories. Now, almost every breath we take is acid-forming.

All these toxic and mucus-forming substances will change the way the body eliminates. In other words, cooked and processed foods slow down body elimination and, in most cases, the toxic by-products of these foods are stored or plaqued in the tissues. This blocks proper cellular respiration, causing a cell to become hypoactive, slowly losing its ability to function.

Many disease symptoms are nothing more than the body's effort to eliminate these stored toxins and mucus, some of which we began storing *in utero*. Most pregnant women consume milk, meat and other toxic foods, thinking that they are building bones and muscle tissue in the fetus. This, however, just adds to her toxicity and acidosis, thus increasing tissue weakness. The same is happening in her fetus.

The body is always trying to keep itself clean and strong by means of detoxification. This is done through sweating caused by fevers, by vomiting, diarrhea, frequent urination, colds, flus, and by simple daily elimination. The more toxic a person becomes, the stronger the purging will be. Take simple bronchitis, for example. If the first time your body had symptoms of bronchitis you went to your doctor and he or she gave you antibiotics, or even extremely high doses of vitamin C, the symptoms of bronchitis would stop. These remedies did not cure the inflammation and congestion, they merely stopped the elimination process or symptoms. Results like these give the illusion that the condition was cured. However, the next time your body tries to clean itself out, it could have symptoms of pneumonia. This is because bronchitis and pneumonia are not diseases but are merely inflammatory/congestive conditions trying to be eliminated by the body. Your symptoms can become worse and penetrate deeper because you did not allow the lungs and bronchi to clean themselves out properly the first time.

Throughout your life no one told you that many of the foods you were eating caused this congestion in the first place. So you continued eating foods that created additional accumulations of mucus and congestion. After a while, the body again reached the point where it needed to clean these congestions, and this caused you to experience an even deeper level of cleansing.

If you always stop your body from eliminating the congestion and toxins that you put into it, eventually you can create lymph node swelling, and then tumors, from holding all these toxins and mucus too long.

Your whole body comes into play during these cleansing cycles—or what we call a "**healing crisis**," which may include fevers, sweats, coughing, mucus discharge, diarrhea, skin rashes and much more (See Module 6.6, *The Healing Crisis*). During these healing crises the functioning of your immune system is enhanced, as well as your eliminative organs, including the skin. This is why it is important never to treat, but to detoxify and regenerate. In the detoxification process the body will clean itself out. Many people, including healthcare practitioners, do not understand this process as they should.

True Naturopathy includes the science of detoxification and cellular regeneration. Because of the status-quo "treatment" mentality, many people use natural products, such as vitamins, minerals and herbs to treat symptoms. I use **only herbs** to assist the body in its detoxification efforts and to enhance the function of cells in related or weakened tissues, organs and glands. Herbs are also highly nutritious, as they are non-hybrid vegetables.

Common sense is, in medicine, the master workman.

— Anonymous

☀ Obstructions and Detoxification

In reviewing acidosis it is important to learn its effects not only on the cells, but also on the nutrients and constituents you consume by eating, drinking and breathing. The word associated with acidosis is **"anionic,"** which means basically **a state or condition of coagulation.** In other words, when the body becomes acidic from what you eat, drink and/or breathe, this sets up a chain reaction causing inflammation and a clustering of the nutrients that are in the blood and tissues of your body.

The reason for digestion is simply to break down and separate food compounds (like proteins or complex sugars) into their simplest forms (amino acids, simple sugars, etc.) so the cells can use them (**catabolic processes**). With this understanding, you can see that by "clustering" these simple elements or compounds, the cells can't use them. They become "obstructions," which are now called "free radicals." These free radicals are like terrorists to the body and can damage your cells.

Added to the above is the accumulated mucus and congestion from the reaction of your mucosa to stimulants, foreign proteins and abrasive foods. This mucus, of course, becomes highly obstructive. Most of us know this well from sinus blockages, sore throats, blurred vision, and other congestive conditions.

Pain is a sign of obstructions or blockages. Pain is a reflex condition wherein the energy that is constantly flowing through the pathways of the body becomes blocked and bottled up. The body will also send additional energy to areas that need healing, since energy is the healer. However, this can create even greater energy blockages. As previously stated, acidosis from acid-forming elements creates inflammation, which in turn can create energy obstructions. Acupuncture, acupressure and therapeutic touch are modalities that "unblock" the "dammed-up" energy and allow it to start flowing again. This unblocking will relieve the pain in most cases, and also increase blood and lymph flow to the related areas.

You must remove the obstructions and acidosis. If you don't, the cause remains, as you've only treated the effect, which can be swelling, pain, or other symptoms. These are nothing more than the natural defenses of the body in response to the cause. Detoxification is the only logical answer that will yield a lasting cure. Alkalization is the method by which detoxification starts. Alkalization neutralizes acidosis. Detoxification not only alkalizes the body, but also gives the body the added energy it needs to clean itself out.

MENTAL AND EMOTIONAL DETOXIFICATION

True detoxification must take place from all levels within you. We have been talking throughout this book about the power that your mind and emotions have upon your health. If you want to be successful in attaining true health and vitality, you must detox your thoughts, emotions *and* your physical body.

All matter is comprised of atoms, which are the basic building blocks of the universe. The movement of these atoms creates electromagnetic energy, which creates magnetism. Movement creates, and is a reflection of, two opposite poles or forces—positive and negative. Energy simply fluxes between these two opposites. These twins are called the *yin* (negative) and *yang* (positive) in Chinese Medicine. These positive and negative energies, although being of the same essence, have different effects upon you and your body.

For example, the emotional states of anger and love will affect your thoughts and your physical body in different ways. Anger creates stress and constricts the blood and lymphatic flow within the body. It shuts down the liver and pancreas, affecting digestion. It overstresses the adrenal glands causing excessive hormone and neurotransmitter release. All this causes acidosis. Love, on the other hand, creates the opposite. It increases the blood and lymph flow. It improves digestion and kidney elimination. And it alkalizes your body. Anger obstructs and restricts, and love opens and expands. You could also say that anger causes "dis-ease" and love heals.

From a spiritual viewpoint each of our emotions is integral to creation, for the whole is merely the sum of its parts. They will each have their own lessons to teach you. You can judge whether one is good or bad for you at any partic-ular time and respond accordingly, or you can merely observe the flow of these emotions and their opposites, not allowing them to affect you in any way, unless you want them to. You must decide what you want in your life and in your body.

I will let you in on a little secret. When you begin to increase the energy of your physical body through detoxification, you will start detoxifying in *all* your bodies. Thoughts and emotions stick like glue to your cells and create subtle obstructions that you can carry for a lifetime (some say for many lifetimes). So, if you start crying or yelling during your detoxification process, this is the reason. Let it all come out. Be observant of your thoughts and feelings, and try not to hold on to anything. Let these obstructions go. In this way, your river of energy and love can dominate inside you once again. This is truly the road to vitality and spirituality.

MODULE 6.3

☼ How Do We Get the Body to Detoxify?

Ours is an alkaline species. Acid-forming foods cause inflammation and congestion in the body, creating an anionic situation. This reaction causes nutrients, blood cells, etc., to start sticking together, and encourages the formation of lipids and oxalate stones of all types. Thus, nutrients become unavailable to cells, which leads to cellular starvation.

Because acidosis is inflammatory and destructive to cells, the body will use steroids, electrolysis, water, lipids (cholesterol), and other things to fight this. This causes dehydration both extracellularly and intracellularly.

The first thing to do is to change the intake from acid-forming foods to alkaline-forming foods. Consumption of alkaline-forming foods, which are mainly fruits and vegetables, will begin the detoxification and rehydration process. If you wish to speed up the cleansing process, these fruits and vegetables must all be raw, i.e., uncooked and unprocessed. If you wish to dig deeper into tissue and speed the process up even further, you can switch to all raw, fresh fruits only. Fruits have the highest amounts of anti-oxidants and astringent properties of all foods. Their sugars are slow burning but powerful, and will enhance the vitality of cells faster than any other food, and with much less digestive effort. They also have the highest electrical properties of any food. The energies in raw fruits are so high that they speed up neuron transport and endocrine function.

TAKE IT EASY

Because raw fruits are so powerful in detoxifying and restoring vitality it is important to note here that **one can detoxify too fast.** This can lead to extreme cleansing symptoms. I have witnessed many severe reactions such as: multiple abscesses popping out in the mouth, tumor-like swellings all over the body, the skin actually opening and oozing pus, and even spitting out tumors. This is only because the individual jumped immediately from a typical diet of dairy foods, flesh foods and toxic chemicals to a highly pure and cleansing one of fresh, raw fruits. A fruit diet will stir up the toxins and mucus in the body in an aggressive manner, leaving you with some very noticeable side effects. However, if you consume an all-raw food diet of both fruits and vegetables for a few weeks first, this will allow for a much slower and generally easier cleansing process.

One of the deepest ways to detoxify yourself is through water fasting. **I do not, however, recommend water fasting in chronic and especially degenerative cases where the patient has little energy in the first place.**

The process of detoxification is not always fun. Most of the more difficult cases are from cancer, HIV, or spinal cord injuries where the individual has become very toxic. Remember, the body will start eliminating anything that should not be in it, even to the point of eliminating weak tissue (like fingernails), and weak muscle tissue. This sounds more gruesome than it is, but you should know what the body will do to clean itself out. The body can tear itself down to a frightening level to rid itself of its weaknesses and toxins. However, rest assured that the body *will* rebuild itself beautifully. If your house burned partially down, you would have to remove the old burned material before you could properly rebuild it.

Your body has to do the same. Most doctors run in fear of this, even though it's a normal process of nature. Nature always eliminates the weak and replaces it with the strong. The same thing can be said of the cells.

If you have toxic chemicals stored in your body you may experience heart palpitations as you cleanse. This is rare, but it can happen. Remember that we have toxins stored deep within us from as far back as when we were in our mother's womb. Don't expect to clean this out overnight. However, I have seen lymphomas disappear in forty-five days, stomach cancer gone in fifty-nine days, and diabetes eliminated in sixty days.

The body will also promote its own diaphoresis (process of perspiration) by increasing its systemic temperature to dilate, sweat and kill parasites. The good thing is that this process does not last long, and the cleaner you get internally, the less cleansing is needed. You may only need to go through one, two or three cycles of this to overcome most disease symptoms.

FOR THE REST OF YOUR LIFE

Life is a constant process of consuming and eliminating. You will be detoxifying for the rest of your life at one level or another; especially if you eat fresh fruits and vegetables on a regular basis. Your body will keep digging deeper and deeper within itself, cleansing and restoring proper functions. Most of this processing then becomes very subtle. You won't know it is even going on, except for occasional symptoms of mucus discharge, cold-type symptoms, or aches and pains.

The body is amazingly designed and highly intelligent. If you learned all that is known about chemistry, biochemistry and physics, you still would not understand much about the human body and how it works. Always ask the question: "What is my body doing this for?" There is always a reason why your body does what it does in any situation. We only have to learn the language of the body to understand what it is doing and why. (See Chapter 5, Module 5.11, *Body Language*). Observation and common sense almost always supersede science. Although science started out by observation and common sense, it has become very biased, yielding to industry and high finances.

To discover the real benefits of a natural healing program or healing modality ask yourself: "What can it do for me in fixing the cause of my problem? Can it help me gain vitality, health, and longevity? Most importantly, does it aid in my spiritual unfolding or awakening?" Vibrant health, in which body, emotions, mind and soul are brought into harmony, is true spirituality.

Remember, true Naturopathy is the study of nature and how nature sustains its own health. When human beings finally learn the basic truths of nature, they too will be able to restore health. Detoxification is the golden key that unlocks the magic door of nature and allows regeneration and vitality to take place. Always keep it simple.

Since detoxification is synonymous with alkalization, the next section will examine this process in relationship to the foods we eat.

MODULE 6.4

☀ Alkaline-Forming and Acid-Forming Foods and Detoxification

It is important to know a little about the foods you eat. As stated earlier, one of the most important factors about food is how it affects the pH of the body. Foods can be divided into two basic categories: foods that have an acid reaction in your body and foods that have an alkaline reaction. This is not necessarily related to the pH of the food itself.

Alkalinity is the great detoxifier of the body, so foods that are alkaline-forming will detoxify the body. The more alkaline-forming they are, the greater and deeper you will detoxify. Fruits, in general, are an example of high alkaline-forming foods. Alkaline constituents are also used to feed the body. They are truly the regenerators.

Acid-forming foods slow, inhibit or stop the detoxification process. They are inflammatory and mucus-forming to your body, ultimately causing tissue failure. Acids can become free radicals, causing tissue damage unless linked to an antioxidant (which is alkaline) and removed.

Acids are necessary, however, for ionization and oxidation.

Don't be fooled. Foods either feed, clean and rebuild you, or they destroy you. Some foods fill you full of mucus, congestion and inflammation, which leads to hypoactivity or failure of cells, tissues, organs and glands. Let your foods be your health and medicine, not the cause of your disease. Now let's discuss the differences between these two food types.

ALKALINE-FORMING FOODS

I compare alkaline foods to winter. They cool and soothe inflamed tissues, heal ulcerations and enhance cellular functions. These foods leave mainly calcium, magnesium, sodium and potassium ash after they have been digested, yielding mainly an alkaline reaction and condition.

The human is predominately an alkaline species. Most of our bodily fluids are (or should be) alkaline, including the blood, saliva, urine, synovial fluids, cerebral fluids and the digestive enzymes (except those in the stomach). If these fluids become acidic, deterioration and death can result. We have only one acid chamber in the body, the stomach. Here proteins are initially broken apart. Your mouth, pancreatic and intestinal enzymes are used for alkaline digestion.

It is vital to consume alkaline-forming foods if you want the detoxification process to take place. Alkalization is the key to your success at regenerating yourself and getting healthy. A good example of the importance of alkalization is found in emergency medicine. In hospital Emergency Rooms, or with other on-the-spot emergency treatments, one is almost always given an IV with normal saline, which is a sodium solution. Sodium is called "the great alkalizer." This helps reverse acidosis, the main reason we get into trouble in the first place. Acidosis equals pain, swelling and inflammation.

Raw fruits and vegetables act the same way that normal saline works, but are much more energizing and nutritional. You cannot alkalize yourself properly if you do not consume raw, ripe, living foods. Alkaline foods, like fresh fruits and vegetables, are the natural food of humans. You should eat at least 80-90 percent alkaline-forming foods.

ACID-FORMING FOODS

I compare acid foods to fire. Acid foods are high in sulfur, phosphorus and nitrogen. They are mainly protein (amino-acid-rich) foods. These foods include all meats, eggs, grains, beans, nuts, seeds, pasteurized dairy products and cooked tomatoes, to name a few.

Most animal protein foods are irritants to the mucosa and cells of the body, invoking an immune response. This causes your lymphatic system and mucosa to respond with mucus and lymph cells. Foreign proteins cause mucus production all through the body, creating congestive

issues. The more we consume, the more congestion we create, and the more we create, the more we store, until our lungs, sinus cavities, ear canals, and throat become saturated. The intestines also become saturated with this mucus. This brings parasites, increases white blood cells, and creates inflammation, all of which affect the body's ability to function properly. This congestion and inflammation eventually leads to cellular death.

The clearest example of this congestion and inflammation problem is seen with dairy products. These proteins are so abrasive to body tissues that many people can feel their lungs, sinuses, ears and throat becoming congested as they drink or eat these foods. Congestion will impair the function of the tissues in these areas as the mucus is stored or pushed deeper within the body. Much of this mucus and these toxins are stored or filtered through the lymphatic system, especially in the lymph nodes. (Lymphatic cancers are extremely high in the U.S.) The body is constantly trying to eliminate this congestion through processes like colds and flus, bronchitis, sneezing, and coughing. The conventional medical profession sees this effort by the body to eliminate these toxins and mucus as "diseases" and tries to stop this effect with toxic-chemical pharmaceuticals which only add to the problem. These preparations suppress the body's elimination of the mucus and/or poisons. The immune system becomes suppressed and overworked as it battles this tremendous insult to the body. Remember: what you don't eliminate, you accumulate. This eventually leads to chronic and degenerative issues, not to mention simple boils or tumor masses.

Many people eat predominantly acid foods. Consequently, notice how many types of inflammation (itis's), ulcerations, congestive disorders, and of course cancers dominate our world today. Because of the high nitrogen or phosphorus content of these foods, we lose our calcium and other electrolytes, as our body uses these alkaline minerals to buffer acid elements.

It is best to only have 10-20 percent of acid foods in your diet. Alkaline foods should especially be eaten in the spring, summer and fall when temperatures are warmer. In the cold alkaline winter, one should increase acid foods somewhat. Remember, opposites attract, creating harmony. When it's hot (acid) outside, you need to consume cold (alkaline) foods, and vice versa.

You may wish to look ahead at the Alkaline/Acid Food Chart now (see Chapter 7, *Module 7.2*). This chart will help you to know which foods are which. This section also explains how the alkaline or acid nature of foods is determined. Remember, because homo sapiens are an alkaline species, our bodies are biologically suited for predominately alkaline-forming foods. These foods will bring health and vitality, whereas acid-forming foods will bring disease and despair. The choice is yours.

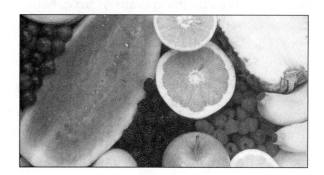

MODULE 6.5

☀ What to Expect During Detox

It is not uncommon to experience many side effects during detoxification. These include cold and flu-like symptoms, changes in bowel movements, pains of various types, fevers, heartburn, lung congestion, energy loss, swelling and itching, and even vomiting. In this section we will examine each of these possible side effects. Sometimes we will suggest ways to help the cleansing process along, or ways to alleviate the discomfort of this "healing crisis" as it is called. In general, we encourage you to continue on through these side effects in the direction of regeneration.

COLD AND FLU-LIKE SYMPTOMS

As the body begins to clean its lymphatic system, the sinus cavities, lungs and most other body tissues will become active in the cleansing process. **Do not stop this natural process.** This is the only true way to increase the function of your cells and to start your body on the path to regeneration.

You will begin to see a lot of mucus being discharged from the body. This mucus can be clear, yellow, green, and even brown or black. Occasionally you might find blood in the mucus. Don't panic. This blood has been there a while. Congestion is acidic and can cause inflammation and bleeding of tissue. The throat can get very sore. This is just mucus and toxins in the tissues trying to get out. It is best not to use cough drops. However, if you must, use only natural cough drops, like those made with Slippery Elm.

The effects of the cleansing process can range from very light (with just a runny nose and minor coughing), to heavy, with deep bronchial and lung expectoration. These deep-cleansing processes can become uncomfortable and sometimes scary. Trust that the body knows what it is doing.

The body will eliminate through any orifice that will be beneficial to it, including skin, ears, nose, mouth, kidneys and bowels. If you detoxify too fast and you're extremely toxic, the body may even open (split) the skin and push toxins out through the opening. An example of this was a patient who detoxified so fast that her skin above the "belly button" opened up and a small tumor popped out. I've seen quadriplegics, who develop a tremendous amount of toxicity because of inactivity, go through the same experience. The skin would open and pour toxins out.

The body can also feel achy all over. Relax. Conserve your energy so your body will do a thorough job of cleaning itself. Welcome these "healing" or "purging" processes. They are essential to well being. Sometimes it can take several months to get your body to have such a response. Keep your detoxification going.

Many people have accumulated sulfur from sulfa drugs, which are a major inhibitor of the lymphatic system. This sulfur must come out of your tissues before your lymphatic system can effectively and freely flow properly. Since your lymph is the vehicle for your immune cells and the sewer system for each cell in your body, you can see how important it is to keep this system moving. Be patient and persevere. It will all be worth it as you feel the life force surge through your body when it is clean.

The detoxification process will always take place as you increase energy and alkalize your body. Allow the body to clean itself out.

CHANGES IN BOWEL MOVEMENTS

It is vital that you have at least one bowel movement per day; however, two or three would be much better. Optimum bowel health means having a bowel movement thirty minutes after you eat. Many people move unnaturally three to six times or more per day from what is called IBS (irritable bowel syndrome), a catch phrase for inflammation within the GI tract.

If you have stools that are too loose or runny (e.g., diarrhea), use a good herbal bowel formula made from Slippery Elm Bark, Marshmallow

---

> ### A FEW DEFINITIONS
>
> - Gastritis is inflammation of the stomach.
> - Enteritis is inflammation of the small intestine.
> - Colitis is the inflammation of the colon or large intestine.
> - Diverticulitis is the inflammation of bowel (intestinal) pockets, which form from our S.A.D. (Standard American Diet).

Root, and/or Chamomile. These types of formulas will help firm your stools, and at the same time remove the toxicity and inflammation that cause diarrhea in the first place. Some formulas have bentonite clay and charcoal in them, which are also acceptable.

A raw food diet is essential to heal, repair, and strengthen the tissues of the GI tract. If you feel you cannot handle the roughage in raw foods, use the herbal bowel formula to buffer the discomfort. This will only be temporary, as it does not take long to reduce the inflammation in the GI tract.

Most people have the opposite problem: **constipation**. Constipation is very hard on the body in many ways, including the absorption of putrefaction from foods that are being held in the intestines. The destruction of the intestinal wall can also begin as a result, especially if these food residues become impacted. Keep the bowels moving with lots of fresh raw fruits and vegetables, and use a good bowel-corrective formula until your colon is clean and healthy.

The best bowel formulas are designed to accomplish the above plus restore and rebuild normal bowel peristalsis. (See Appendix C—*Resource Guide*—for companies that supply the best bowel formulas.) A good formula will strengthen and tone the bowel without addiction. It will also heal the inflammation and ulcerations from acid-food eating.

Chamomile or peppermint tea is great for inflamed bowels. Both teas soothe smooth muscle tissue. The consumption of 2-ounces of aloe vera juice three times a day is also very helpful. However, aloe may cause a little diarrhea. Two other botanicals that can reduce inflammation of the gastrointestinal tract are Slippery Elm and Marshmallow Root. Make a tea out of these by using 1 teaspoon of herb to 1 cup of water. Boil the tea for 8 minutes, then let it steep for another 5 minutes. Strain and drink. Taking 1 cupful, 3-6 times per day, would be an appropriate dose. NOTE: In case of severe constipation, you may need to add a more powerful purgative herb. This should be for short-term treatment, as these formulas can be very addicting. Also, colonics are highly recommended in these cases. (More on the use of colonics later in this chapter, see Module 6.12.)

ACHES AND PAIN

There can be many aches and pains during the cleansing and healing process. Wherever there is a weakness in the body, it will show itself through aches and pains. The body will tug, draw and pull the toxicity out of itself. This process can also cause pain in degenerative areas. These aches and pains are normal and should not be feared. Most will last anywhere from a few hours to a week. After the crisis (healing crisis), you will notice that particular area becoming much stronger than before.

Pain is a result of acidosis that has created inflammation. This can stimulate or degenerate the nervous system. Pain also develops where energy becomes blocked in the body from toxins, splinters, clots, cholesterol, acid crystalline deposits (uric, calciumate, etc.) and chemical medications.

We have been taught to treat the pain or get rid of the symptom. But, drugs that block pain may also block the healing process. In the science of natural health, however, we learn that the cause, not the symptom, must be eliminated.

Pain is our warning sign to stop and cleanse our bodies naturally. Masking the symptoms of pain by unnatural means can set the body up for future degenerative problems, as the cause of the pain is ignored. This allows for a continuation along the path of degeneration of tissues.

Pain can have many different levels depending on the degree of inflammation or tissue degeneration. However, in bone cancer, other types of cancer, shingles, and certain other conditions, it may become necessary to use a pain medication. Too much pain can weaken the spirit and the body to the point of death. Since pain medications cause constipation, the person taking them will want to stay on a bowel formula to enhance bowel management. It is necessary to always keep the bowels moving, especially when detoxifying, as this process creates an extra burden of toxins to be eliminated.

Working with the Detoxification Pain

For painful situations, alternating hot and cold compresses can be used. Arnica oil, used topically, can also help. Castor oil packs are also beneficial. When these methods are not enough, painful situations should be monitored closely by a healthcare professional. Remember that pain is acid. Alkalize yourself always.

VOMITING

Most people do not vomit unless they are extremely toxic or have been on many chemical medications, which can accumulate in the tissue of the stomach. Vomiting is quite normal when the stomach needs to eliminate toxins and mucus quickly. Some people will even vomit worms or parasites that have developed in the upper GI tract. However, vomiting is rarely experienced on this program.

What to Do For Vomiting

Vomiting is the natural way the body uses to clean the stomach when too many poisons, mucus, toxins or parasites have accumulated within its tissues. Ginger, Mint or Chamomile tea will help soothe the stomach and ease the spasms. These teas will help promote liver and intestinal function, aiding in your relief.

FEVERS (THERMOTHERAPY)

Fevers are a natural process that your body uses to eliminate toxins quickly, including pus, mucus, parasites and even unwanted cells. Your skin is your body's largest eliminative organ. According to the American Medical Association, the body eliminates upwards of two pounds or more of wastes per day through the skin under normal circumstances. When the body is cleansing even more elimination is needed.

Most adults will develop fevers under or around 103° Fahrenheit. Always drink plenty of pure water and fresh fruit or vegetable juices during times of cleansing. Never let the body dehydrate. You can use cold showers, baths, or a cold wash cloth on the forehead or on the back of the neck to cool yourself down a little.

Children can naturally have fevers of 104° to 105° Fahrenheit, so don't panic. Again, the most important issue in these cases is hydration. Many parasites are killed during these high fevers through both heat and the increase of white blood cells.

It has been stated that fevers above 106° kill cancer cells. At 110° Fahrenheit, you begin to kill your healthy cells. Elevated temperatures are created from the thyroid gland and hypothalamus by the cellular release of interleukin-1, which then stimulates and releases the prostaglandin E2 (PGE2) from the hypothalamus, which in turn creates diaphoresis (sweating). This dilates the vascular system and creates activity in the sweat glands. Sweating pushes the toxins out through the skin; these toxins are then oxidized (eaten by skin mites) or washed away. This is vital in assisting the body in proper elimination. Fevers stimulate the immune sys-

tem to increase white blood cells and interferon. This enhances the immune system considerably, calling out its army to do battle.

The body has its own intelligence; we only need to understand it. Never fear a natural process that the body uses to help itself stay healthy. Fevers are just one of the mechanisms used to accomplish this. Don't fear a fever—understand it! If you fear anything about fevers, it would be dehydration. Most people, through acidosis, are always dehydrated to some degree. Learn all you can about the ways of nature. This will help you immensely on your journey toward health and vitality.

Working with a Fever Caused by Detoxification

In case of high fever, keep yourself hydrated. Drink plenty of distilled water, fresh fruit juices or vegetable juices. You can place a cold cloth on the back of the neck and forehead, and you can also take a cold bath. Do not suppress this natural reaction of the body. NOTE: Liquid minerals may be added to your water or juice for better hydration. This can be very important in highly depleted cases.

GENERAL INFLAMMATION

Inflammation does not always need to be eliminated. Inflammation from a histamine response is one method the body uses to dilate the vascu-

---

FACTS ABOUT DEHYDRATION

- Acidosis leads to dehydration, and dehydration leads to acidosis.

- Eating predominately cooked food leads to dehydration.

- Dehydration leads to hypoactivity of tissue, eventually leading to tissue death.

lar system, which brings in additional blood and immune factors during a crisis or when an irritant is involved. Hot and cold compresses can help. There are many anti-inflammatory botanicals available, e.g., Wild Yam Root, Marshmallow Root, Slippery Elm, Comfrey (leaves and root). Inflammation is always acidic, so alkalize, alkalize and alkalize! Raw fruits and vegetables are your best alkalizers. Sodium is called the "Great Alkalizer."

HEARTBURN

Heartburn is a result of acidosis of the stomach and intestinal tract. Wrong food combinations cause fermentation and putrefaction, bringing on this acidosis or over-acid condition. Eating too much acid-forming food also creates heartburn. This is especially true in meat eaters where hydrochloric acid is over-produced. Eating too many grain products and/or cooked tomatoes can cause severe heartburn. A lack of pancreatic enzymes causes poor digestion, which can also create heartburn and gas.

Poor production of sodium of bicarbonate from the pancreas, as well as poor bile flow or production from the liver/gallbladder also causes acid reflux. Many times, gallstones block the bile duct so that the bile flow is restricted. Additionally, a weak sphincter muscle (like a door) between the esophagus and stomach allows stomach acids to regurgitate back up the esophagus yielding acid reflux.

The detoxification and regeneration program recommended in this book does not cause heartburn. However, because the nature of raw foods is "energy," you may experience some stimulation of these conditions temporarily.

Working with Heartburn During Detoxification

Ginger tea is excellent for heartburn. In this situation, food combinations must be scrutinized. If improper eating, including improper food combining, has occurred, an apple will help. Apples contain strong digestive enzymes and will aid digestion greatly. You can also make a tea from other soothing herbs: Chamomile flowers, Gentian Root, Slippery Elm Bark, or Marshmallow Root to help heal the gastric walls. Alkalize, alkalize, alkalize! It's the only true way to health.

LUNG CONGESTION

The lungs will attempt to clean themselves out of mucus and toxins. In asthma, emphysema, and C.O.P.D. (chronic obstructive pulmonary disease) where the adrenal glands are also involved, tissue spasms can be a problem. This can block or inhibit one's ability to breathe. This is when an herbal antispasmodic is invaluable. It will stop the spasms, but allow your lungs to expectorate the congestion.

If one really wants to cure lung condition and he or she is using an inhaler, success will be moderate. I recommend the use of an herbal antispasmodic in place of an inhaler. However, if you are advanced in your condition, you may need to use your inhaler periodically. Some people are on four or more different inhalers, which is potentially a very dangerous situation. Some current research has even indicated that inhalers may be carcinogenic.

The main problem with inhalers is their lymphatic-inhibiting properties. They not only dilate your breathing passages, but they do so by inhibiting expectoration. On the other hand, herbal antispasmodics dilate and allow for proper breathing, but they also allow for expectoration. Expectoration is the removal or elimination of congestion within the tissues of the lungs. This is vital for greater oxygen exchange. Many herbs, like Comfrey Root, Chickweed, Marshmallow Root and Yerba Santa Leaf, can help rebuild lung tissue.

Chronic asthmatics and those who have chronic lung problems must be careful as they approach detoxification. Better to start out with

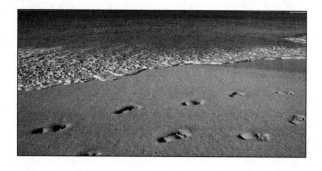

70 percent raw foods and 30 percent cooked, which will allow cleansing to proceed slowly and gently.

Remember your adrenal glands. They play a vital role in why your lungs spasm. Underactive adrenal glands can create low neurotransmitter production, which weakens the nervous system to the lungs. This can result in sensitivity and irritability of the nervous system. Add to this a hypofunction of the thyroid, which causes low calcium utilization, and you have spastic conditions of your tissues. Clean your lungs out. Enhance the function of your adrenal glands, and check the basal temperatures of your body to determine thyroid involvement (calcium utilization). It is highly suggested that a health care professional closely monitor this process in advanced lung conditions.

Working with Asthma and Lung Congestion During Detoxification

Asthmatics and people with lung congestion may use a castor oil pack with hot cayenne compresses placed over the lung area on the chest. (Directions for making and administering a castor oil pack are given in Chapter 10.) Drinking a cup of Peppermint tea followed every ten minutes with a teaspoon of the tincture of Lobelia (up to 6 teaspoons). Lobelia is an antispasmodic at low doses and an emetic at higher doses. This might induce vomiting in some individuals. Vomiting will compress the lungs and expel the phlegm.

Alternating hot and cold compresses are also good—apply a hot compress for 2 minutes, followed by cold compress for 2 minutes, then another round or two of each. You may wish to use an antispasmodic herbal formula. This will control the spasms allowing you to breathe and to expectorate the mucus.

LOSS OF ENERGY OR EXHAUSTION

As stored toxins are broken up and released from the tissues into the blood system, the side effects of that particular toxin or poison may be re-experienced. Generally speaking, the older the individual, the greater the accumulated toxins. Glandular weaknesses, lowered immune system functioning, unhappiness, chronic lung involvement, thyroid and adrenal weakness, and malabsorption are all factors that can cause serious energy loss. Sugar imbalances can also cause energy changes. More rest is needed at different times, especially when all stimulants (like coffee, tea, and refined sugars) are removed from the diet.

We are a society that relies on stimulants for energy. This eventually weakens our true energy centers, the glands. When we stop our intake of stimulants, we can experience a whiplash effect and feel quite fatigued. This will soon pass with the ingestion of living foods and juices. It is important to understand that the S.A.D. (Standard American Diet) is weakening your physical body, not strengthening it. Those foods create a lot of inflammation and toxicity in tissues. When you add stimulation to this package you can begin to see why we develop tissue failure.

Most cases of "Chronic Fatigue Syndrome" *are not* the Epstein-Barr virus. This virus can cause fatigue. However, it is an easy virus to kill. (If, in fact, a virus is an organism. Because viruses are so small, an electron microscope must be used to see them. "Viruses" are considered by many scientists to be more of a protein, which involves an immune response, instead of a single-celled living organism, like bacteria.)

The real cause of so much fatigue in our society is thyroid and adrenal weaknesses. When these two endocrine glands are weak, the results can be fatigue, depression and anxiety. These glands must be regenerated if you truly wish to overcome chronic fatigue. This will not happen overnight, but if you persist you will be successful. A raw food diet and herbal formulas are the secret.

Working with Lack of Energy or Fatigue During Detox

The stoppage of all stimulating foods can cause a large energy loss. This is especially true if a person has hypoactive thyroid or adrenal glands. These are your energy glands, which become weakened from acidosis and toxicity. Stimulating foods actually have a negative effect on these glands making them weaker instead of stronger. The constant stimulation from coffee, tea, etc., hides this fact from you. Most of our energy throughout our lives comes from stimulated cellular activity.

Energy should be dynamic, not stimulated. Drinking 3–6, 10-ounce glasses of carrot, spinach and celery juice per day will help increase energy levels. Eating as much fresh, ripe fruit as possible will help. Panax Ginseng extract, Royal Jelly, Alfalfa, Barley Green Complex, and/or a well-balanced super-food complex, will also aid in increasing energy levels. (See the Resource Guide for where to find the finest super-food blends.) Rest and time are also great healers.

SWELLING AND ITCHING

There can be many swellings that erupt from the skin during detox. Tumors can even become larger before they are dissolved. Most swellings are short-lived, however, so it is important to keep up the fruit during these times.

Itching is another factor in detoxification. This is mostly caused by a fungal or Candida involvement. An individual can develop itching and redness of the skin anywhere.

Remedies for Itching During Detoxification

Angelica Root, Aloe Vera, or Chickweed applied topically can ease the itching. If itching continues, the fungal infestation needs to be killed and the lymph they live in must be cleaned. This requires herbal lymphatic and parasite formulas and a raw food diet.

OTHER SIDE EFFECTS DURING DETOXIFICATION

Other side effects may include, but are not limited to: excessive menstruation; frequent or deep coughing; frequent urination; headaches; diarrhea; numbness; tingling of the arms, legs, hands and feet; skin eruptions and gas.

During this cleansing and healing process, old symptoms of past diseases or weaknesses may return and then disappear as the body heals that particular area. These are old, toxic problems that were originally suppressed; and now the body has worked its way into these areas to rebuild and restore normal tissue function. In one case, an Amish woman who had poison ivy over twenty years ago had treated it with chemical medications and "cured" it (supposedly). On her detoxification program, her poison ivy came back in exactly the same places where she had treated it before. This was amazing even to me. You can clean out old, suppressed toxicity from when you were a child, or even from when you were still inside your mother's womb.

LIMITING OR STOPPING THE USE OF PHARMACEUTICALS

If you are taking chemical medications and you wish to limit their use, or stop them completely as you approach this process of detoxification and regeneration, here are some of the things that I, personally, would do:

FIRST — This program normalizes blood sugars. If I were a diabetic, I would watch my sugars daily and adjust my insulin accordingly or have my doctor help me.

SECOND — This program lowers blood pressure when it is too high, and raises it when it is too low. If I were taking medications for high blood pressure I would monitor my blood pressure regularly. I would not want to give myself hypotension or low blood pressure. This could make you faint, have equilibrium problems, or worse. It's not wise.

THIRD — I would always reduce my use of medications slowly. However, high blood pressure and diabetes may require a more rapid termination of medication and can be done without side effects.

Some medications "lock" you in and cause your body to become addicted to them. This is especially true with neurological medications and some steroids like prednisone. Always ask your doctor to help you. If he or she refuses, then you have no choice but to do it for yourself. Many medical doctors get angry and upset if their patients try to help themselves. Many if not most allopathic doctors have no training and education in detoxification and regeneration; therefore they tend to disparage what they don't know. This viewpoint leaves many disgruntled people to seek their own ways. This is one reason why this book is being written. Remember, it's always your choice. Live healthy, live medication free.

Note: It is rare to have reactions between herbs and medications. However, it is always possible. Simply observe yourself and how you feel. You will know if the things you are taking are reacting with each other or not. Use common sense and work with your natural health practitioner.

Summary

Most individuals do not experience many of the previously explained symptoms. In general, the more toxic the person, the stronger the "healing crisis" that may occur. Always remember that a healing crisis is very important and extremely beneficial. The symptoms or discomforts are all part of the cleansing process, as the toxins and poisons in the body must be expelled.

Generally the healing crisis is short-lived, so give it time and be patient. Be sure you are eating all raw foods—mainly fresh fruits and fresh juices. Most fruits have strong antioxidant and astringent properties for helping the body rid itself of toxins. If you do not feel like eating, do not eat. Let the body rest and be sure to drink plenty of fresh juices or pure water. Do not let the body dehydrate.

If your diet is 80 percent or more of fresh, raw, uncooked fruits and vegetables, **all your symptoms will be due to the "process of detoxifying"** that your body is putting itself through. If your diet is 50/50, your symptoms may be more of an acid condition. This can keep your healing crisis hanging on for days.

You may also wish to use botanical formulas to assist the cleanse. Resting and having a positive mental attitude are essential as well. If the healing crisis has lasted more than two to three weeks and you need a break from this process, just begin eating cooked foods again. This will lower the body's energy causing the cleansing action to stop. However, it is highly recommended to push the cleansing as long as possible. Detoxification *always* leads to vitality. **In the end, detoxification will bring vibrant health, vitality and spirituality.**

☀ The "Healing Crisis"

The following are some examples of the "Healing Crisis" that can happen during the cleansing processes. During my thirty years of detoxification experience I have witnessed so many different types of healing "crises" that I do not have the space to cover them all. This section deals with the most common side effects, many of which I have undergone from my own detoxification efforts.

I have divided these cleansing side effects into three categories: Mild, Moderate and Strong. Each of these levels may be experienced at one time or another. However, most people do not experience the strong levels. It all depends upon one's level of toxicity, combined with his or her systemic (total body) energies or strength.

MILD CLEANSING EFFECTS

- Cold and flu-like symptoms
- Low-grade fevers (99°–100° Fahrenheit)
- Coughing with or without discharge
- Clear and yellow mucus discharge from nose or throat (lungs, bronchi, etc.; this mucus may include blood)
- Minor aches and pains
- Mucus in stools
- Mucus in urine
- Loss of energy (may go up and down)
- Rashes and itching
- Disease symptoms increasing temporarily
- Mucus from eyes
- Mild headaches
- Minor blurred vision
- Minor vertigo
- Weight loss (average 8-15 lbs. in two weeks. Depends upon level of thyroid weakness. Can be as little as 2 lbs.)

- Chills
- Emotions rising up, such as mild crying, anger or even laughter
- Short term nose bleeds
- Some rectal bleeding (hemorrhoids or lesions)
- Minor blood in urine

MODERATE CLEANSING EFFECTS

- Symptoms of bronchitis or pneumonia
- Heavy discharges of green to brown mucus from nose and throat (lungs, bronchi, etc.)
- Pain in joints
- Heavy discharge from kidneys (urine color changes to brown, orange or dark yellow, etc.)
- Pain in old injuries or in degenerative areas of the body
- Minor paralysis of limbs
- Chronic fatigue symptoms
- Nosebleeds
- Spasms of the lungs in asthma/emphysema/C.O.P.D.
- Moderate shortness of breath (asthma, emphysema, C.O.P.D.)
- Temporary increase in tumor size
- Disease symptoms magnifying (short-lived)
- Sores appearing on the skin
- Oozing of innumerable substances from the skin, especially from the hands and feet
- Bruising
- Weak muscle breakdown (muscle built from meat protein)
- Heavy mucus discharge from eyes and ears
- Vomiting
- Diarrhea
- Cellulitis "clumping"
- Dizziness and/or vertigo

- Minor heart palpitations
- Loose teeth (minor)
- Minor abscesses in mouth
- Migraines
- High-grade fever (103° to 105° Fahrenheit)
- Deep coughing (sometimes dry). Use herbs to loosen and eliminate (expectorate) the impacted mucus.
- Depression or anxieties
- Emotional releasing (crying, anger, laughter, etc.)
- Heavy thoughts (lack of clarity)
- Skin splitting where heavy toxins exist
- Excessive itching
- Mercury tooth fillings can be pushed out by the body
- Rectal bleeding from past or present hemorrhoids or lesions

You may experience one or several of the above cleansing effects. Don't panic. You want these. I love to see dark-green mucus coming out of my patients. That's an excellent sign that they are doing the program correctly and are benefiting from it.

It is always smart to work with a qualified healthcare practitioner who has had advanced experience with detoxification and its side effects.

STRONG CLEANSING EFFECTS

- Paralysis of any part of the body
- Black mucus discharges from the lungs
- Heavy brown discharge or blood in the urine with associated kidney pain
- Heavy black discharge from the bowels with diarrhea
- Tumors popping out all over the body
- Loss of sight
- Loss of hearing
- Severe dizziness (or vertigo)
- Severe fatigue
- Abscesses developing all through the mouth
- Loss of fingernails or toenails

- Excessive weight loss (this can result when a pancreatic weakness exists)
- Severe shortness of breath (use an antispasmodic or inhaler)
- Temporary deep depression, released through crying, anger, laughter, etc.
- Mental confusion
- Skin cracking open
- Teeth becoming loose (major)
- Old suppressed symptoms (like the case of "poison ivy") reappear

Most people do not experience this severe level of detoxification. It depends upon the individual and how toxic he or she is. How many medications a person is taking is also a factor. A few people who have chosen to suppress their body's need to cleanse itself (through steroids like prednisone) will have some deeper issues. However, those who are more likely to experience the severe effects are the chronically toxic from birth, who manifest cancer, H.I.V. and/or other serious illnesses.

TWO CASES OF CLEANSING

Let's examine two cases that exemplify the healing crisis.

Case #1

A thirty-six-year-old female with pancreatic cancer. This was the degenerative type of cancer that shut her pancreas down. Very little of any digestive activity was left. When she ate any food, it came out in her stools the same way it was eaten. Her gastrin levels were extremely high. During her program she had at least forty golf-ball-size tumors "pop" out all over both legs. The medical doctor told her that her cancer had spread throughout her body. However, I kept her on a fruit diet and within three weeks or so the leg tumors were all gone.

A month later she went to the dentist because one of her teeth became loose. The dentist told her it was abscessed and pulled it. When she found a second loose tooth, the dentist again recommended pulling it. Luckily, her monthly appointment to see me took place before the second tooth extraction. I told her it was just a symptom of her healing crisis and to be patient.

By the following week her mouth was full of abscesses and most of her teeth were loose. But a week or so later, all the abscesses were gone. All her teeth were tight and her mouth felt "clean" and healthier than ever. Her sense of taste improved dramatically as well. After eleven months there was no cancer left, and she is alive and well today.

Case #2

A thirty-two-year-old female who had a C3-C4 cervical spine severation from a head-on collision. She had been immobile for twelve years. Besides the standard healing (cleansing) processes, she went through some tough emotional releasing. One night she might call me crying deeply. The next night she would call me laughing uncontrollably. This emotional release went on for almost two months. Her caregiver wanted to hang me! However, I assured him that this was her emotional body cleaning itself out. The car crash that left her paralyzed in her late teens had also resulted in the death of the other driver. For twelve years she had held in all the feelings that you can imagine would be associated with such a situation. To make a long story short, in eleven months she had total neurological reconnection, with free and conscious movement of any part of her body, with total feeling. Because the cleansing had assisted her in removing this deep grief, she also became more emotionally stable and her healing process was accelerated.

These two cases are among thousands that I have witnessed in my thirty years as a healer, yet they represent extremes. Some healing crises deserve the "Wow" factor, as these two did, but most are the "Oh, that was nothing . . ." type.

Most of you will probably have mild to moderate symptoms at most.

No matter what your healing crisis looks like, never lose sight of your goal: total health. Achieving your goal will be worth the discomfort of any symptoms.

Never fear a healing crisis or cleansing, as these are as natural as the sunrise every morning. Look forward to these cleansings. With each one you will feel better, and you'll be much healthier for your efforts.

END RESULTS OF A CLEANSING PROCESS

- Increased energy—many times more dynamic and dramatic
- Deeper breathing (greater lung capacity)
- Increased sense of smell, taste, and hearing
- Tumor reduction or elimination
- Loss of lymphatic swelling
- Greater strength in previously weak areas
- Increased circulation

- Gray hair begins to disappear (goes back to natural color)
- The skin begins to tighten and become softer
- Clarity in thinking
- Improved memory
- Disease symptoms disappear
- Blood sugars normalize
- Blood pressure will normalize
- Deeper relationship with God and Nature
- Higher sense of happiness, joy and well-being
- Skin blemishes (like pimples, rashes, etc.) disappear
- Bowels move better
- Improved kidney function
- Voice strengthens
- Heart arrhythmias disappear
- Improved eyesight
- Overall sense of well-being and vibrancy comes back
- Reversal of the "aging" process
- Never get "sick" or "catch" what's going around
- And much, much more.

WHAT TO AVOID DURING A HEALING CRISIS

DEHYDRATION — Keep yourself hydrated with fresh mineral water or freshly juiced fruit and vegetable juices.

OVEREXERTION — During a healing crisis try to conserve your energy.

TOO MANY PESTICIDES — Pesticides can cause shortness of breath and "hypo" conditions of the endocrine gland system and nervous system.

PUSHING IT TOO FAR — If you need to slow down or stop the cleansing process temporarily, start eating some cooked foods. Try to make do with the minimal amount, if possible, like some steamed vegetables or whole grain rice. This will lower the body's systemic energy for a time and it will stop the intense cleansing. As soon as you can, resume the cleansing program.

FEVERS ABOVE 103° FAHRENHEIT — In adults and children such fevers should be controlled by cool baths and the like. Children can naturally have high fevers, especially around 104° and 105°. Keep the child cooled down with cold washcloths and cool baths. There's a fine line between interfering with the body's effort to clean and heal itself and simply allowing your body freedom to do as it chooses. However, a slight fever would be no cause for concern, and require no control. But with higher fevers we want to carefully monitor the body and control those situations that could cause more severe side effects. Remember, always keep the body hydrated by drinking plenty of water or fresh fruit juices. But don't over-hydrate yourself either. Balance is key.

IMPATIENCE — When you start energizing and alkalizing your body, it will start to clean itself out. Always remember that the body is doing this cleansing. You can use herbal formulas to increase the cleaning action of congested lymphatic systems, to kill parasites, and to enhance the function of your organs and glands. However, your body has its own rhythm of healing and cleansing itself. Be patient.

DON'T OVEREAT — Animals generally don't eat at all when they're sick. Your body was designed to heal itself and clean itself out, as God is at work in all its mechanisms. All you have to do is feed the body properly.

SMART CLEANSING

It is important to be smart in helping your body to detoxify itself. Again, there can be a fine line between helping or hindering it. Have some common sense about this whole process of detoxification. Each person is unique. What an asthmatic goes through may be totally different than a case of uterine cancer.

The healing process is truly magnificent. It's part of a "Letting Go" that frees you on so many levels, yet few understand that. Embrace Life, Health and God!

If as you cleanse you experience side effects such that you feel you need to go to an Emergency Room—GO! I spent many years working in them. They are there to help in a crisis. It's just too bad that most ER personnel don't understand about the detoxification process and the "healing crisis." During these times, which are generally rare, review Module 6.5, *What to Expect During Detox*.

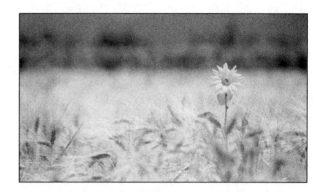

ITEMS FOR YOUR HOME FIRST AID KIT

Below is a list of First Aid items to have in your home to aid your comfort level during a detoxification process.

CASTOR OIL PACKS
See Chapter 10 for what is needed to prepare these.

OLIVE OIL
Used like or instead of castor oil.

CAYENNE PEPPER
Used to dilate the skin and/or vascular system; for high blood pressure or castor oil packs.

PLEURISY ROOT, MULLEIN LEAF AND/OR FENUGREEK SEED
Lung expectorant

A HEAT SOURCE
Hot water bottle or heating pad, etc. Used to dilate or "drive" herbs through the skin.

AN ANTI-SPASMODIC (AN HERBAL TINCTURE)
Spasms, convulsions, cramping and pain

HERBAL PAIN FORMULA
Tincture, preferably

SLIPPERY ELM AND/OR MARSHMALLOW ROOT HERBAL TEAS
For acid reflux

ARNICA OIL
Use externally for sprains, pulls, stiff or sore muscles, etc.

HERBAL HEALING SALVE
Should contain a variety of healing herbs like comfrey, horsetail, lobelia, marigold, etc. Used for sprains, muscle pulls, pain in joints, wounds, etc.

PLANTAIN TINCTURE AND SALVE
Used for insect bites, snake bites, and other poisonous bites.

"HEAL-ALL TEA"™
From God's Herbs™, (see Resource Guide) or another alternative. Used for tumors, snake bites, abscesses, infections, anything and everything.

HERBAL INTESTINAL CORRECTIVE LAXATIVE

ALOE VERA
An "all-heal" for burns, itching from fungus, intestinal soother, etc.

TEA TREE OIL
Herbal antiseptic, itching from fungus, etc.

AN HERBAL PARASITIC FORMULA
Bacterial infections, E-coli, Candida, etc.

☀ Fasting in Detoxification

Fasting, in some form or another, has probably been practiced since the beginning of history, by humans and animals alike. Fasting is instinctual and is associated with rest and energy management. I enjoyed a six-month orange fast back in 1972. This turned out to be one of the most incredible experiences in my life. I had so much energy that I kept having tremendous out-of-body experiences that took me right into the heart of God.

There are basically two forms of fasting. The first one, known as "forced fasting," is literally forced upon us because of disease. You simply can't eat. Or if you try, you simply can't keep the food down. This is the body's own mechanism to divert much-needed energy from digestion to the immune, lymphatic and endocrine systems. This gives our bodies energy to expel the intruder, the obstruction or the congestion.

The second form of fasting is "conscious fasting," which is done to cleanse and restore the body. Conscious fasting builds self-discipline and self-confidence. These are two important attributes to develop on the road to good health.

Both forms of fasting are energy management for the body. Most of the foods that humans eat rob their bodies of energy instead of giving it. Health and vitality is energy; disease is a lack of energy. Fasting is the way the body can rest from extensive digestive and metabolic issues. It uses that same energy, instead, to clean itself out of acids and toxins, thus allowing itself to heal.

Our digestive and eliminative systems become overworked and weakened on a typical diet of meats, grains, dairy products, and the like. Fasting allows the pancreas, stomach, liver, intestines, and even the kidneys to have somewhat of a rest. This gives more energy to the immune, glandular and lymphatic systems. **Fasting at one level or another is vital in getting well.**

There are many types of fasts you can do. Let's explore four basic types of fasting and then discuss how to properly stop or "break" a fast.

TYPES OF FASTS

All Raw-Food Fast

This of course is not really a fast since you are still eating food. But to most people who eat heavy, cooked foods, this is definitely considered a fast. Remember: no other animal cooks its food before eating it. Take this fast a day at a time, and try to eat all raw food that day. Try this fast for 5, 10, 30 or 60 days in succession, eating only all raw foods, the longer the better. This type of fast would include fresh raw fruits, fruit juices, vegetables and vegetable juices. No "protein" type foods like nuts or seeds.

All Fruit Fast

I highly recommend this type of fast. Being frugivores, this fast would be more harmonious with our physiological and anatomical processes and design. Grapes should be the focus, organic if possible. If not organic, they must be thoroughly washed as they would contain a high level of pesticides. However, any fruit or combination of fruits, or melons, will do. As you will learn in the next chapter, on food combining, "Eat melons alone or leave them alone." You could eat grapes alone, or watermelon, or apples, whatever you like or crave. I've helped a lot of souls clean cancer out of their physical bodies with grapes and grape juice fasts. Eat as much as you want. We do not count calories on this program.

Juice Fasting

This is high-level fasting which gives your GI tract and digestive tract a rest. Juice fasts are high-energy fasts that stimulate much-needed cleansing and lymphatic movement, while keeping the kidneys flushed out. Juices still supply glucose and fructose to cells for energy. Juices can be vegetable or fruit; however, the power is within the fruit juice, especially fresh grape juice.

There are always exceptions to any rule. In a pancreatic cancer case I worked with, the individual had stopped digesting food completely. I started her on fruit juices only. Then I added vegetable juices, and finally, after a short period of time, I added first raw fruit and then vegetables. The reason I chose this method is simple. First, her pancreas had stopped digesting her food. When she ate any food it came out in her stools undigested. I needed to maintain her systemic energy but give her something that took little, if any, effort for the pancreas to digest. A freshly-made fruit juice is the best choice in this solution. I added vegetable juices after awhile, even though they are harder to digest, but her pancreas had improved enough to handle them. I also used liquid botanical extracts to enhance various organs and glands in her body, especially the pancreas. I finally added solid foods starting with fruits, again because of their high energy levels and ease of digestion. Finally in eleven months, she was cancer free!

Water Fasting

This is the fourth and ultimate type of fasting. Water fasts should only be done with R/O (reverse osmosis) or distilled water. At this level, your digestive energy is totally given to the immune, lymphatic and glandular systems. A water fast creates a high level of body cleansing and purging. The body, in its tremendous wisdom, will focus on removing stored toxins, mucus and inflammation.

To the average individual, water fasting can give energy. However, in weakened or depleted conditions the goal is to give energy to the body by elevating the systemic energy. **I do not recommend a water-only fast for highly depleted and weakened individuals**, especially those with cancer. This is because one is not feeding the body energy, per se, so the body must work with the energy it has.

Even though fasting gives most individuals energy, when you're dealing in advanced tissue weakness, raw foods, especially fruits, will empower the body with nutrition and energy. Consuming high-energy fruits or fruit juices will begin to bring one's cellular and systemic energies up, at the same time allowing for detoxification. Water fasting in highly-depleted cases can enervate the body and lead to death. After the individual is built up, then water fasting would be appropriate.

PREPARATION BEFORE FASTING

If you intend to "go all the way" up to juice or water fasting, you would want to prepare yourself by eating raw foods for a week, spending the last couple of days on fruits only. This helps clean the bowels of putrid matter, flushes the liver and kidneys, and sets the body in proper motion for your fast.

Fasting can be fun and self-empowering. Its role in helping the body to cleanse and restore itself has been proven over and over again. **For long, extended fasts, seek the advice of someone who is experienced in fasting and detoxification.**

WHEN TO "BREAK" A FAST

The best time to "break" a fast will be discovered by listening to your inner guidance or intuition. You know your body better than anyone. Listen to it. You'll know when you have had enough. (But also, be fair and honest with yourself, knowing that desire can creep in even though you may not actually be hungry.) After about three days or so, one generally loses the desire for eating. This is because the body is starting to use that digestive energy for cleaning and healing. When you start feeling hungry again, this is a good sign that you are ready to start eating. Remember to start with fruits only.

Another way to determine how long to fast is the tongue-examination method. This is the old-fashioned method that I've used for years. When you start fasting, your tongue will become coated with a thick white, yellow, green, or brown substance. The more toxic you are, the thicker and darker this coating becomes. Of course the healthier you are, the less your tongue will coat when you fast. If you fast until your tongue becomes pink again, you will have done a tremendous job of cleaning your body out.

Detoxification is an ongoing process that can take years. That sounds worse than it is. Health should become one of your hobbies. Spend a good year or so aggressively working on yourself; then set your new lifestyle in motion with balance and harmony. This will be the new, healthier, vibrant, cleaner and more aware you. As you grow spiritually, always seek to balance your lifestyle and eating habits with your spiritual awareness. The more you expand your awareness, the healthier and more energetically you will want to eat. You want your physical body to keep up with you. Have fun on your journey of health, vitality, and spirituality; there is nothing like it.

HOW TO "BREAK" A FAST

It is very important how you break a fast, and depends on how long you've fasted and what type of fast you did. A general rule of thumb would be: **Break most fasts with a day or two** **of eating fresh, raw fruit, only, for every three days of fasting you have done.**

This is especially true after juice or water fasting. The longer you fast, the more days you should spend eating just fruits before you start with heavy vegetables. I have known of a case or two through the years where an individual died from breaking a fast incorrectly. One man died from breaking an extended fast with boiled potatoes. Being a sticky, gluey starch, I can understand how it locked his bowels up.

Always try to keep your bowels moving. When you're on a juice or water fast, this is not always possible. In Module 6.9 we will discuss bowel health and management.

Please Buy a Juicer

N.W. Walker lived to be a healthy 107 from juicing. What more proof do you need? Try a glass of carrot, spinach and celery juice today.

Raw fruit and vegetable juices are a powerhouse of nutrition. A glass of carrot juice contains 6–8 carrots, giving 6 times the nutrition of a simple carrot. This is what I call a "High Electrical" Drink, a powerhouse of energy and amino acids.

Drink 2–4 glasses each day of your favorite vegetables or fruits.

Read *Vegetable and Fruit Juices* by N.W. Walker.

☀ Two Great Fruit Juice Fasts

LEMONADE FAST

HOW TO MAKE LEMONADE:

- 2 tbsp. lemon or lime juice (approx. 1/2 lemon)
- 1/2 to 3/4 tbsp. genuine Maple Syrup (not maple-flavored sugar syrup)
- pinch of Cayenne Pepper (optional)

Combine the juice, maple syrup, and cayenne pepper in a 10-ounce glass and fill with medium/hot distilled or R/O water. (Cold water may be used if preferred.) Use fresh lemons or limes only; never use canned lemon or lime juice, or frozen lemonade or lime juice.

Cayenne Pepper may be used with this formula as it adds extra vitamin C and B-complex. It also increases warmth for an additional lift. For those not used to hot peppers, start with a dash and increase it as you are able. You may eliminate the pepper if you wish. Pure sorghum, black strap molasses or honey may be used as a lesser replacement when maple syrup is not available. You might wish to make a quart of lemonade for the whole day.

FOR A FULL QUART OF LEMONADE:

    10 cups distilled water
    1 1/2 cup of fresh lemon juice
    1/2 cup of pure maple syrup
    Shake well and refrigerate

HOW TO TAKE THE LEMONADE:

Drink this lemonade as much and as often as you want, but **drink only this lemonade, no other foods or drinks.** This fruit juice fast can be done for 1, 2, 3 or up to 10 days easily.

GRAPE JUICE FAST

HOW TO MAKE GRAPE JUICE:

- A juice extractor or juicer is necessary.
- Juice a quart of grapes (seeds and small stems as well).
- Any type of grape is okay; however the dark, seeded ones are the best. And always try to use organic grapes.

HOW TO TAKE THE JUICE:

Drink this grape juice as often and as much as you want. Grapes are high in antioxidant and astringent properties, which help remove toxins from the body. Eating grapes and drinking Grape Juice only makes for an excellent fast. I have "fasted" people for over twenty days on just grapes. A 5- or 10-day grape or grape juice fast is superb and extremely beneficial.

Grapes and lemons are two of nature's greatest lymphatic cleansers and "tumor busters." I have seen lymphomas gone in forty-five days and stomach cancer gone in fifty-nine days using these fruit juice fasts in combination with herbal therapy and a raw food diet.

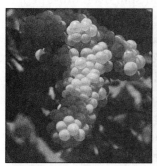 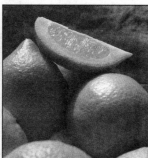 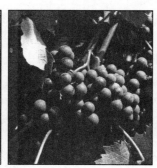 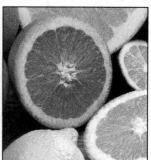

☀ Healthy Bowel Management

Poor bowel management lies at the root of most people's health problems. I have been teaching colon health for the last thirty-five years. My friend, the late Dr. Bernard Jensen, was teaching this for well over sixty years. Having worked with over 300,000 clients, Dr. Jensen's research has concluded: "It is the bowels that invariably have to be cared for first before any effective healing can take place." As a matter of fact, the natural health field mainly got *started* around matters of the gastrointestinal tract.

Bowel wisdom is generally a topic that few people desire to discuss. Yet, keeping the bowels (intestinal tract) healthy and in good shape is one of the best ways to keep out of the grip of toxicity and cell enervation.

Your gastrointestinal tract is the center or hub of your body, just as the hub of a wheel is the supporting part of a wheel. It is one of the main organ systems of your body. Now the real question should be, "How do we save and regenerate the GI tract, which is as important as the heart?" Without digestion, absorption *and* elimination we die. This canal—mouth through anus—is how you introduce energy and chemistry from foods into your body. From the colon on is where and how we eliminate our wastes, which is vital to the survival of your body. The proper elimination of wastes from food digestion and cellular metabolism is as important as the ingestion of your foods.

As we learned in Chapter 2, the small bowel is divided up into three parts: the duodenum, where digestion takes place, which is about 10 inches long; the jejunum, for both digestion and absorption, which is approximately 9 feet long; and the ileum, for absorption, which is approximately 13 feet long. The large intestine is called the colon, which is 5 feet long and divided up into the cecum, ascending, transverse, descending, sigmoid and rectal sections. Each section of the colon has been linked to different organs and glands of the body and has an effect upon these tissues, good or bad. When you were in the embryo stages of life, this colon plus the spinal cord were the first two areas of the body that were formed. You will find all your genetic weaknesses in the colon first, then reflected to organ, gland, nerve, or other tissues within the body.

Your bowels take the brunt of abuse from acidic-toxic foods and drinks. Many of these foods inflame and weaken their structure. Some foods act like glue and actually adhere to its walls. Many other foods are so abrasive that they cause excessive mucus to be produced from the intestinal walls to protect itself. This mucus is stored along the bowel walls and interstitially in its structure. All of the above affect your GI tract's ability to digest food and absorb nutrition.

Your GI tract also plays a valuable role with the lymphatic system. The lymphatic system is your sewer system. It must have a way to eliminate wastes from the body. The kidneys, GI tract and the skin are its main avenues for this purpose. When the skin, kidneys, and especially the colon become impacted or obstructed, the lymphatic system becomes backed up. You can imagine what would happen in your home if your septic tank became blocked. The wastes from your toilet would back up and spill over. Most people would leave their house at this point.

The sympathetic and parasympathetic nerves of the autonomic nervous system control your digestive tract through the neurotransmitters produced from the adrenal glands. Weak adrenal glands can cause nerve weakness, causing constipation. Many overlook this relationship that the adrenal glands have to both nerve weakness (which can cause constipation) and their steroid production in response to inflammation. It always pays to strengthen your adrenal glands at the same time that you are regenerating your GI tract.

The importance of keeping your intestinal tract clean and healthy cannot be overstated. Remember that this is your main canal of digestion, which is where the breakdown of your foods into fuels and building materials takes place. After your food is digested, it is then absorbed through the lining of the intestines through the villa. Absorption of the nutrients from the foods you eat is just as essential as the digestive process. The billions of cells that comprise the body depend upon the absorption from the bowels for their nutrition. As previously stated, proper nutrition can be blocked from the cells by retained waste in the colon. This leads to a toxic buildup and the accumulation of a gluey substance throughout the intestines called "mucoid plaque." This plaque causes inflammation and the breakdown of the tissues of the intestinal walls.

Mucoid plaque is mostly a by-product of refined starches, sugars and dairy products. When the walls of the intestines are coated with layers of sticky plaque, the nutrients the body needs to properly function and perform to its highest potential cannot be absorbed. In addition, the sticky mucoid plaque is a breeding ground for parasitic infestation. These destructive parasites consume any remaining nutrients left in the GI tract.

We require certain intestinal parasites (known as intestinal flora) for positive and beneficial breakdown of various by-products of digestion. A great example of this is B-vitamins, which are created by intestinal flora action upon starches. Generally your intestines are colonized by non-harmful organisms which aid digestion and the breakdown of foodstuffs into other nutrients. However, there are many destructive parasites that can flourish in the intestines. This is especially true in the case of meat consumption, which can perpetrate the formation and growth of all types of worms (pin, hook, tape, etc.) and

proteolytic (protein-splitting) microorganisms. It is important to clean the intestinal walls and heal the inflammation at the same time that the elimination of toxic substances is taking place.

A healthy diet will create a bowel movement approximately thirty minutes after you eat. It is important to move your bowels two-to-three times per day. If your bowels become sluggish, this will cause additional fermentation and putrefaction of your foods. We absorb these toxins and gas particles directly into our blood stream. This can cause headaches, cloudy or foggy thinking, bloating, abdominal pain, and even heart arrhythmias. I've known people to go thirty days without moving their bowels. Don't miss even one day!

Diarrhea is just as bad as constipation—moving your foods too quickly through the GI tract is just as bad as holding your foods too long. Some say diarrhea is just another form of constipation. The former creates lack of proper breakdown of your foods, yielding poor absorption; and the latter causes fermentation and putrefaction of your foods yielding alcohol, acidosis, gas and inflammation. Both create starvation within the body.

FOUR WAYS TO CLEANSE THE BOWELS

Herbal Bowel Formulas

A good bowel formula (a preparation of herbs that you take on a daily basis during your cleanse) will help break down mucoid plaque, kill only the destructive parasites, remove the inflammation and strengthen intestinal walls.

When I designed my stomach and bowel formulas, I wanted ones that would gently move you. A formula that would be anti-inflammatory (removing the inflammation), and would clean the mucoid plaque off the walls, as well. My formulas would also clean out the pockets (diverticulum) that were formed from impactions.

I wanted a formula that would also strengthen the GI tract, eliminating these pockets, as well as the ballooning and/or the spastic conditions that we all suffer with. The problem with most bowel formulas is that they have heavy Cayenne Pepper, Aloes, Buckthorn or other stimulating and habit-forming herbs that cause gripping, cramping, or excessive mucus production. These types of formulas can cause a great deal of abdominal discomfort and are oftentimes hard to regulate. Many intestinal formulas can become addicting; that is to say, the body becomes dependent upon these as it does with other stimulants, leaving the opposite effect when you stop taking them—constipation.

A good bowel formula will not be addicting. It will gently move you, clean you, remove the inflammation, and strengthen—all at the same time. Additionally, it will stimulate lymph flow and circulation within the intestinal wall tissues themselves. (See Chapter 8, Module 8.3 for herbal formulas for the stomach and bowels; also see Resource Guide for companies that make good bowel formulas.)

Colonics

Colonic therapy may also be used to assist the cleansing of the colon (large intestine). However, the small intestine must be cleaned and cared for as well—which is why an herbal bowel formula is also recommended. Colonics are like a "high" enema, but have a "washing" effect upon tissue. Colon therapists, who are generally licensed massage therapists, perform colonics. (In my opinion, every Emergency Room should have a colonic machine and a trained colon therapist on staff.) Colonics are great at removing impactions of the large bowel, aiding in relief of acidosis, distention of the abdomen, lower back pain, sciatic pain, kidney pain, headaches and fevers, to name a few conditions. They can also help clean out diverticula or bowel pockets.

Colon therapy is a gentle procedure, yet it can have aggressive results, as it can break loose plaque that has been impacted upon the colon wall for years. I've seen impactions removed by colonics that have been in the body for fifty years or more.

Many years ago, a chiropractor-friend of mine had a registered nurse on his staff, who performed colonics. One of the nurse's patients, who had gone home when the colonic was finished, started feeling pain in her sigmoid bowel a short while later. The patient waited several hours until she felt she needed to determine what was causing her discomfort, and finally went to the Emergency Room. There they discovered that she had cancer of the sigmoid bowel. The colonic did not cause this, of course, her lifestyle did. However, the colonic did expose the cancer. This was a good thing because the woman then could do something about it. If she had not had the colonic the cancer could have spread throughout her body without her knowing it, until it was too late to achieve an effective cure.

Exposing inflammation, such as happened in this case, can be painful and yield some discomfort. Generally, this is why I prefer to recommend a good intestinal (bowel) herbal formula that is designed to be anti-inflammatory and restorative, not laxative. Herbal restorative bowel formulas will slowly loosen and remove the plaque that has impacted upon the walls. They will also reduce the inflammation behind this plaque and heal the bowel wall. In this way, your healing experience becomes much smoother and less traumatic.

Colonics are great for colon obstructions, as long as they're not tumors or adhesions. Colonics are good for the large bowel. My preference in terms of the administering of colonics? I personally recommend Dr. Jensen's Colema Board® concept as the best option. I've seen some real success through this process with eliminating the mucoid plaque build-up in the GI tract. The Colema Board is designed to fit over your toilet at one end, with the other end resting on a chair or stool. By lying on this board (while at the same time using a five-gallon bucket of skin temperature water), you give yourself a high enema. However, this procedure is much more relaxing than an ordinary enema, because you just lay there and allow the water to slowly and gently clean you out.

Dr. Jensen has created a whole bowel management program that can't be beat (see his book, *Tissue Cleansing Through Bowel Management*, 1981). His procedures help to clean the small bowel as well as the large bowel, whereas professional colonics only affect the large bowel. With some self-discipline, the Colema System can be done at home with the purchase of a Colema Board. For information about his program, and for purchasing and using a Colema Board, see www.colema-boards.com.

I'm not against professional colonics. To maximize the benefits, change your diet to a 100 percent raw food program and add intestinal restoratives for a month or so before your start your colonic regime. Three to five colonics should be sufficient.

Enemas

Enemas are another great way to help yourself out in time of need, or to assist in colon-rectal conditions such as hemorrhoids or cancer. There are many types of enemas that one can use to help clean and open this channel.

LOW ENEMAS — These generally clean and strengthen the descending, sigmoid and rectal areas of the large intestine (colon). They require about one-half to one quart of skin temperature water in an enema bag (these are available in most pharmacies; oftentimes they are labeled as "enema/hot-water bottle," or "enema/douche/hot water bottle" combination).

Any number of the following herbs can be made into tea, strained, and used in place of plain water in the enema bag. These herbs will clean and strengthen the colon walls: Cascara Sagrada, Marshmallow Root, Slippery Elm Bark, Plantain

Leaf, Comfrey Root, Burdock Root, Gentian, etc. See, *How To Do An Enema*, instructions below.

HIGH ENEMAS — A high enema is necessary to achieve results higher up in the colon, e.g. in the transverse, ascending and cecum portions of the large intestines. What distinguishes the high enema from the low enema is often a function of the way it is applied and the amount of water/mixture used, which determines how far the water/mixture will go up into your colon. The same herbs can be used as stated above. In cases of debility where extreme fatigue is involved, high enemas can be given using fresh green juices like wheat grass, spinach, kelp, alfalfa, barley, etc., instead of water or herbal tea. These juices are readily absorbed through the colon wall and are electrifying to the body, bringing much needed energy into the system. Chlorophyll is another constituent that can be introduced into the colon via the enema method to assist the healing and cleansing process.

COFFEE ENEMAS — Many people use coffee enemas as these are very stimulating to the bowels and liver. However, I never recommend them unless your colon is "locked" and you can't have a bowel movement. The continual use of coffee enemas has a whiplash effect causing extreme enervation of the colon and inflammation of the liver and kidneys.

Coffee enemas also have a negative effect upon the nervous system creating hyper- or hypoactivity of this system. This then will have a residual effect upon the whole body in numerous ways including nerve disorders, severe constipation, diarrhea, bloating, edema, and acidosis.

HOW TO DO AN ENEMA

1. Purchase an enema-bag / "hot water bottle" combination from a pharmacy.

2. Fill the bag with 1/2 quart to 2 quarts of skin temperature water or herb-water mixture. Always use skin temperature water no matter what you mix it with.

3. Hang the hot water bottle at least two feet above you.
4. Lay on your left side as you start your enema.
5. Use a healing herbal salve to lubricate the tip for easy insertion.
6. Let the water (or herbal mixture) flow slowly into your colon; stopping the flow periodically while you rest and do some deep breathing.
7. After a few minutes, move from your left side to lying on your back, and continue to let the water flow into your colon; then turn over to your right side.
8. You may wish to massage the region of your colon as it is being filled with the mixture. This will help loosen impacted "plaque" for removal.
9. Retain this water (mixture) somewhat, then allow elimination.
10. Repeat until the bag/hot water bottle is empty.

Use enemas wisely and when needed. There is no need to over use them. A diet of raw fruits and vegetables along with a good intestinal rejuvenator will work much better in the long run at reestablishing the health of the GI tract.

Healing Clay

A fourth method of cleansing the bowels involves the use of clays. These are not used as much in America as in Europe. In many countries, like Portugal, health professionals use clay packs over the abdomen to accomplish the same results we get with colonics. The late Dr. John Christopher has a great intestinal powder (*Intestinal Corrective #2*®) that includes bentonite clay and charcoal. This has a highly cleansing and absorbing effect within the intestines. This formula is beneficial in cases of irritable bowel syndrome and with uncontrolled diarrhea.

Summary

Our intestines (GI tract) are so vital that God made them one of the first things formed when a cell initially becomes an embryo. In this early stage, the spinal column and "gut" tissue is formed, and the gut tissue later becomes the GI tract. Your very survival depends upon its proper functioning. Nutrients, building materials, and fuels are absorbed from its walls, and the GI tract also creates white blood cells, various vitamins, and amino acids. The synergistic role of the GI system with the lymphatic system is not totally understood. But its essential relationship to every cell in your body (via the lymphatic system) should give you an indication of just how vital it is to keep it functioning properly. You should "feed it" only alive, easy-to-digest foods with electrically alive fiber so it can maintain its health.

Physicians pour drugs of which they know little, to cure diseases of which they know less, into humans of which they know nothing.
— Voltaire, French satirist (1694-1778)

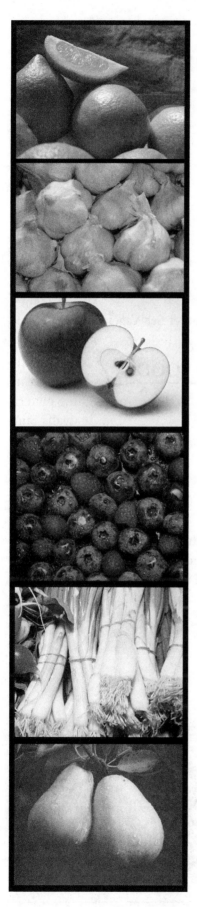

CHAPTER SEVEN

Eating for Vitality

Up to this point we have looked at how the body works, the processes of disease, detoxification and regeneration. We have examined our species and the types of foods that best suit us. We have also looked at foods and their effects on tissue.

In this chapter we will discover what to eat and how to eat it. It is important not only to know what to eat, but *how to mix* these foods properly to get the optimum benefit from them—the art of food combining.

Here, too, we will offer a series of menus that you can begin to use immediately to start yourself in the direction of detoxification and regeneration. These menus will address your needs, whether you consider yourself a timid beginner or a bold adventurer.

Further topics covered will include the amazing health value of raw fruit and vegetable juices, and the subject of beans, soybeans and grains as they relate to detoxification and regeneration.

In the concluding pages of this chapter you will find a number of excellent recipes for both raw and steamed foods that will strengthen you on your journey and make your meals more varied and delightful.

☀ What Foods to Eat

The following is a list of acceptable raw fruits, vegetables, nuts, and seeds. Always buy organic if possible.

MOST FRUITS AND BERRIES

Grapes
Bananas
Strawberries
Mangoes
Oranges
Grapefruit
Apples
Peaches
Pears
Pineapple
Dried fruits of all kinds (unsulphured)
Flowers are acceptable

AVOID—Cranberries, Prunes and unripe fruits

VEGETABLES

Romaine Lettuce
Spinach
Carrots
Celery
Green Peppers
Cucumbers
Sprouts
Avocados
Green Leafy Vegetables
Squash
Green Beans
Peas
Raw Tomatoes
Kelp, Dulse and other Sea Vegetables

OTHER RAW FOODS

Pecans
Almonds
Sunflower Seeds
Sesame Seeds
Pumpkin Seeds
Coconuts
Pine Nuts

NOTE—Eat moderately of this category. Too many of these foods can be acid-forming, energy robbing, and will slow or stop the cleansing process.

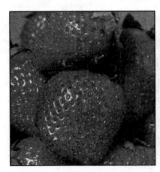
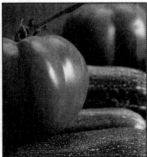
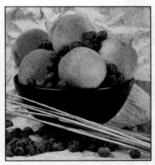
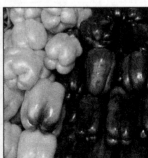

☼ Acid/Alkaline Food Chart

All foods contain both acid-forming and alkaline-forming elements. It is not the organic matter of foods that leave these acid or alkaline residues in your body. It is the inorganic matter or minerals that determine the acidity or alkalinity of the body fluids and tissues. Potassium, sodium, magnesium and calcium are considered the alkaline-forming electrolytes. Phosphorus, sulfur and manganese are the acid-forming elements.

Several processes can be used to determine whether a food is more acid-forming or alkaline-forming. Generally, if a food has dominant acid-forming elements over alkaline-forming elements it's considered acid-forming. The reverse is also true. If a food has dominant alkaline-forming elements, then the food is considered to be alkaline-forming.

Titration is the laboratory method used to measure acidity vs. alkalinity. There are two stages to this process. First, the appropriate amount of food is burned to ashes. This takes the place of digestion. Secondly, we add approximately one liter of distilled water to 100 grams of these ashes, which now makes a solution. The solution is then tested for its acidity or alkalinity.

Another method of determining the acidity or alkalinity of a food is its nitrogen or proteid (chemical compounds comprising a protein structure) content. Since nitrogen has an acidic influence, all protein-rich (nitrogen-rich) foods are considered acid-forming. This, however, is an older method and is not as accurate because it has been determined that vegetable matter supplies more available nitrogen and proteid material than meats do.

The following Acid/Alkaline Food Chart is based upon a combination of the above methods, and will help you on your journey toward alkalization. Remember, a diet of 80 percent alkaline and 20 percent acid-forming food is essential for greater health. A diet of 90 percent or more of alkaline-forming foods means vibrant health.

Keep it simple. People always ask me: "What can I *add* to my diet?" My response is: "What can I take away?" Believe it or not, the simpler you eat the healthier you'll be. This statement drives nutritional scientists nuts. That is because the focus has been on deficiencies, leading to the use of high dosages of amino acids, vitamins and minerals. Mega-dosing like this can make some symptoms disappear, but they will only reappear when these supplements are stopped. This is not true regeneration or healing, but treating symptoms while ignoring the causes. It is not the high level of nutrients consumed that is the key. It is the power and synergistic action of ripe, raw, whole food. The power of raw food to clean and rebuild the physical body is little understood in our pharmaceutical scientific communities.

Look at the diets of most wild herbivores, e.g., elephants, horses, or cows. They eat predominantly grass and leaves. Look at the wild silver-back apes. Their diet is very simple as well, consisting of sweet things including fruits, sweet tubers, berries and flowers. Seventy percent or more of the diet of a grizzly bear is grass. These are among the strongest animals on this planet.

I can tell you from my own personal experience that when I fasted for six months on organic navel oranges, I never felt better and more in tune with God and nature. Always trust nature, God and your inner intuition to know the truth.

The Alkaline/Acid Food Chart shows what foods are alkaline-forming and what foods are acid-forming. It is best during detoxification to eat ALL raw fruits and vegetables only.

Alkaline Forming Foods

FRUITS

Apples
Apricots
Bananas
Berries
Cherries
Coconut, fresh
Currants
Dates
Figs
Grapefruit
Grapes
Guava
Kumquats
Lemons, ripe
Limes
Loquats
Mangos

Melons, all
Nectarines
Oranges
Passion Fruit
Papaya
Pears
Peaches
Pineapple, fresh
Pomegranates
Prickly Pear
Raisins
Sapotes
Strawberries
Tamarind
Tangerines

VEGETABLES

Alfalfa
Almonds
Artichokes
Asparagus
Avocados
Bamboo shoots
Beans—green,
  string, wax
Beans, lima
Beets
Bell Peppers,
  all colors
Broccoli
Brussels Sprouts
Cabbage, red
  and white
Carrots
Celery
Cauliflower
Chard
Chestnuts
Chicory
Chives
Collards
Corn, sweet
Cucumber
Dandelion
Dill
Dock, green

Eggplant
Escarole
Garlic
Horseradish
Kale
Kohlrabi
Leeks
Lettuce
Okra
Olives
Onions
Parsley
Parsnips
Peas
Pumpkin
Radish
Rhubarb
Sauerkraut
Sorrel
Spinach
Sprouts
Squash
Sweet Potato
Tomatoes,
  orange only
Turnips
Watercress
White Potato

OTHER

Apple Cider Vin-
  egar
Buttermilk, raw
Dulse and Kelp
Grains—
  Amaranth,
  Millet, Quinoa
Milk, raw
Miso

Molasses
Olive Oil
Spices, natural
Tea, herbal
  and Chinese
Whey
Wine, organic
Yogurt, raw

Acid Forming Foods

Alcoholic
  beverages
Artichokes
Asparagus, tips
  (white only)
Aspirin
Barley
Bananas, green
Beans, dried
Blueberries
Breads
Cakes
Candy

Cereals,
  breakfast
Crackers
Cheeses, all
Chocolate and
  Cocoa
Coffee
Cola and soft
  drinks
Colorings,
  artificial
Condiments, all
Corn, cooked
Corn starch

Cranberries
Crackers
Custards
Dairy products
Dressings
Doughnuts
Eggs, whites
Flavorings,
  artificial
Flour products
Fruits, canned
Garbanzos
Gelatin

Grains, most
Grapenuts
Gravies
Grits, hominy
Ice Cream
Jams and Jellies
Lentils
Mayonnaise
Meats, including
  fish, shellfish
  and fowl
Oatmeal
Oils, processed

Olives, pickled
Nuts
Pasta
Pastries and Pies
Peanuts
Pepper, Black
Plums
Prunes
Rice cakes
Rice, white and
  brown
Salt
Soda water

Soybeans
Soy products
Spaghetti
Sugar, refined
Tapioca
Teas, Indian
Tobacco
Vegetables,
  canned
Vinegar
Yogurt

Remember . . .

Pleasure, laughter, happiness, rest and sleep are all *Alkaline* forming.
Worry, anger, hate, envy, gossip, fear and lack of sleep are *Acid* forming.

☀ The Vital Role of Proper Food Combination

Throughout this book I have taken you on a simplified journey into the body, its many systems, and how they work. We have covered disease processes and their causes. You have learned the importance of the pH of the body. We've examined the two pillars of chemistry: alkalies and acids; and we looked at the role of acidosis in disease. You are learning the power of raw foods and their effects on tissue. Now it is time to put these factors together and examine proper food combinations.

According to the American Dietetics Association, it doesn't matter how we combine our foods, as long as we eat proteins, carbohydrates, and some fat at each meal. This philosophy is ridiculous and unscientific, and we have all suffered with gas, bloating and acidosis as a result. Chemistry does not support this approach. As a matter of fact, chemistry becomes our friend when we look into proper food combinations. For a diabetic, particularly, it is vital to follow proper food combinations if he or she wants to regulate blood sugars.

Many great books have been written about proper food combinations, and I would suggest studying a little about this important subject. (See: *Food Combining Made Easy* by Herbert Shelton, and *Proper Food-Combining Works* by Lee DuBelle.)

Chemistry tells us that when we combine a base (or alkalie) with an acid, they neutralize each other. Fermentation and putrefaction then become the digesters, instead of digestive enzymes. This causes improper food breakdown and many unwanted chemical changes, all leading to malabsorption, acidosis and cellular starvation. Protein-dominating foods when mixed with starches fall into this category.

The two most important food-combination tips are, first, to never mix proteins (acid foods) with carbohydrates (alkaline foods), and second, to separate your consumption of fruits or melons from any other type of food. These two tips will be discussed in more detail below.

If you observe proper food combinations you will end the acid regurgitation, ulcerations, bloating and gas commonly caused by violating these natural rules. Keep in mind that the fewer types of foods you combine, the better the digestion of your foods will be. If I ask you to think of ten different things at the same time you would become confused, as the mind can attend fully to one thing at a time. Remember this when you are planning to eat ten different foods at one meal. Simplicity is always best. It's not *how much* you eat, but whether you can digest, absorb, utilize and eliminate what you have eaten.

Keep your diet simple and keep your life simple. Be happy when you eat. Never eat when you're angry or upset, as this causes elevated stomach acids that can neutralize your digestive efforts and create acidosis. Relax and enjoy what you are eating. Chew your foods well, as the first stage of digestion takes place in your mouth. Try not to drink with your meals, as this only dilutes or neutralizes your digestive enzymes.

THE TWO MOST IMPORTANT FOOD-COMBINING TIPS

Do Not Combine Proteins (acid) and Carbohydrates (alkaline)

In chemistry we learn that we cannot combine acid digestive enzymes with alkaline digestive enzymes because they will normally neutralize each other, causing proper digestion to stop and putrefaction and fermentation to begin.

Carbohydrates begin their digestive process in the mouth with amylase, ptyalin and other alkaline digestive enzymes. Protein-type foods, including meat and nuts, start their digestive process in the lower stomach with the release of HCL (hydrochloric acid), which in turn releases pepsin. These substances are both acidic in nature.

When a predominant starch combines in the stomach with a predominant protein, you have a clash. You know this by the bloating and the full feeling you get after you eat a meal like this. Fermentation of sugar creates alcohol. This alcohol can stimulate or decrease our energy levels, cause over-acidity, mucus congestion, protein toxicity and inflammation of the tissues. The liver, pancreas and adrenal tissues get hit the hardest. It is difficult for diabetics to regulate their blood sugars eating this way.

Separate Your Fruits or Melons from All Other Foods

Fruits and melons digest very quickly. When combined with foods that digest slowly, their sugars are held up in the stomach. This results in the fermentation of the undigested sugar, which then yields alcohol. This alcohol from fermentation of food sugars raises blood alcohol levels and has even caused plane crashes, car wrecks and DWI arrests.

Make a whole meal of fruits or melons by themselves. These are high energy and cleansing meals that are very important to the detoxification process.

There are many other important concepts in proper food combinations, such as, "Don't combine two different types of proteins at the same meal," or "Certain fruits can combine with certain proteins." The subject can be quite vast, and the details are beyond the scope of this book. For more information see the recommended books listed above.

The simpler you eat, the better it is for your digestive processes. The better your food breaks down, the more energy you will have. The following chart provides an overview of proper (and improper) food combinations.

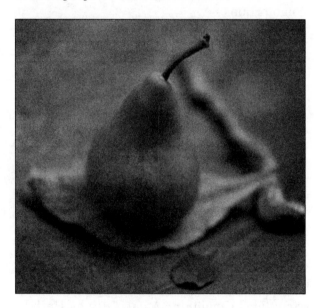

Simple Food Combining

MELONS

Cataloupe
Honey Dew
Papaya
Watermelon

*Eat melons
alone or leave
them alone.*

 NO

FRUITS

ACID	SUB-ACID	SWEET
Citrus Fruits	Apples	Bananas
Pineapples	Cherries	Dates
Strawberries	Grapes	Figs
Sour Fruits	Mangos	Raisins

*Eat more fruit meals high in energy, antioxidants,
astringents, and nutrition. Great brain and nerve foods.
Do not combine with other types of foods.*

 NO

 NO

VEGETABLES

Avocados	Cauliflower	Green Beans	Radish
Beets	Cabbage	Herbs	Romaine
Bell Peppers	Celery	Kale	Spinach
Broccoli	Cucumbers	Peas	Sprouts
Carrots	Greens	Onions	Zucchini

*Vegetables are full of nutrition, fiber, amino acids and minerals.
Great for building a weakened body. Vegetables are more
muscular/skeletal foods than fruits.*

 YES

 YES

STARCHES

Breads*
Cereals*
Corn
Potatoes
Pumpkin

*Starches are very mucus-forming, hard
to digest and gluey to the bowels. Rarely
eat starches or only in winter.*

 NO

*Not fit for
humans.*

PROTEINS

Dairy Foods*
Cheeses, raw
Meats*
Nuts
Seeds

*Proteins are very concentrated foods. Eat
in moderation depending upon the time
of season and the location you live in.*

☀ The Detox Miracle Menus

I created the following dietary program after thirty years of clinical and personal use. I call it the "Detox Miracle Diet" because I have seen it heal and rebuild tissue for thousands of people. I also call this "God's Rainbow Diet" because it consists of all colors of fruits and vegetables. Each food and its color feeds, energizes and heals the body in its own special way. Fruits feed the brain and nervous system, whereas vegetables feed the muscles and skeletal system. Nuts and seeds are structural foods.

The more raw, uncooked and unprocessed food you eat, the more vital you become. Challenge your self-discipline. Try a 100 percent raw food program, which is to say, nothing cooked. It makes a huge difference in the level of vitality you can achieve. One should at least consider eating 80 percent raw foods and 20 percent cooked.

Here are a few things to keep in mind as you begin this process:

1. I do not recommend any kind of animal products at all, due to their huge toxicity and acidic factors. They cause disease instead of rebuilding your body. If you are going to eat meat, you should not eat it more than three times a week, and only at lunch. This will allow the bulk of the digestive process, which is acidic, to take place. Some believe that the body doesn't produce hydrochloric acid after 2:00 P.M. I personally have never seen any scientific evidence to support this theory. However, light alkaline meals in the evening will give you more energy, better sleeping, and better healing potential.

2. Never eat meat with a starch. If you enjoy that heavy feeling, I suggest you replace meat with a baked potato. You can use real butter, or natural oils like olive oil, but no salts, sour cream or cheese. A baked sweet potato would be preferable to an ordinary potato.

3. If you just want something hot, I would suggest a cup or bowl of homemade vegetable soup (no tomatoes), steamed vegetables, or stir-fry vegetables, along with a salad. (See our recipe section at the end of this chapter for various soups you can make.)

4. Demand organic, vine-ripened foods that are chemical-free and irradiation-free. We cannot allow the destruction of our foods or we will all die. In a world where cancer is soon to be in every other person, it is time for every individual to stand up and take charge of their own health. No one else will.

5. The focus for the first two or three months of detoxing should be on low-protein, or "no-protein" type foods. This includes avoiding meat, beans and nuts. Nuts, of course, are your best source of amino acids, and would be my choice if you felt that you needed this type of food.

ONE DAY AT A TIME FOR FIVE DAYS

Take each day as it comes. Try to eat all raw fruits and vegetables that day. The next day, try again. Keep trying each day until you have eaten all raw, uncooked fruits and vegetables for **five days straight**. Feel the difference between all raw and just some cooked foods. The difference is like night and day.

Some days you may only want to eat fruits, which is great. Fruits have the greatest cleansing power of all foods. Their high energetics makes them an unmatched nerve and brain food.

Another method I've found to be successful is to eat all raw foods from Monday through Friday. Then on Saturday and/or Sunday, if you must, have your cooked vegetables with rice, etc. Get a cycle going for yourself. Your body loves cycles. It loves habit. It actually depends and functions better on routine.

As time goes on you may want to incorporate some fasting into your program. This will accelerate the detoxification process. Give fasting your best shot. The longer you last, the healthier you will get. Recondition yourself by retraining your eating habits.

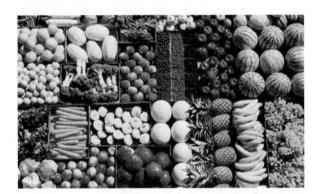

I designed this menu in our "Getting Healthy" program to be easy and yet effective. Enjoy the clean feeling and the sense of vitality that raw foods offer. You will never regret this journey into vibrancy, longevity and spirituality.

HOW MUCH FOOD AND HOW OFTEN?

There has always been the question of: "How much and how often should a person eat?" It is my personal opinion that we should **eat only one-to-three different foods at a time, and eat as often as we like, but only when we are hungry**. Our society recognizes eating only three times a day: breakfast, lunch and dinner. Because of this, we tend to overeat and combine many different types of foods at the same meal. This only serves to overwork the GI tract and digestive organs, causing mal-digestion and malabsorption of our nutrients. Thus, people in our culture "live" mostly on fermentation and putrefaction by-products.

Lack of Funds? Make Food Your Medicine

Lack of funds is a common problem that most of us have experienced. My answer to this is simple: "You must always eat." But *what* you eat has everything to do with your health. Instead of buying meats, which can be expensive, spend that money on fruits and vegetables. Your goals and priorities should always include your health.

Disease can be extremely expensive compared to getting healthy. A good example of this was a young man who came to me with stomach cancer. He had just been diagnosed at a cancer center in Tampa, Florida. The oncologists there told him that they needed to remove two-thirds of his stomach. He also needed some chemotherapy, and I believe radiation therapy as well. The cost would be somewhere around $100,000 for all of this, after which he had a twenty-five percent chance to live. They charged him $5,000 just to diagnose him and report their findings. It took me fifty-nine days to help him cure himself of stomach cancer, at a cost of $1800.00. So if you think natural health is costly, think again.

Instead of buying items of desire, buy only out of necessity. Use any funds you have left for good quality herbs or herbal formulas that will help you achieve your health goals. Disease can leave you penniless; health will leave you rich.

☀ The Detox Vitality Menu

This menu is set up for a **four-week transition from heavy toxic food to pure, more alkaline food, leading to detoxification and regeneration** of your system. While this menu is designed for beginners in this process and for "social eaters," meaning those who eat out a lot, it is not necessary to use the cooked vegetable and grain alternatives that are offered. Instead, for those who want to engage this process more dynamically right from the beginning, or those who are under the care of a health professional for particular medical conditions, including cancer, MS, Parkinson's, spinal cord injuries, Alzheimer's, and other conditions, this menu can simply be replaced at any time with the choice to eat only raw fruits and vegetables (See **Menu for the Bold**, which follows). Remember, you have the freedom to make your life what and how you want it. OK, now let's have fun and eat.

TODAY'S SPECIALS

Always feel free to eat only fresh, raw fruits and/or vegetables in place of this menu for greater detoxification and regeneration.

Breakfast

Choose one.
1. Fruit
2. Melon

Pick any single or combination of fruits or melons that you like. Some dried fruit or coconut may be added to the fruit meal.

Between Meal Juice

Drink an 8 oz. to 10 oz. glass of freshly juiced vegetable or fruit juice.

Lunch

Choose one.
1. Large Salad, with a side of:**
   Vegetables, steamed or raw
   Vegetable soup, no tomato
   Stir-fry vegetables
2. Fruit
3. Melon

Between Meal Juice

Drink an 8 oz. to 10 oz. glass of freshly juiced vegetable or fruit juice.

Dinner

Choose one.
1. Large Salad, with a side of:**
   Vegetables, steamed or raw
   Vegetable soup, no tomato
   Stir-fry vegetables
2. Fruit
3. Melon

Snacks

In between meals, snacks must consist of fresh fruits, dried fruits and fruit or vegetable juices only.

** Do not mix starches and proteins at the same meal. Pick one or the other.

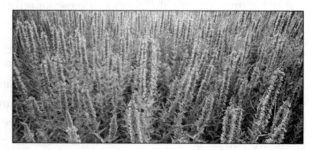

☀ The Detox Menu for the Bold

This menu is for the serious-minded individual who truly wants to achieve dynamic health and vitality. This menu should also be followed by those with chronic and especially degenerative conditions or injuries, like cancer, diabetes, MS, Parkinson's, spinal cord injuries, or Lou Gehrig's disease.

Try to acquire organic foods if possible. If not, wash, wash, wash your produce! Place two capfuls of hydrogen peroxide and the juice of two fresh lemons in about a sinkful of water. You could also add a pinch of salt. Let your fruits or vegetables soak for about five minutes, then rinse. You may scrub them if you wish with a vegetable brush.

Be happy when you eat, and relax. Try not to drink when you eat. Keep your eating simple and fun.

TODAY'S SPECIAL

Breakfast

Choose one.
1. Fruit
2. Melon

Pick any single or combination of fruits or melons that you like. Some dried fruit or co-conut may be added to the fruit meal.

Between Meal Juice

See recommended juices.

Lunch

Choose one.
1. Large Salad
2. Fruit
3. Melon

Salad may consist of any raw vegetables. (*See* additional salad suggestions among recipes in Module 7.9.)

Between Meal Juice

See recommended juices.

Dinner

Choose one.
1. Large Salad
2. Fruit
3. Melon

Salad may consist of any raw vegetables. (*See* additional salad suggestions among recipes in Module 7.9.)

Snacks

In between meals, snacks must consist of fresh fruits, raw vegetables, and fruit or vegetable juices only.

Recommended Juices

Vegetable juices:
carrot, spinach, parsley, dandelion greens. (*See* Module 7.7, which follows, for more juice combination suggestions.)

Fruit juices:
grape, apple, pear, fresh-squeezed orange or lemon. I do not recommend pineapple juice (bottled), cranberry juice or prune juice.

☀ Raw Fruit and Vegetable Juices

The highest nutritional and electrical-energy foods on the planet are fresh raw fruits, vegetables, herbs, seaweeds, nuts and seeds. These are the foods for humans. It is essential that you eat at least 80 percent of your diet from fresh, ripe, raw, fruits and vegetables. These foods carry the power of life in them. They are full of enzymes, vitamins, minerals (tissue salts), amino acids, antioxidants, simple sugars, water, electricity and much more. However, being frugivores, the fruits and nuts are more suited for us. Remember, the human gastrointestinal tract is only twelve times the length of the spine, whereas an herbivore's GI tract is thirty times the length of its spine. Herbivores also have numerous stomachs because vegetable fibers are much more difficult to break down than fruit fibers.

Fruit fiber is the easiest fiber for our GI tract to handle, consequently it keeps our intestinal walls clean. Because the energy from fruits is much higher than that of vegetables, the power to enhance the nervous system is higher. This increases bowel peristalsis, as well. Vegetables, on the other hand, have more minerals, chlorophyll and amino acids, which are great in building up a depleted body. You've probably observed that children will eat fruits long before they will eat their vegetables.

By now in our society practically everyone has heard of, or tasted, freshly-made vegetable or fruit juice. This is thanks to Norman W. Walker, Paul Bragg, Herbert M. Shelten, Bernard Jensen, and "The Juice Man," a few of the pioneers and practitioners of juicing for health.

If you are weakened or depleted, especially in the digestive tract, or if you *do* not want high fiber but do want nutrition, juicing is the answer. Juicing takes the fiber out of the food and gives you all the rest in a drinkable form, thus bringing concentrated power to your body. While you might only eat one whole carrot, you can drink the juice of five or six carrots. The importance of this in cancer, injuries, or any disease or depletion issue is obvious.

When you're healthy, drinking fresh raw juices just makes you healthier. It is important to realize, however, that raw roughage from fruits and vegetables is essential for good bowel health. When refined grains, mixed with other cooked foods and meats became the staple diet in the U.S., bowel cancer in this country went from being the fourth highest incidence of cancer to being the first. Currently it is #2, only surpassed by lung cancer.

Thirty years ago I used to fight the medical establishment over the importance of fiber. Their claims were that my program damaged and irritated conditions like gastritis, enteritis, colitis or diverticulitis. They didn't realize that the reason for these inflammatory conditions, including the "pocketing" of the intestines, was from a lack of fiber. Nowadays however, most doctors realize the importance of fruit and vegetable fiber. Grain fiber, on the other hand, can be too rough for our GI tract. We learned that by using too much bran in the 1960s and 70s.

There are many books on the market on vegetable and fruit juices. I recommend, *The Complete Book of Fresh Vegetable and Fruit Juices* by N.W. Walker; *Juicing* by Michael T. Murray; and *Juicing Therapy* by my friend Bernard Jensen, Ph.D. Keep it simple, but do explore and enjoy the tremendous power of these juices.

I would suggest at least two to four 10-ounce glasses of vegetable or fruit juice a day, along with a raw food diet. The best time to prepare fresh juice is just before you intend to drink it. However, in our busy society, I find people get tired of juicing because of the clean-up issues. I suggest juicing for the whole day, storing the juice in a glass container, and keeping it in the refrigerator for no more than two days.

Please refer back to Chapter 6, Modules 6.7 and 6.8, and read about juice fasting for more encouragement about the tremendous benefits of juices. Remember fruit juices are great brain, nerve and glandular foods. They are the cleansers of the body as well. Vegetable juices rebuild the structure of the body, especially bone, muscle and connective tissue.

Your body will go through cycles in which you will crave fruit juices and fruits only. Then there will be a time when your body craves vegetable juices and vegetables. Listen and flow with these cravings. The body knows what it is doing and what it needs. One of our greatest shortcomings is that we don't listen. People don't listen to God or to their own bodies. We think that the mind and emotions control us. However, these are only conditioned tools that we can use to create our lives. Tradition, social belief systems of right or wrong, our schooling, and the like, are what condition the mind and the emotions. Today, especially, with major corporations and associations focusing on money and control, we are taught and sold a toxic way of life. Become free and return to God's way of vitality and vibrancy.

Juicing is an art and somewhat of a science. Read, learn and keep it simple. Enjoy the way these juices rebuild and cleanse the body. You will find you can't live without them. Find yourself an easy-to-clean juicer (like the Champion® brand) and start juicing now.

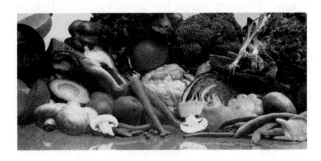

"Power House" Juice Suggestions

Two of the best single-fruit juices are grape juice and apple juice. These will supply loads of calcium, while they clean the liver and kidneys, and feed the nerves and glandular system.

GRAPE JUICE
Juice the seeds and stems, too.
Effects: Tumor buster; lymph stimulation; free-radical eliminator; toxicity removal, including heavy metals and minerals. Strengthens the heart and vascular system.

APPLE JUICE
Effects: Enzyme-rich juice aids digestion; supplies amino acids; a free-radical eliminator; strengthens the body.

VEGETABLE JUICE COMBINATIONS
The following vegetable juice combinations are power packed for the liver, kidneys and adrenals. They are also high in electrolytes, including calcium, magnesium, potassium and sodium. These drinks are rich in chlorophyll ("plant blood" or "green blood") for purifying the blood and lymphatic system. Chlorophyll is one of nature's best heavy-metal and chemical detoxifiers.

- Carrot + Beet +Parsley
- Carrot + Beet + Spinach
- Carrot + Alfalfa Sprouts + Parsley
- Carrots + Spinach + Celery + Parsley
- Wheat grass + Alfalfa sprouts
- Juicing cabbage and the cruciferous vegetables is very beneficial for cancer cases.

☼ Beans and Grains: Good or Bad?

Beans and grains are dormant foods. Enzyme inhibitors block the germination process by blocking enzyme action, which allows for long-term storage without spoilage. Even though beans are more protein-rich and grains are starches, they are both acid-forming and very hard to digest. I have always said that it takes more of your body's systemic energy to digest, assimilate and excrete these foods than they give back to you. Simply put, they rob the body of energy in the final analysis.

Why do we give grains to hogs and cattle? To fatten them up. And these foods will do the same to you. Dried beans and grains are very concentrated, making digestion long and difficult. It is also possible that the enzyme inhibitors will affect your body's enzyme action.

Sprout For Life

If you **sprout beans or grains** you release the "life force" within them—the enzymes. Their nutritional content then becomes more balanced and more usable by the body. They become chlorophyll rich. Chlorophyll has been called "green blood," as its composition is close to that of human blood. Not only does it give you energy, but it also acts like an antioxidant, removing toxic metals and mucus from the body. Read: *Love Your Body* and *Survival into the 21st Century* by Viktoras Kulvinskas; and *Sprouts* by Kathleen O'Bannon, CNC.

If you want true bodily vitality and regeneration, avoid unsprouted beans and grains. If you must eat them, do so in cold climates and never together, as you don't want to combine protein and starch at the same meal. This causes even greater body enervation from fermentation and putrefaction (see Proper Food Combinations, Module 7. 3). Animals in the wild do not consume such foods. If they did, it would make them sluggish and vulnerable as prey to other more robust animals.

Health is energy and energy comes from life, not death. As you begin to eat more "alive" foods you will know firsthand the effects that beans and grains will have on your energy levels and your agility. We must look beyond our limited, culturally-determined, nutritional ideas to see the vast array of foods that nature supplies for us.

The seasons have a great impact upon us, especially in the northern climates where more drastic weather changes are experienced. In summer, being acidic, we need mostly alkaline foods. However, in the cold of winter, which is alkaline, we tend to desire acid-type foods like beans and grains. This is a natural process. However, these foods should always be kept to a minimum. Remember, the healthier your glands are, the more the body will naturally create its own internal heat regulation.

An example of this heat-regulating factor can be seen in the operation of the thyroid gland. Since the thyroid gland regulates metabolism, your body's temperature can be greatly affected if these tissues are weak. Beans and grains, even though warming in nature, in the long run can make the thyroid weak. This can then have the opposite effect to warming, instead causing you to be cold all the time, especially your extremities.

THE SOY MYTH

As with every aspect of life, one always needs to question and investigate the truth behind the propaganda that fills the press concerning issues of nutrition and health. If you learn the basics of health as set forth in this book you will be better prepared to recognize fact from fiction. Use the facts and truths presented here as your template.

Ask yourself and try to investigate who might benefit from whatever information is being given. The current "soy fad" is one area that definitely deserves your attention. To understand who might be behind what I consider a horrendous and highly-calculated myth, let's first examine some of the facts about soy.

Properties of Raw Soy Beans

- Acid-forming
- Extremely high in phytic acid (blocks mineral absorption, especially zinc)
- Full of enzyme inhibitors
- Extremely hard to digest
- 85 percent genetically modified (also called Round-Up Ready Soy Beans®) where the cell DNA and structure are combined with herbicides and bacteria to create resistance to these factors for better yield
- Full of excessive amounts of hemaglutin—a clot-causing compound
- Allergy causing
- Extremely high in levels of aluminum (very toxic to brain and nerve tissue)

Facts about Cooked and Processed Soy Beans

- Over 80 percent of the oils and fats used in the U.S.A. are from processed soy beans
- Over 80 percent of the margarine made in the U.S.A. comes from soy beans
- Soy beans, as most beans, have enzyme inhibitors and also are high in phytic acid. They must be processed at high temperatures to break these metabolism-blockers down.

The Basic Processes in Obtaining Soy Bean Oil and Soy Protein

1. COOKING

Heated to between 225°F and 250°F, which:
- Destroys all nutrients
- Bonds proteins to minerals
- Bonds proteins to lipids and starches
- Causes free-radical formation
- Creates trans-fatty acids (which are hardening and obstructing as well as mutagenic to DNA)
- Encourages rancidity (toxic for the bacterial action needed)
- Is extremely acid-forming
- Possibly promotes formation of acrylimides (carcinogenic compounds)

2. PRESSING

Cold pressed or solvent extraction involves:
- Exposure to light and air causing free-radical formation through oxidation
- Rancidity, causing further breakdown (mostly stored in clear containers allowing a continuation of this process)
- Cold pressing only after cooking
- Solvent extraction method that creates many toxic and carcinogenic compounds, lysinealine being a major carcinogen
- Solvent extraction, which requires: alkali soaps, hexane (petroleum distiller), phosphoric acid and sodium hydroxide (the primary ingredient in Drano)

3. HYDROGENATION

- A process of heating the oil to over 400°F, forcing hydrogen gas (in the presence of a metallic catalyst) through this oil for over five hours
- Not only "super kills," it literally renders a food substance "dead and toxic"

As you can see from the short overview above, soy is not a food, but a toxin, especially if it is cooked or processed. If it indeed has any estrogenic properties this adds to its destructive side effects, especially in 80 percent of the females who are estrogen dominant.

Soy is not a health food, but an industry brain child from chemical, bio-tech mega-corporations posing as food producers. It is shameful when companies put money first and God and life last.

Over 60 percent of the foods manufactured in the U.S. have some level of soy involvement —from natural flavorings, vegetable shortening, hydrolyzed protein, textured vegetable protein and soy bean oil to soy protein.

Many people are consuming some form of soy: protein powders, soy milk, soy candy bars, health bars and even baby foods. Soy products account for close to $100 billion a year in business. What does that tell you about why soy is being presented as the greatest thing since white bread?

Remember: If it's not a fruit, vegetable, seed, or a nut, you don't need it and it is probably toxic to you.

NOTE — A great web site to visit on this subject and more is www.thedoctorwithin.com

MODULE 7.9

☀ Recipes to Enjoy

This small collection of raw-food and cooked recipes will give you some idea of the many simple dishes you can prepare for yourself. The different vegetable combinations in salads, soups, stir-fried or steamed dishes are endless. Prepare these combinations of either fruit dishes or vegetable dishes according to your taste. Keep it simple. Heavy creams and sauces were created to cover up the dead taste of cooked foods. Enjoy the rainbow of colors, energies, smells and tastes of nature's foods. These foods are designed for our species.

RAW MENU

The Master Salad

Combine any or all of the following:
    Romaine lettuce
    Peas
    Spinach
    Cucumbers
    Olives
    Bell peppers (all colors)
    Tomatoes
    Onions
    Asparagus
    Avocado
    Cabbage (red or white)
    Green beans
    Carrots
    Sweet corn
    Any dark green leafy vegetable

Make your salad fun and filled with a rainbow of colored vegetables. Use only small amounts of dressing. (*See* Raw Dressing recipe in this section.) For those who wish oil on the salad use only raw organic olive, coconut or grape seed oil. Enjoy the natural flavors of vegetables.

Relish

    2 cups sweet corn, cut right from the cob
    1/4 cup sweet onions, chopped
    1/4 cup red bell peppers, chopped

Mix all ingredients together. If you want your relish creamier, put your ingredients into a blender and blend to your desired consistency.

Raw Dressing

Avocado
Garlic
Cucumbers
Olive oil (optional)
Bell peppers (all colors)
Sweet onion
Apple cider vinegar

Place ingredients in a blender and blend them until a semi-liquid is formed. Pour over your salad as desired.

Guacamole

2 cups of diced avocados (remove skin)
4 diced green onions
Freshly squeezed lemon juice to taste
    (1/2 lemon)
1/2 cup of tomatoes
1/4 cup of chopped bell peppers (optional)

Chop or mash the ingredients until desired texture, and then mix together.

Veggie Sandwich

Lettuce (romaine or any dark green
    leafy vegetable)
Black olives
Sprouts
Tomato
Avocado*
Sweet onion
Pickles
Bell peppers (all colors)
Cucumbers
Bread, all natural sprouted multi-grain
    or millet bread**

*You can mash your avocado and use it like mayonnaise. You can sprinkle some of your salad dressing on your sandwich as well.

**We recommend millet bread because it is more alkaline to the body while most other grains are acid-forming.

Rainbow Fruit Salad

Fruit bowls are extremely delicious and loved by all ages. Certain fruits, however, do not combine well together. **Generally your acid type fruits, like oranges and pineapples, do not mix well with your sweet type fruits, like bananas.** The following are some suggestions for fruit bowls. Be creative.

Bananas, Peaches
Bananas, Blueberries
Bananas, Strawberries
Bananas, Mangos
Bananas, Apples, Strawberries, Grapes
Bananas, Blueberries, Apples, Grapes
Bananas, Strawberries, Apples
Bananas, Apples, Grapes

Melons

Remember "Eat them alone or leave them alone." All varieties are acceptable.

Watermelon
Cantaloupe
Honeydew
Papaya

Almond Nut Milk

1 cup of raw almonds
1/2 cup of maple syrup
3 1/2 to 4 cups of distilled water
1/2 tsp of almond extract (or vanilla extract)

For a spicy Indian version, add the following to the above ingredients:

1/4 tsp of cardamom
1/4 tsp of nutmeg
1/2 tsp of cinnamon

Place all ingredients into a blender and blend on a high speed for three minutes. For a smoother consistency, strain through a large strainer layered with a piece of cheesecloth.

Almond milk is a protein and should not be combined with starches. Use rice milk if you wish to combine with a starch.

Banana Ice Cream

    4 to 6 bananas
    1 to 1 1/2 cups of apple juice
    1 tsp. of vanilla
    1/2 cup of raw almonds

To make any frozen treat you will need some frozen fruit and fresh fruit juice. Organic fresh juice and fruit is always preferred. However, glass-bottled organic juice may be substituted.

Peel 4 to 6 bananas and freeze overnight in a zip-lock baggie. Put about 1 to 1 1/2 cups of apple juice and 1 tsp of vanilla in a blender. Break off pieces of frozen banana and add to the apple juice as you blend them (a few pieces at a time) until you get a creamy consistency. If you want a thicker blend simply add more frozen banana, or, first add 1/2 cup of raw almonds to blender and blend to small pieces or powder, then add your apple juice, vanilla and frozen bananas.

Date/Coconut Rolls

    2 cups of dates
    1 cup of raisins
    1/4 cup of coconut
    1 cup of nuts—pecans or
        almonds (optional)

Remove pits from the dates. Put dates and raisins through a food grinder. Chop nuts to medium size. Mix all ingredients together and then form into balls. Roll in grated coconut or finely ground nuts. Keep in the refrigerator.

Frozen Bananas

    Bananas
    Sesame seeds
    Honey
    Melted carob (optional)

Peel your bananas and roll them in the honey, then roll them in the sesame seeds or drizzle with or dip into melted carob. Place the bananas on a plate, cover and freeze.

Smoothies

    1/2 cup Blueberries
    2 Bananas
    4 Dates
    Organic Grape Juice (fresh or bottled)
    Chopped Ice (4 to 6 cubes)

Add your juice, dates, ice, bananas and blueberries to a blender and blend to desired texture. Any fruit and fruit juice combination can be used. Fruit smoothies are like milkshakes, but very healthy.

COOKED MENU

Vegetable Soup

    Carrots
    Sweet corn
    Pearl onions
    Green beans (optional)
    Peas
    Garlic (optional)
    Cauliflower
    Potatoes (sparingly)

Use a water base when making this delicious soup. You may add any herbal spice like Herbamare® or Spike® toward the end of the cooking process or after the soup is cooked. Fresh raw spices are preferable. No salt or pepper of any type because they are irritants and mucus-forming.

Cauliflower Soup

    2 cups chopped cauliflower
    3 cups of distilled water
    1 large sweet onion
    2 Tbs. of olive oil
    1/2 cup bell pepper (red or yellow)

Sauté onion in olive oil until translucent. Bring water with cauliflower and pepper to a boil and simmer for 10 minutes. Add sautéed onion, stir. Take out 2 cups of soup and blend in blender. Add back to pot, stir and enjoy!

Carrot/Squash Soup

1 sweet onion, chopped
3 lbs butternut squash chopped
    (peeled, with seeds removed)
10 chopped carrots
4–5 chopped garlic cloves
3–4 tablespoons of olive oil
1/3 bunch parsley, chopped

Sauté onion until translucent in 2 tablespoons of olive oil, set aside. Add the squash and carrots to water (make sure that they are covered) and bring to a boil. Cook over medium heat until carrots and squash are slightly soft. Add the cooked onion. Add the chopped garlic and parsley and boil for 1 minute longer. Remove from heat. Serve.

Steamed Veggies

Broccoli
Cauliflower
Bell peppers (all colors)
Onions
Asparagus
Pea pods (optional)
Green beans (optional)

Place your desired veggies into a stainless steel steamer, and steam for 5 to 7 minutes. You may wish to put these steamed vegetables over whole grain brown rice with an onion or veggie sauce.

*Stainless steel "leaf" steamers are inexpensive and can be purchased at any department store that carries kitchen utensils. They are made to fit down into saucepans. Avoid all aluminum cookware.

Stir-Fried Veggies

3 tablespoons olive oil
Chopped vegetables of your choice
    (including bean sprouts)

Add olive oil to skillet. Heat oil and add chopped vegetables (the sky is the limit where your choices are concerned). Stir-fry for approximately 5–10 minutes, but don't overcook. Season to taste with your favorite herbal spices.

Short-Grain Whole Brown Rice

1 cup of short-grain brown rice
2 cups of water

Rinse rice and put into a pot with 2 cups of water. Bring to a boil, cover and cook on low heat for 45 minutes until all water is absorbed.

Millet Cereal

Use this once a week only. Prepare according to package directions, or as you would oatmeal. Use rice milk only. Sweeten with honey, molasses or maple syrup.

Your food determines in a large measure how long you shall live – how much you shall enjoy life, and how successful your life shall be.
— Dr. Kirschner, *Live Food Juice*

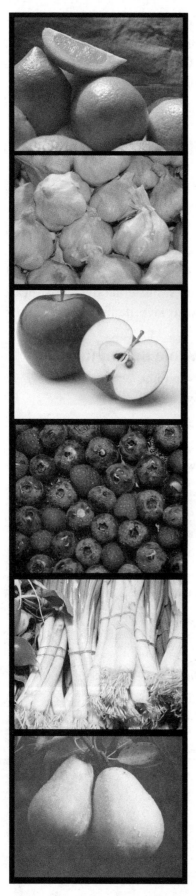

CHAPTER EIGHT

The Power of Herbs

When I started using herbs and herbal formulas over twenty-seven years ago, my success in my clinic skyrocketed. I began to see much deeper cleansing and healing—true regeneration and vitality—in tissues. Previously, with supplements, I would see *some* improvement, and maybe some symptoms eliminated. However, these symptoms would return when the supplementation was stopped.

Today, the use of herbs (botanicals) is vital to the restoration of the human race. Their power to invoke the cleansing and regeneration process can't be equaled by manufactured supplements or chemical medications. Where chemical medications suppress and hold toxins in the body, herbs pull and clean these toxins out as well as strengthen the cells. Because herbs haven't been hybridized they haven't lost their powerful nutritive and electrical properties.

From a spiritual viewpoint, herbs carry the "original awareness" with which they were created. When an herb's "consciousness" or awareness unites with the consciousness of a human cell, this empowers the cell to function as *it* was originally created. As DNA and cellular activity changes, this yields greater vitality to cells, tissues, or glands. With their powerful cleansing actions, herbs empower the body to clean itself out of all obstructions, thereby enhancing blood, lymph, and neuro (energy) flow to the cells.

The original power (consciousness), nutrition, and active ingredients that herbs have can make the difference between life and death. We have come to a point genetically in our cellular patterns where treatment is no longer effective. The chemical toxicity levels in our air and from our foods is so high that acidosis and deterioration is affecting everything—our buildings, statues, water supplies, animals, and especially ourselves. In the last 100 years humans have done what no other animal has ever done in billions of years: we have destroyed the earth. If you wish to survive this, changing your approach from treatment to detoxification is essential. If you do not alkalize and clean out the poisons that are killing your body, your chances of getting healthy remain very low.

This book is aimed at changing your viewpoint about treatment. It has been my life's work not to treat, but to detoxify and regenerate. This is especially true in chronic and degenerative disorders, such as diabetes (type I), cancer, arthritis, and MS. One cannot just treat these conditions. The tissues (organs and glands) that are failing must be restored.

Herbs have been used for ages by humans and animals for the treatment of disease as well as for nutrition. Herbs are non-hybrid vegetables. Their nutritional, electrical, and medicinal content is much greater than most hybrid, garden vegetables. The uniqueness and superiority of herbs lies in their strong medicinal compounds, or what I call their restorative properties, which include acids, alkaloids, saponins, flavonoids, coumarins (clotting factors), tannins, (astringent properties), antioxidants (immune), bitter principles and much more. A list of many of these herbs and their effects upon tissues will be found in Module 8.2, *Power Herbs*.

The restorative principles in herbs can enhance, cleanse and provide nutrition to cells and tissues, thus affecting cell and tissue response. Herbs increase the blood and lymph flow within tissues, which increases nutrition to cells and allows them to eliminate their wastes.

Herbs are "tissue-specific" in that each herb was designed by God to affect a specific type of tissue or part of the body. The beauty of God's herbs is that they can and do affect many different types of tissues at the same time. Examples of this would be Licorice Root, Saw Palmetto Berries, and Chaste Tree Berries. These herbs not only affect the endocrine gland tissues but also have a broad range effect upon the body. They strengthen the vascular system, enhancing male and female organs, and are anti-inflammatory as well. Parasite herbs such as Black Walnut Hull and Pau d'Arco not only kill parasites but enhance the immune system and the endocrine gland system. They have a broad range effect, killing all types of parasites, including, but not limited to yeasts, fungi, molds, bacteria, viruses, flukes and worms. Antibiotic drugs, on the other hand, only kill bacteria, and at the same time stimulate yeast growth. Because antibiotics are sulfur-type drugs, this inorganic sulfur accumulates in body tissues causing tissue impairment. The parasitic herbs are also cellular proliferators, which means that they rebuild and strengthen cells. The true beauty and importance of using botanicals is that they affect the whole body in a positive manner.

I have used huge amounts of herbs in my career (many times on just one client), and have seen only positive results in my thirty years of practice. Our clinic has become world renowned for its successes, where others have failed. We have not seen any negative interaction with herbs and chemical medications, but this is always a possibility. The goal, of course, would be for the patient to become free of all chemical intakes.

It is my opinion that herbs are mainly meant to be consumed raw and uncooked, or in a tincture form, whereby digestion is minimal and absorption is optimal. However, the roots, barks, and tubers can be boiled and still have a great affect upon liver, pancreatic and GI tract function. Boiling, of course, destroys the water-soluble constituents such as the vitamin C-complexes (flavonoids), the B-vitamins, and the like. Boiling or heating the herbs can also saturate (bond) the fats. However, most of the time, when you are using boiled teas, you are treating symptoms and are trying to promote an immediate action in the body. Most of the active medicinal properties are not destroyed by heat.

I use herbs to promote detoxification and for tissue enhancement through nutritive and energetic stimulation, not abrasive stimulation. We are living beings who require living foods and herbs to heal ourselves. The power of a raw herb to accomplish this is a hundred times that of its cooked counterpart.

Remember that herbs are food. They are made of proteins (amino acids), carbohydrates (starches and sugars) and fats. They also have lots of fiber (cellulose) which is vital for the health of the intestinal tract. The immortal words of Hippocrates, the famous Naturopath and Father of Medicine, apply here: "Let your food be your medicine and your medicine be your food."

In religious and spiritual texts from many world traditions you will find mention of the power and importance of herbs. God did not create chemical medicines, but God did create herbs.

Herbs are fun to use and remarkable to experience as they clean and rebuild your body. There are only a few herbs to approach with caution, such as Peruvian Bark (Cinchona calisaya). This herb is beneficial at low dosages, but toxic at high dosages. I would leave herbs like this alone.

This chapter begins with a short essay (Module 8.1) on the common and traditional uses of botanicals, and then in Module 8.2 provides a detailed list of some of the strongest and most effective herbs that nature has to offer. These herbs have been clinically tested for many years. The results of these herbs in supporting tissue regeneration have been miraculous. We humans have a lot to learn when it comes to the power of botanicals to rebuild the body.

Herbal formulas, consisting of combinations of herbs, can have a much stronger effect upon the body than single herbs. There are many things to consider when combining herbs, such as compatibility, synergistic actions and effects to related tissues. In Module 8.3 I will suggest an ideal herbal tincture or blend for each of ten major conditions, including adrenal gland enhancement, parasite cleansing, and kidney and bladder functioning.

In Module 8.4 you will find the body systems listed once again (Cardiovascular, Digestive, etc.), with suggestions for herbal detoxifiers and strengtheners for each system. Finally, we will close with an important consideration of pharmaceutical antibiotics vs. nature's anti-parasitics in Module 8.5.

Have fun with herbs and herbal formulas, for their power and strength is much needed in today's world. With the use of herbs to clean and rebuild the body, vibrant health can be achieved by anyone who is willing to put his/her heart into it. Do not be afraid of what God created for your use. Simply learn which herbs are for what purpose. Herbs are easy to use. Don't let those who have no education in herbology tell you that herbs are bad. That's like saying God is bad. God created herbs for everything from bone growth and repair to nerve regeneration. Herbs are God's greatest healers, especially when used in conjunction with a raw food diet.

The June 1992 issue of the *Food and Drug Law Journal* contained the following: "The results of an extensive review on botanical safety conducted by the Herbal Research Foundation (a non-profit organization of leading experts on pharmacognosy, pharmacology and toxicology), confirmed there is no substantial evidence that toxic reactions to botanicals are a major source of concern. The review was based on reports from the American Association of Poison Control Centers and the Center of Disease Control." (McCaleb, R.S.)

☀ Common and Traditional Uses of Botanicals

Each country has its own fantastic herbs. I always recommend using the herbs that grow in the country that you live in. These tend to have a more powerful effect upon your body, because your body adapts to and becomes harmonious with its predominant environment.

There are thousands of herbs in use worldwide. I recommend studying as much as you can about 50 to 100 of the best and strongest herbs known and used in your country. These herbs will take good care of you, and you won't become confused or overwhelmed trying to learn about all the herbs there are to choose from. Exceptions exist for every rule, however. Even though you may live in the U.S., don't neglect some of the remarkable herbs from China, Brazil and India, for instance, like Ginseng, Ginkgo Biloba, Ginger, Pau d'Arco, and certain medicinal mushrooms. When I use herbs from other countries, I only use the best and strongest that each country has to offer.

Herbs should be organically grown or "wildcrafted." Unfortunately, the demand for herbs has become so great that wildcrafting has depleted many of the wild herbs. Organic herb farms are needed, similar to organic fruit and vegetable farms. Such farms are the only hope we have of regenerating and saving our species.

Herbs may be consumed as teas, capsules or tinctures. I prefer the teas and tinctures. This is especially true where poor digestion and malabsorption exist.

MAKING TEA

Teas are simple to make. For each cup of single-herb tea desired, place one heaping teaspoon of the herb and one cup of distilled or reverse osmosis (R/O) water into a glassware pot or saucepan. I recommend using glass instead of any metals, including stainless steel. Even stainless steel releases copper into your teas or foods. When using several herbs, use one cup of water for each different herb and one heaping teaspoon of each herb.

If the herb consists of leaves and flowers, boil them in the water for approximately 3–6 minutes, and let them steep for another 5–10 minutes. If the herbs are roots, tubers or rhizomes, boil them for 10–15 minutes and let them steep for 10–15 minutes. If your tea is too strong, add more water to your mixture. Drink 1 cupful, 3–6 times a day, or use as a douche, enema or poultice depending upon the desired results.

TINCTURES

Herbal tinctures are made by distilling herbs in alcohol, vinegar or glycerin. The strongest, most potent method of making tinctures is accomplished by using 1 part herb to 3–4 parts pure grain alcohol, mixed with equal parts of distilled water. Place the mixture in a glass container and let set in a darkened area for 30 days or so. Start on the new moon and finish on a full moon. Shake this tincture every day. On the last day put your mixture in the sun for at least 4 hours of sunlight. If there is no sunshine on one day, wait until there is, or leave this step out. Now you're ready to bottle your tincture. Use some sort of a press to squeeze this distilled mixture into pure liquid. Take one full dropperful 3–6 times a day.

There are so many ways to use herbs for your benefit, but it is not the purpose of this book to cover them all. Those who are interested can consult my other book, *Power Botanicals and Formulas* (available from God's Herbs, www.godherbs.com), which is a more comprehensive guide to the chemistry and use of botanicals. There are also a multitude of books on the market that are excellent to further your information on herbs and their uses. Some of these are referenced for you in the Bibliography.

Unfortunately, there are also many books on herbs that are not worth the paper they're printed on. These books are written by so-called herbalists or individuals who know little about the true use of each of these herbs. They merely contain information that is referenced from other sources. Some of them copy what the FDA says about herbs, along with the misleading information being fed to the public from pharmaceutical companies to instill fear in people about the use of God's natural foods and medicines. Never fear nature or its products. Simply learn what others have been using and doing for hundreds of thousands of years.

Always fight to keep your right to eat and use God's foods. Estimates are that over 2 million deaths (some estimates as high as 5 million) occur each year needlessly as a result of procedures and products supported by the allopathic medical and pharmaceutical industries. Rarely do we hear of a death from the use of herbs. When one occurs, it's almost always from misuse. Read…Study…Experiment…Lose the fear…Become alive again.

MODULE 8.2

☼ Power Herbs: A Reference Guide

The following herbs are some of the best herbs you can find in the Northern Hemisphere. As you study this section be sure to check the Glossary for definitions of unfamiliar terms.

Alfalfa

- A great alkalizer of the body.
- High in chlorophyll and nutrition.
- High in minerals and trace minerals.
- A body cleanser.
- Enhances the endocrine glandular system, especially the adrenal and pituitary glands.
- Helps eliminate retained water and carbon dioxide.
- Helps with alcohol, smoking, and narcotic addiction.
- Helps eliminate toxic chemicals and heavy metals (lead, aluminum, mercury, etc.) from the body.
- Bonds (chelation) to inorganic minerals for elimination.
- Infection fighter and acts as a natural deodorizer.
- Strengthens the body.
- High in chlorophyll, helps rejuvenate the blood.
- Pulls mucus (catarrh) out of the tissues.

Scientific name: *Medicago sativ*

Parts used: Whole plant, (leaves, seeds, and flowers).

Actions: Astringent, diuretic, nutritive.

Aloe Vera

- Internally, aloe heals ulcerations and inflammation of the GI tract.
- Aloe and Burdock are the "burn botanicals." First, second, third and fourth degree burns

all respond to aloe's tissue-healing and rebuilding properties.

- Used as a bowel mover in heavy constipation cases. (Avoid prolonged usage for this.)
- Aloe Vera is known as the First Aid Plant. It is great for cuts, wounds, and the like.

Scientific name: *Aloe vera linn*

Parts used: Pulp (gel) from inside leaves and powder of the leaf.

Actions: Abortifacient (when used in high doses), alterative, anthelmintic, anti-arthritic, antifungal, antibacterial, anti-inflammatory, antiseptic, astringent, bitter tonic, bitter, cathartic, cell proliferant, cholagogue, decoagulant, demulcent, depurative, emmenagogue, emollient, insecticide, laxative, nutritive, purgative, resin stimulant, stomachic, tonic, vermifuge, vulnerary.

Astragalus

- Astragalus is a tremendous cellular proliferator (strengthens cells).
- I especially like this herb for its effect upon the adrenal tissues.
- Astragalus is a superb immune builder, strengthening the bone marrow, the endocrine glandular system (thymus, etc.), and the spleen.
- Aids in shortness of breath.
- Strengthens the nervous system.
- Increases energy to cells, especially in the spleen and GI tract (stomach, in particular).
- Strengthens prolapsed conditions, e.g., uterus, stomach, intestines and bladder.
- Has mild diuretic properties and helps tone the lungs.
- Brings tone and balance to tissues.

Scientific name: *Astragalus membranaceus*

Parts used: Roots

Actions: Anhydrotic (stops sweating), cellular proliferator, diuretic.

Bilberry

- Tremendous in strengthening the vascular system (arteries, capillaries, and veins); great for varicose veins.
- Helps reduce inflammation (flavonoids) in the vascular walls, hence reduces arteriosclerosis (obstruction of the vascular walls with lipids).
- Inhibits coagulation of platelets in the blood.
- Helps with edema, aids in diarrhea.
- Bilberry helps tone the skin.
- Helps prevent cataracts and protects eye tissue from effects of diabetes.
- Used in formulas to help control blood sugar levels.
- A great anti-inflammatory for all tissues.
- Helps to control stress and anxiety.
- A great aid in night blindness or any vision weakness.

Scientific name: *Vaccinium myrtillus*

Parts used: Leaves and fruits

Actions: Antidiabetic effect, antidiarrheal, astringent, anti-inflammatory.

Black Cohosh

- This herb stimulates estrogen receptors and has estrogenic properties itself.
- Used in female conditions where vaginal dryness, lack of menstruation, and infertility is present. Stimulates estrogen production.
- Not suited for estrogen dominant females, where excessive bleeding and cysts, fibroids, and fibrocystic conditions exist.
- Said to help loosen and expel mucus from the lungs.
- Contracts the uterus and increases menstrual flow.
- Said to be a tonic for the central nervous system (CNS).

Scientific name: *Cimicifuga racemosa*

Parts used: Rhizomes, fresh and dried root

Actions: Alterative, antiseptic, antispasmodic, anti-venomous, arterial, astringent, cardiac stimulant, diaphoretic, diuretic, emmena-gogue, expectorant, sedative, stomachic – tonic.

Black Walnut Hull

Black Walnut Hull is one of my favorite herbs for many reasons.

- It's one of nature's most powerful antiparasitics.
- It will kill microorganisms (bacterium, fungi, yeasts, etc.) to larger parasites including all worms and flukes.
- It is a cellular proliferator (strengthens cells).
- It increases the oxygenation of blood cells.
- It is a detoxifier used to balance sugar levels and disperse fatty materials.
- Black Walnut Hull is excellent for any condition and weakness of the body.
- Promotes healing of all tissues and is said to help restore tooth enamel.
- Strengthens and stimulates the immune system.
- Promotes lymph movement and bowel peristalsis.
- Strengthens the bones (high in calcium).

Scientific name: *Juglans nigra*

Parts used: Inner hull (can use the bark)

Actions: Alterative (leaves) bitter, Anthelmintic (vermifuge), astringent, cholagogue, deter-gent, expectorant, hepatic, laxative, mild cathartic, purgative, tonic (fruit).

Bugleweed

- A specific for the thyroid gland, especially when enlarged or when a goiter exists.
- Said to be a detoxifier, and especially valuable at removing heavy metals.
- Bugleweed is said to offer protection against radiation.
- Beneficial in irregular heartbeat and palpita-tions.
- Improves thyroid and adrenal function.
- Restores tooth enamel.

- Possibly enhances neurotransmitters.
- Also said to resemble digitalis in its actions.
- Has a strengthening effect upon tissue.

Scientific name: *Copus virginicus*

Parts used: The aerial portions of the herb

Actions: Antigonadotropic, anti-inflammatory, anti-thyrotropic, astringent, cardiac tonic, diuretic (mild), narcotic (mild), and sedative.

Burdock

- The leaves are considered by many to be one of the top "burn healers" of all times. This includes first, second, third and fourth degree burns.
- A strong blood and liver cleanser and tonic.
- Reduces swelling in the body, especially around the joints.
- A great aid in detoxification.
- Burdock rids the body of toxins and mucus.
- Promotes urine flow and perspiration.
- Number one in skin conditions of all types.
- Promotes kidney function and helps remove acid build-up within the body, especially sulfuric, phosphoric and uric acids.

Scientific name: *Arctium lappa*

Parts used: Leaves, roots and seeds

Actions: Alterative, anti-inflammatory, antiscor-butic, aperient, astringent (mild to medium), demulcent, depurative, diaphoretic, lipotropic, stomachic, tonic, sedative.

Butcher's Broom

- A great circulatory herb.
- Has anti-inflammatory properties (flavonoids and tannins) which help remove plaque in the vascular system. Used in cases of phlebitis.
- Tones and strengthens the vascular walls (arteries, capillaries and veins), thus used for varicose veins, hemorrhoids and post aneurysms.

- Increases circulation throughout the body, especially to the peripheral areas (e.g., brain, hands and feet).
- Antithrombotic (use to prevent postoperative thrombosis).
- Strengthens bones and connective tissue.
- Aids alkalization of the blood.

Scientific name: *Iuscus aculeatus*

Parts used: Herb and rhizome.

Actions: Anti-inflammatory, aromatic, cellular proliferator, diuretic, laxative (mild), vasoconstrictor.

Cascara Sagrada

- A great herb in low dosages to strengthen the GI tract.
- Helps tone and strengthen the intestines.
- Increases and strengthens peristalsis.
- Increases secretions of the liver, pancreas, stomach and intestines.
- Strengthens the autonomic nervous system of the alimentary canal.
- Use for constipation, but better used in a cleaning and rebuilding formula for the GI tract.
- Helps clean and strengthen the liver.
- Promotes bile secretion.
- Improves digestion in small dosages.
- Use in cases of gallstones, piles and hemorrhoids.
- Can be used for intestinal worms.

Scientific name: *Rhamnus purshiana*

Parts used: Aged, dried bark.

Actions: Alterative, anti-bilious, antidiabetic, bitter tonic, cathartic, emetic, febrifuge, hepatic, laxative, nervine, peristaltic strengthener, purgative, stomachic.

Cayenne (Red) Pepper

- Used in high blood pressure cases because of its vascular dilation properties.
- Increases circulation. Excellent in cold conditions.

- Stimulates lymph flow. However, it also creates mucus. I do not recommend long term use of cayenne or any hot peppers because of their stimulating and mucus-forming properties.
- Can be an irritant to the mucosa of the GI tract in prolonged usage.
- Used to heal ulcers.
- Used with castor oil packs to help drive oils and herbs into tissues.
- Used as a homeostatic externally and internally (stops bleeding).
- A must for strokes and heart attacks.
- Treats shock.

Scientific name: *Capsicum annuum*

Parts used: Fruit

Actions: Alterative, anti-rheumatic, antiseptic, antispasmodic, astringent, carminative, condiment, emetic, expectorant, hemostatic, pungent, rubefacient, sialagogue, stimulant, stomachic, sudorific, tonic.

Chaparral

- Chaparral is one of God's top herbs in the Northern Hemisphere.
- Its greatest power lies in its ability to move the lymphatic system.
- Used for removal of tumors, boils and abscesses.
- Has strong antimicrobial properties (bacterial, viral, fungal, etc.).
- Very useful in rheumatic and arthritic conditions. Also excellent for gout.
- Has analgesic properties (for pain).
- Stimulates peripheral circulation.
- Stimulates liver function and increases bile production and flow.
- Works as an anti-inflammatory.
- Somewhat of a cellular proliferator (strengthens cells).
- Use in all cancers and HIV.
- Use for all types of stone formation.
- Prolapsed conditions, especially of the uterus.
- Poisonous bites including snakebites.

- Chicken pox, mumps, and the like.
- Useful in all types of female conditions.
- Very useful for stomach and intestinal conditions, including hemorrhoids.

Scientific name: *Larrea tridentata*

Parts used: Leaves and small stems

Actions: Alterative, analgesic, anti-arthritic, anticancer, anti-inflammatory, antioxidant, anti-rheumatic, anti-scrofulous, anti-tumor, anti-venomous, aromatic, astringent, bitter, depurative, diuretic, emetic (large doses), expectorant, laxative (mild), tonic, vasopressor (mild).

Cleavers

- One of the great lymphatic herbs. Helps move and dissolve lymphatic congestion.
- Use in swollen lymph nodes, abscesses, boils and tumors.
- A great blood cleanser.
- Has diuretic properties and helps dissolve kidney and bladder sediment.
- A strong herb for cleansing the skin.
- Excellent for eczema, dermatitis and psoriasis.
- Helps eliminate upper respiratory congestion (sinus, throat, lungs, etc.).
- Helps clean, tone, and strengthen the body.
- Use for all cancers.
- Use in urinary tract obstructions.
- Has anti-inflammatory properties, and is used for any "itis" (inflammatory) condition.

Scientific name: *Galium aparine*

Parts used: Whole herb, especially leaves

Actions: Alterative, anti-inflammatory, antipyretic and laxative, antiscorbutic, antitumor, aperient, astringent, blood purifier, diuretic, hepatic (mild), lipotropic, refrigerant, tonic.

Comfrey

- For centuries considered one of nature's top healers.
- Nicknamed "knit bone" for its powerful effect upon rebuilding the skeletal structure.

- Strengthens connective tissue. Used for hemorrhoids, varicose and spider veins, prolapsed conditions (uterus, bowels, bladder, etc.), muscular degeneration, osteoporosis, hernia, aneurysms, etc.
- A powerful wound healer.
- Useful in sprains, fractures, and the like.
- A good astringent used to detoxify and clean tissue.
- Helps move the lymphatic system.
- Very beneficial for respiratory issues, both for its expectorant properties and its antibacterial properties.
- Comfrey is a tonic to the body, strengthening cells and tissue.
- Checks hemorrhages, especially in the GI tract, urinary tract and lungs.
- Comfrey is used to help regulate blood sugars.
- Said to aid protein through increasing the secretion of pepsin.
- A great lung tonic.
- Excellent as a poultice for any injury.
- Promotes the formation of epithelial cells.

Note: Because of a strong alkaloid called pyrrolizidic acid, the FDA considers this herb dangerous to the liver. However, generations of use do not bear this out. If you were to extract this alkaloid and take it by itself in large dosages it would cause liver damage. However, in Herbology we never extract individual constituents.

Scientific name: *Symphytum officinalis*

Parts used: Root and leaves

Actions: Alterative, anti-inflammatory, antiseptic (mild), astringent, cell proliferant, demulcent, essential oil, expectorant, hemostatic, inulin, mucilage, nutritive, pectoral, primary constituents, starch, styptic, tannins, tonic (yin), vulnerary.

Corn Silk

- A powerful cleanser of bladder and kidney tissue.

- Helps clean toxins and mucus from the urinary tract.
- Helps lower blood sugar.
- Gently stimulates bile flow, aiding in improved digestion and alkalization.
- Used for bedwetting and edema.
- Used for prostatitis.
- Helps remove inorganic minerals from the body.
- Used for both gallstones and kidney stones.
- Excellent for cystitis.
- Useful in hypertension and C.O.P.D.

Scientific name: *Zea mays*

Parts used: Inner silk (stylus).

Actions: Alkaloid, antiseptic, antispasmodic, cholagogue, diuretic, lipotropic, vulnerary.

Corydalis

- The "Great Corydalis" is valued as one of the top non-addictive pain herbs of the world.
- Used for all types of pain including nerve, joint, abdominal, menstrual, muscular, heart.
- Use for arthritis and rheumatism.
- As a bitter, it has beneficial effects upon the liver and GI tract.
- Use for spasms, convulsions, and seizures.
- Use to relax and calm the nervous system.
- Useful for asthmatic attacks.

Scientific name: *Corydalis yanhusuo*

Parts used: Root.

Actions: Analgesic, antispasmodic, bitter tonic, emmenagogue, diuretic.

Dandelion

- One of nature's top herbs.
- A liver and gallbladder tonic.
- Aids in pancreatic function.
- A kidney and bladder tonic and cleanser.
- Said to have the same diuretic strength as Lasix© (trade name for furosemide).
- Promotes the formation of bile.
- Improves the enamel of the teeth.
- A great alkalizer.

- Effective in liver conditions including hepatitis, jaundice and cirrhosis.
- High in iron, and other minerals, which increases the oxygen-carrying capacity of the blood.
- A natural source of protein.
- Aids in blood sugar issues including diabetes and hypoglycemia.

Scientific name: *Taraxacum spp.*

Parts used: Whole plant: leaves, roots and flowers.

Actions: Alterative, anti-rheumatic, anti-tumor, aperient, bitter, blood purifier, cholagogue, deobstruent, depurative, diuretic, hepatic, immune enhancer and rebuilder, laxative (mild), liptotriptic, nutritive, stomachic, tonic.

Devil's Claw

- One of nature's great anti-inflammatory herbs. (Promotes prostaglandin production and activity.)
- A specific for arthritis and rheumatism.
- Great for any inflammatory condition: joint, muscular, neuro, or other.
- Use in prostatitis.
- Valuable in diabetes (pancreatic) or liver conditions.

Scientific name: *Harpagophytum procumbens*

Parts used: Roots and tubers.

Actions: Alterative (blood purifier), analgesic, anodyne, anti-arthritic, anti-inflammatory, anti-rheumatic, astringent, bitter tonic, cholagogue, hepatic (mild), sedative.

Echinacea Angustifolia

- Echinacea is another one of God's greatest herbs.
- It is known as the "immune herb."
- Strengthens and stimulates the immune system.
- It enhances tissue function, especially bone marrow, thymus gland and spleen tissue.

- Has strong antibiotic and antiseptic properties.
- A blood purifier and anti-inflammatory.
- Useful in cases of arthritis and rheumatism.
- Useful in colds, flu, pneumonia, and similar conditions.
- Strengthens cells.
- A blood purifier.
- Very useful in sepsis of the blood or any toxic blood conditions.
- A must in all cancers, tumors, boils and abscesses.
- Great in urinary tract infections and inflammation.
- Useful in prostate conditions.

Scientific name: *Echinacea angustifolia*

Parts used: Roots, rhizomes.

Actions: Alterative, antibacterial, anti-inflammatory, anti-putrefactive, anti-venomous, antiseptic, antiviral, deodorant, depurant, aphrodisiac, sialogogue, diaphoretic, aromatic, carminative, bitter, stimulant, vulnerary.

False Unicorn (Helonias)

- One of nature's top tonics, especially for the male and female reproductive organs and glands.
- Strengthens the endocrine glands.
- Use in prolapsed conditions of the intestines, uterus, hemorrhoids, veins, etc.
- It revitalizes and regenerates tissue, especially the reproductive tissues.
- Increases the ability of conception.
- Strengthens the mucous membranes, especially the genital-urinary tissues.
- Use for diabetes.
- Use for ovarian, uterine or prostate weakness or conditions.
- Helps prevent miscarriages.
- Use for sterility problems.
- Use for relaxed vagina.

Scientific name: *Chamaelirium luteum*

Parts used: Root and rhizomes.

Actions: Anthelmintic (vermifuge), cellular proliferant, diuretic, emetic (high doses), emmenagogue, oxytocic, sialogogue (fresh), stimulating, tonic, uterine tonic.

Fenugreek

- Fenugreek is a great expectorant.
- It softens, loosens, and helps expel mucus (phlegm), especially from the bronchial and lung tissues.
- Helps dissolve cholesterol and other lipids.
- A great blood cleanser and antiseptic.
- Fenugreek is a medium range parasite killer.
- Has some diuretic properties.
- Excellent for diabetes (helps regulate sugar and insulin levels).

Scientific name: *Trigonella foenum-graecum*

Parts used: Seeds.

Actions: Alterative, antiparasitic, aphrodisiac, aromatic, astringent, carminative, demulcent, deobstruent, detergent, detoxicant, emollient, expectorant, galactagogue, laxative, nutritive, stimulant, stomachic, tonic.

Garlic

- Garlic is one of the great blood cleansers.
- It has antiseptic, antiparasitic, antibacterial, antiviral, antifungal properties.
- Especially good for intestinal parasites.
- A great immune enhancer.
- Stimulates the action of the liver and gallbladder.
- Excellent for colds, flu, bronchitis and any congestive conditions.
- Great for yeast infections of all types.
- Garlic can be too strong and pungent for fruitarians.
- Stimulates digestive enzymes.

Scientific name: *Allium sativum*

Parts used: Bulbs

Actions: Alterative, antibacterial, anticatarrhal, antifungal, antiparasitic, antiseptic, antispasmodic, antisyphilitic, anti-venomous, antiviral, aromatic, carminative, cathartic, cholagogue, depurative, diaphoretic, digestant, disinfectant, diuretic, emmenagogues, expectorant, hypertensive, hypotensive, immuno-stimulant, nervine, rubefacient, stimulant, stomachic, sudorific, tonic, vulnerary.

Gentian

- One of nature's best bitter tonics for the GI tract (gastrointestinal).
- Strengthens the entire body.
- One of the best herbs for the improvement of digestion.
- Increases liver and pancreatic function.
- Increases gastric secretions, while toning and strengthening the stomach.
- Has antiparasitic properties, kills plasmodia and worms.
- Strengthens the liver, spleen and pancreas.
- Has a toning effect upon the kidneys.
- Increases circulation.
- A revitalizer of the body; used for fatigue, exhaustion and low energy levels (anemia).
- Used in all female weaknesses.
- Use for indigestion, dyspepsia and gas.
- Can be used for lightheadedness, dizziness, etc.
- Can be used for infections and toxic conditions of the body.
- Also can be used for poisonous bites and malaria.

Scientific name: *Gentiana lutea*

Parts used: Root.

Actions: Alterative, antacid, anthelmintic (vermifuge), anti-bilious, anti-inflammatory, antiperiodic, antipyretic, antiseptic, antispasmodic, anti-venomous, bitter tonic, cholagogue, emetic (large doses), emmenagogue, febrifuge, hepatic, laxative (mild), stimulant, stomachic, tonic, sialagogue.

Ginger

- Used throughout the world as a digestive aid and for circulation.
- Used as a catalyst with other herbs.
- Increases circulation to peripheral areas (brain, hands and feet) of the body.
- Great for indigestion and nausea.
- Increases lymph flow and aids elimination of mucus from the upper respiratory areas, especially the lungs.
- Effective in motion and morning sickness.
- Lowers cholesterol and blood pressure.
- Prevents blood clotting.
- Useful in post strokes.
- Aids in the cleansing of congestion (mucus) in the cerebral and sinus areas.
- Increases perspiration and elimination through the skin.

Scientific name: *Zingiber officinale*

Parts used: Dried rhizomes and root.

Actions: Analgesic, anodyne, antacid, antiemetic, antispasmodic, aperitive, aphrodisiac, aromatic, carminative, cholagogue, condiment, detoxicant, diaphoretic (whole), diffusive stimulant, diuretic, emmenagogue, expectorant, nervine, pungent, rubefacient, sialagogue, sternutatory, stomachic, sweet, tonic.

Ginkgo Biloba

- One of the best herbs for the brain and nervous system.
- Improves cerebral vascular insufficiency.
- Used throughout the world for memory loss and vertigo (dizziness).
- Strengthens the heart and vascular system.
- Increases blood flow to the tissues.
- Useful in cases of asthma.
- Used for tinnitus (ringing in the ears).
- Has been proven beneficial for fibromyalgia.
- Very beneficial for hemorrhoids, spider and varicose veins.
- Has been useful for carpal tunnel syndrome.
- One of nature's great tonics, especially to the "neuro" system.

Scientific name: *Ginkgo biloba*

Parts used: *Leaf*—promotes blood circulation, stops pain, benefits the brain, and is astringent to the lungs. *Seed*—considered astringent for the lungs, stops nocturnal emissions, stops asthma, enuresis, excessive leukorrhea and increases energy.

Actions: Adaptogen, alkalizer, anti-aging, antifungal, anti-inflammatory, antioxidant, antispasmodic (mild), astringent, bitter tonic, cardiac tonic (mild), expectorant (mild), nervine, sedative (mild), tonic, vasodilator, vulnerary.

Goldenseal

- One of nature's greatest "heal-all" herbs.
- A true tonic for the body.
- Not for long term use because of its accumulative properties.
- It increases gastric juices and digestive enzymes. It also increases the production and secretion of bile.
- Used to strengthen and tone the pancreas.
- Helps regulate blood sugars.
- Considered a source of natural insulin.
- Strengthens the nervous system.
- It has homeostatic properties, especially for the uterus.
- Tones the vascular system and helps increase circulation.
- A great anti-inflammatory, especially for the glandular system.
- Use for gastric and intestinal problems.
- Use in cancerous conditions.
- A gentle laxative.
- Use for drug and alcohol dependency.
- Helps eliminate catarrh (mucus) in the body, especially in the respiratory and GI tract tissues.
- Use in cystitis, prostatitis and nephritis.
- Excellent for hemorrhoids and hemorrhages.
- Use for HIV and venereal diseases.
- Has antiparasitic properties, and is antiseptic.
- Use for infections, wounds, sores, fissures, etc.
- Use in chronic skin conditions, eczema, dermatitis and psoriasis.
- Use in all types of prolapsed conditions, (uterus, intestinal, etc.).
- Makes a great eyewash.
- Tones and cleans the liver. Use for jaundice, hepatitis, etc.
- Use for ulcerated tissue.
- Use for tonsillitis, typhoid fever, malaria, meningitis, and mononucleosis.
- Use for boils, abscesses and tumors.
- Use as a mouthwash for gum conditions and canker sores.
- Great for ringworm and amoebic dysentery.

Scientific name: *Hydrastis canadensis*

Parts used: Root and dried rhizomes.

Actions: Alterative, anti-diabetic, anti-emetic, anti-inflammatory, antiparasitic, antiperiodic, antiseptic, aperient, astringent, bitter tonic, cholagogue, deobstruent, depurative (antifungal), detergent, diuretic, heal-all, hemostatic (urine esp.), hepatic, laxative, nervine, ophthalmic, oxytocic (stimulates uterine contractions), stomachic, vulnerary.

Gotu Kola

- One of God's finest herbs for brain and nerve regeneration.
- A tremendous herb for spinal cord injuries.
- A cellular proliferator (strengthens cells).
- Increases oxygen to cells.
- Strengthens the immune system.
- Helps with difficult menopause issues.
- Aids in weight loss.
- Used for depression and endocrine glandular weaknesses.
- Promotes blood flow in lower extremities.
- Strengthens the vascular walls, therefore excellent in cases of varicose or spider veins, hemorrhoids, venous insufficiency or any vascular distensibility.
- Shows healing potential in ulcerated conditions.

Scientific name: *Centella asiatica*

Parts used: Whole plant or root.

Actions: Adaptogen, alterative, antipyretic,

antispasmodic, aphrodisiac, astringent, cellular proliferator, diuretic, nervine, sedative, stimulant (mild), tonic (brain and nerve).

Hawthorn Berry

- Hawthorn berry is "the great heart herb."
- This flavonoid-rich fruit is tissue specific for the heart and vascular system. It strengthens these tissues and removes the inflammation.
- It aids in dissolving lipid deposits, therefore increasing circulation.
- Has vasodilating properties, which also aid in increasing circulation.
- Use in high (hypertension) or low (hypotension) blood pressure cases.
- Considered a cardiac tonic for all heart-related issues.
- Also used in cases of insomnia (consider adrenals as well).
- Strengthens vascular walls, therefore excellent for regeneration of varicose and spider veins, hemorrhoids and prolapsed conditions of the body.
- Has strong antioxidant power to help remove acids from the body.
- Hawthorn berry is an excellent anti-inflammatory and should be used in all cases of inflammation.

Scientific name: *Crataegus spp.*

Parts used: Berries and leaf.

Actions: Anti-inflammatory, antioxidant, antispasmodic, astringent, cardiac tonic, cellular proliferator, digestant, diuretic, emmenagogue, hypertensive, hypotensive, sedative, tonic, vasodilator.

Horse Chestnut

- This is another one of God's great circulatory herbs.
- Horse Chestnut strengthens and tones the vascular walls.
- It has anti-inflammatory properties, thus it helps dissolve plaqued lipids.

- Both of the above actions together greatly increase circulation.
- A "must" for varicose and spider veins as well as hemorrhoids.
- Reduces vascular swelling.
- A strong astringent, similar to witch hazel and white oak bark.
- Useful for ulcerated conditions.
- Helps remove toxins from the body.
- Useful for prostatitis.
- Use in cases of rheumatism.

Scientific name: *Aesculus hippocastanum*

Parts used: Bark, dried horse chestnut seeds, dried horse chestnut leaves.

Actions: Anti-inflammatory, anti-rheumatic, astringent, bitter, cellular proliferator (especially to the vascular walls), expectorant, febrifuge, mild narcotic, nutritive.

Horsetail or Shavegrass

- Horsetail is one of the greatest herbs for bone and connective tissue weaknesses.
- It is very high in silica, which is converted into calcium by the liver.
- This herb has great healing powers to all tissues of the body.
- It is an extremely good herb for the urinary tract (kidneys and bladder).
- Use to strengthen any prolapsed condition of the body, e.g., bladder, bowels, uterus, veins, skin and the like.
- Has some minor antiparasitic properties.
- One of the greatest helps for increasing platelet production by the spleen.
- A very good herb for prostate inflammation and weakness.
- Used in the detoxification of the body.
- Has diuretic properties, therefore very beneficial in relieving kidney congestion.
- Used to strengthen fingernails (check thyroid/parathyroid).

Scientific name: *Equisetvense*

Parts used: Whole plant.

Actions: Alterative, anti-inflammatory, antiparasitic (mild), antispasmodic (mild), anti-tumor, astringent, carminative, cellular proliferator, diaphoretic, emmenagogue (mild), galactagogue, hemostatic, lithotriptic, nutritive, tonic, vulnerary.

Juniper Berry

- Juniper Berry is considered one of the great kidney herbs.
- It has a very strong action upon the kidneys. Use caution in cases of extreme kidney damage.
- It is anti-inflammatory and has some antispasmodic properties.
- It has antiseptic properties, which are useful in killing fungi, bacteria and yeasts.
- Great for UTIs (urinary tract infections) and parasitic overgrowths in the GI tract. It is also a natural diuretic, and relieves excess water.
- Said to aid in restoring the pancreas, and beneficial in cases of diabetes, as it has natural insulin properties.

Scientific name: *Juniperus communis* or *species*

Parts used: Usually the berries, also the oil (from the berries and wood), leaves, bark.

Actions: Anodyne, antiseptic, aromatic, carminative, diaphoretic, diuretic, emmenagogue, stimulant, stomachic.

Licorice

- A definite power herb for the adrenal glands.
- A powerful endocrine glandular herb.
- Acts as a natural anti-inflammatory steroid (cortisone, etc.) without inhibiting the adrenal production of steroids.
- Helps increase neurotransmitters and steroid production.
- Has antifungal and antibacterial properties.
- Aids in the regulation of blood sugars.
- Promotes tissue healing, especially of the GI tract.
- A great blood cleanser and detoxifier.
- Use for hypoglycemia and diabetes.

- Use for ulcerated tissues.
- Can be used for Candida albicans.
- Useful in infections and respiratory congestive issues.
- Helps break up and remove mucus.
- Used as a laxative.
- One of the top herbs for hemorrhoids.
- Good for healing up the whole GI tract.
- High in phytosterols.

Scientific name: *Glycyrrhiza glabra*

Parts used: Root and dried rhizome.

Actions: Aperient, demulcent, emollient, expectorant, flavoring, pectoral, sialogogue, and slightly stimulant.

Lobelia

- One of nature's greatest antispasmodics.
- Useful in spasms, cramping, convulsions, epileptic seizures, spinal cord injuries, and the like.
- A very powerful nervine.
- Has a relaxing effect.
- Very useful in cases of asthma, emphysema, and C.O.P.D., where spasms of the bronchi and lung tissue blocks proper breathing. Action is similar to inhalers, but allows for expectoration (which is vital).
- Lobelia has some expectorant properties, therefore very beneficial in removal of congestion, specifically in the respiratory system.
- It is also a hemostatic (stops internal and external bleeding).
- Great for angina pectoris or infarctions (heart attacks).
- Useful in cases of equilibrium or fainting issues.

Scientific name: *Lobelia inflata*

Parts used: Fresh and dried herb and seeds.

Actions: Alkaloids, antispasmodic, anti-venomous, astringent, cathartic, chlorophyll, counter-irritant, diaphoretic, diuretic, emetic, fixed oil, gum, isolobeline, etc., lignin, salts of lime and potassium. Lobelia also contains sulfur, iron, cobalt, selenium, sodium, copper and lead, lobelic and chelidonic acids, lobeline, nauseant, relaxant (in large doses) and stimulant (in small doses), resin.

Marshmallow

- A great anti-inflammatory and healer of the gastrointestinal tract (stomach and intestines).
- A specific for gastritis, enteritis, colitis, diverticulitis, ulcers and cancers of the GI tract.
- Being high in mucilage it coats and protects from free radical (acids) damage to the mucosa.
- It neutralizes over-production of stomach acids, therefore allowing improved digestion.
- Superb for cystitis and urinary tract inflammation.
- A great aid in prostatitis.
- Heals wounds, especially good in burn cases.
- Works well in cases of bronchitis and sore throats.
- Great for inflammation of the vascular system, liver and pancreas.
- Aids digestion and is a mild stimulant to the GI tract.
- High in calcium and lime. Excellent for the skeletal structure.
- Has been used very successfully in gangrene.
- Especially useful for coughs, laryngitis, swollen tonsils (tonsillitis), respiratory congestion and inflammatory conditions.
- Excellent for arthritis and rheumatism.
- Useful for diabetics.
- Great in eyewash formulas to help soothe and heal irritated eyes.
- Superb for vaginal issues of all types.
- Useful for boils, abscesses and skin conditions.
- Very useful as a mouthwash for swollen, inflamed and infected gums.

Scientific name: *Althaea officinalis*

Parts used: Root (greater potency), leaves and flowers.

Actions: Absorbent, anticomplementary, anti-inflammation, demulcent, diuretic, emollient, immune stimulant and hypoglycemic, laxative, mucilage, nutritive, protective, vulnerary.

Milk Thistle

- The great "liver protector."
- Milk Thistle protects, tones, strengthens and detoxifies the liver, like no other.
- It has high antioxidant properties and is considered one of the best to protect against free-radical damage.
- Aids in the regeneration of the liver and pancreas (stimulates new liver cell production).
- Superb for hepatitis A, B and C and in cirrhosis of the liver.
- Increases the production and flow of bile.
- Increases formation of new liver cells.

Scientific name: *Silybum marianum*

Parts used: The ripe seeds.

Actions: Cholagogue, diaphoretic, emmenagogue.

Motherwort

- Motherwort is a great heart tonic.
- It helps to eliminate palpations and arrhythmias.
- Used for any heart condition, including atrial fibrillation, V-tach, PVCs, PACs, tachycardia, and CHFs.
- Helps to enhance the adrenal glands.
- Used in female conditions, including menstrual cramps and hot flashes.

Scientific name: *Leonurus cardiaca*

Parts used: The aerial portion of the herb.

Actions: Antispasmodic, cardiac (tonic), cathartic (aperient), diaphoretic, diuretic, emmenagogue, hepatic, nervine and tonic.

Mullein

- Mullein is one of the great expectorants (removes mucus and congestion).

- Used especially for bronchial and lung conditions including bronchitis, asthma, emphysema, pneumonia and allergies.
- Mullein is also strongly anti-inflammatory, aiding in all types of inflammatory conditions.
- A great herb for the endocrine glandular system, especially the thyroid.
- Used for coughs and sore throats.
- Mullein has strong astringent properties as well.
- Aids in the movement of the lymphatic system.
- Helps reduce tumors and boils.

Scientific name: *Verbascum thapsus*

Parts used: Leaves, flowers, root and fruit.

Actions: Absorbent, anodyne, anthelmintic (vermicide), anti-asthmatic, anticatarrhal, antiseptic, antispasmodic, astringent, demulcent, diuretic, emollient, germicide, hemostatic, narcotic, nutritive, pectoral, vulnerary.

Nettles (Stinging)

- A highly nutritive herb with a broad range of actions.
- Nettles has an alkalizing effect upon the body.
- Used to increase circulation.
- A specific for arthritis and rheumatism.
- Great for the joints.
- Used in pain and inflammation issues.
- One of the few herbs for the thyroid gland.
- A strong detoxifier of the skin.
- Being alkaline it neutralizes acids (like uric and sulfuric acids).
- Somewhat of a hemostatic (stops bleeding).
- Feeds the body nutrition, especially potassium and iron (although it is also full of minerals).
- Useful in circulation issues, somewhat of a vasodilator.
- Promotes the flow of urine and is useful for kidney stones.
- Shrinks swollen tissues.

- Excellent for pregnancy, nutrition, and for anti-abortive issues.
- Used in cases of bronchitis especially asthma, emphysema and C.O.P.D.
- Nettles is an expectorant (removes mucus) and has antispasmodic properties.
- Used for anemia.
- A great blood purifier and body regulator.

Scientific name: *Urtica dioica*

Parts used: Leaves.

Actions: Astringent, diuretic, expectorant, galactagogue, hemostatic, nutritive and tonic.

Oregon Grape Root

- One of the great blood purifiers.
- Has a powerful effect upon the liver, spleen, skin and blood.
- It is one of the greatest herbs for stimulating, strengthening and cleansing of the liver.
- Specific for skin conditions like psoriasis, eczema or dermatitis.
- Increases immune response.
- High in iron; aids in increasing red blood cells and hemoglobin.
- Excellent for anemia, jaundice and hepatitis A, B or C.
- Has a fair amount of antimicrobial action. Shown to kill various fungi and bacteria including: staphylococcus, streptococcus, chlamydia, salmonella typhi, corynebacterium, vibrio cholerae, trichomonas vaginalis, shigella, giardia, treponema pallidum, pseudomonas, pneumococcus, and candida albicans.
- Has some larger parasitic activity as well.
- Also used against protozoas.
- A nerve tonic.
- Slightly laxative.

Scientific name: *Mohonia spp.*

Parts used: Root and rhizome.

Actions: Alterative, antiperiodic, antiscorbutic, anti-scrofulous, antisyphilitic, depurant, diuretic, hepatic, laxative, nerve tonic, stimulant (slightly), tonic.

Parsley

- A tremendous herb for the urinary tract and adrenal glands.
- Has a strengthening and cleansing effect upon the bladder and kidneys.
- High in chlorophyll, therefore it enhances the blood and cleans and moves the lymphatics.
- Excellent for heavy metal and chemical toxicity.
- Enhances nerve and heart function.
- Superb for the endocrine glands.
- Increases the iron-carrying capacity of the blood.
- Used to fight infections.
- Used in cases of jaundice and dropsy (edema).
- Excellent for upper respiratory congestion and infections.
- Also used in conjunctivitis and inflammation of the eyelids.

Scientific name: *Petroselinum sativum*

Parts used: Whole herb; leaves, root and seeds.

Actions: Antiperiodic (juice), antispasmodic, aperient, aromatic, carminative (seeds), culinary, diuretic, emmenagogue (seeds), febrifuge (seeds), tonic, vulnerary.

Pau D'Arco

- A tremendous Brazilian "friend." A true tonic.
- Considered a top cellular proliferator (strengthens and enhances cells).
- A top parasitic herb used for microorganism infestations (bacterial, viral, and protozoa).
- A great immune builder.
- Used especially in cancer cases.
- Has a powerful effect upon the lymphatic system.
- Helps eliminate tumors, boils, abscesses, and the like.
- Used in skin conditions including eczema, dermatitis, and psoriasis.

- Also considered a nutritive and resolvent.

Scientific name: *Tabebuia impetiginosa*

Parts used: Bark.

Actions: Antimicrobial (bacterial, etc.), anti-viral, cellular proliferator/strengthener), nutritive, alterative (cooling), anti-tumor, tonic, hypotensive, anti-diabetic, astringent, bitter (digestive), stimulant, restorative, somewhat decongestant.

Pipsissewa

- A great alkalizer of the urinary tract system.
- Helps clean and remove sediment from the bladder and kidneys.
- An excellent diuretic.
- Used in urinary tract infections.
- Lowers blood pressure when kidneys are involved.

Scientific name: *Chimaphila umbellata*

Parts used: Leaf, stem, aerial portions.

Actions: Alterative, astringent and diuretic.

Plantain

- The great Plantain can't be beat for pus and septic conditions of the blood and body.
- Great for boils, abscesses and tumors.
- Known for its anti-venom properties in snake-bites.
- Has a strong astringent action (pulling and cleansing) upon tissues.
- Useful for inflammation and for its healing abilities.
- Neutralizes stomach acids and helps restore proper gastric action.
- Has mild expectorant properties (therefore aiding in bronchial and lung congestion).
- Used in venereal diseases.
- Use topically and internally for all skin conditions including eczema, dermatitis and psoriasis.
- Great in an eyewash, especially for cataracts and glaucoma.

Scientific name: *Plantago spp.*

Parts used: Root, leaves, flower spikes and seeds.

Actions: Alterative (cooling), anthelmintic (vermicide), antiseptic, antisyphilitic, anti-venomous, astringent, deobstruent, depurant, diuretic, emollient, refrigerant, styptic and vulnerary.

Poke Root (a.k.a. Pokeweed)

• The tumor buster. One of the best for abscesses, boils and masses.
• Encourages movement in the lymphatic system.
• Used for enlarged or hardened organs and glands (thyroid, spleen, liver, etc.).
• Has some mild cardiac-depressant qualities.
• Skin cleanser especially good for eczema, dermatitis and psoriasis.
• Increases bile and digestive juices.
• Promotes kidney function.
• Has some anti-inflammatory properties.
• Helpful in chronic rheumatism and arthritis.
• Stimulates thyroid and adrenal function.
• Used for all cancers and HIV.

Scientific name: *Phytolacca americana*

Parts used: Fresh root, berries and leaves.

Actions: Alterative, anodyne, anti-sorbic, anti-syphilitic, antitumor, cathartic, detergent, emetic, leaves: anodyne, cardiac-depressant, nutritive and resolvent.

Red Clover

• Another one of nature's great herbs.
• Similar to cleavers and sassafras.
• A tremendous blood purifier.
• Use in all cancers, especially leukemia.
• Helps dissolve tumors and masses. Also great for abscesses and boils.
• Cleans and strengthens all liver conditions.
• Strengthens red blood cells.
• Excellent for all skin conditions, including eczema, dermatitis, and psoriasis.
• Great for syphilis and venereal diseases.

• Has some antispasmodic properties and soothes the nerves.

Scientific name: *Trifolium pratense*

Parts used: Flowers and leaves.

Actions: Alterative, antispasmodic, somewhat depurative, antitumor, deobstruent, detergent, expectorant, nutritive, sedative and stimulant (slightly).

Red Raspberry

• One of nature's top female herbs.
• Considered a nutritive tonic.
• A specific in pregnancy, and produces a far less painful and more natural delivery.
• Strengthens both mother and fetus during childbearing.
• Checks hemorrhages, especially during labor.
• Enriches mother's milk.
• A great herb for cleansing the male and female reproductive organs.
• Excellent for cleansing and strengthening the blood.
• Decreases excessive menstrual flow.
• Used for prolapsus of the uterus, anus, intestines, bladder, etc.
• Used for piles and hemorrhoids.
• Somewhat of a nerve tonic and nervine.
• Increases healing in wounds, sores and ulcerated conditions.
• Used to relieve excessive labor pains (uterine cramps).
• Used as a mouthwash for bleeding and infected gums.
• Used in eyewashes for inflammation, congestion or swelling.

Scientific name: *Rubus idaeus*

Parts used: Leaves, root bark and fruit.

Actions: Alliterative (mild), anti-abortive, anti-emetic, anti-gonorrheal, anti-leukorrheal, anti-malarial, antiseptic, astringent, cathartic, hemostatic, parturient, stimulant, stomachic, tonic. *The fruit* acts as an antacid, esculent, mild laxative, parturient, refrigerant. *The leaves* are alliterative, anti-abortive, anti-emetic, anti-gonorrheal, anti-leukorrheal, antimalarial, antiseptic, astringent, cathartic, hemostatic, parturient, stomachic stimulant, tonic.

Reishi Mushroom

- A powerful immune stimulator.
- Helps lower cholesterol and increase circulation.
- Helps lower blood sugar levels.
- Helps the body restore itself in degenerative issues.
- Stimulates T and B cell production (NK = natural killer) cells.
- Said to improve heart and liver functions.
- Used in cancer and AIDS cases.
- Used where abscesses, boils and tumors exist.
- Helps reduce swollen lymph nodes.
- Increases fibroblasts, macrophages and lymphocytes.
- May help steroid production by its positive effect upon the adrenal glands.

Scientific name: *Ganoderma lucidum*

Parts used: Whole mushroom.

Actions: Immune system support.

St. John's Wort

- One of the great herbs for the nervous system.
- Has a fairly strong regenerative effect upon the nervous system.
- Also has a balancing effect upon the tissues.
- Used for depression, anxiety and irritability.
- Great for insomnia. (Insomnia and anxiety are the effects of adrenal gland weakness.)
- A great aid with headaches and cramping of all types, including menstrual.
- Has antiparasitic properties, including antibacterial, antifungal and antiviral.
- Shown to have a very positive effect against the HIV virus.
- Has anti-inflammatory properties.
- Will help somewhat in sciatica.

- Used in colds and respiratory congestive issues.
- Helpful in Parkinson's Disease.

Scientific name: *Hypericum perforatum*

Parts used: Herb, flowers, aerial portions.

Actions: Alterative, anti-spasmodic, anti-inflammatory, astringent, vulnerary.

Saw Palmetto

- One of God's great endocrine gland herbs (thyroid, adrenal, pancreas, pituitary, etc.).
- Called the "male herb" for its anti-inflammatory and healing effect upon the prostate. (Inhibits the production of dihydrotestosterone.)
- A strong herb for both female and male reproductive disorders.
- Enhances sexual function and desire.
- Beneficial in inflammation of the respiratory system (nose, throat, bronchi and lungs).
- Has a strong effect upon the adrenal glands, thus increasing neurotransmitters and steroids.
- Aids in sugar issues involving the pancreas and adrenals.
- Helps increase urine flow and kidney function.
- Useful in urinary tract infections.

Scientific name: *Serenoa repens*

Parts used: Berries (fruit).

Actions: Antiseptic, aphrodisiac, diuretic, expectorant, roborant.

Skullcap

- One of the greatest herbs for the brain, spine and nervous system.
- Strengthens the brain and nervous system.
- It's a powerful nervine, sedative and anti-spasmodic.
- Used for spasms, cramping, convulsions, and the like.
- Aids in cases of insomnia and restlessness.
- A specific for multiple sclerosis, Parkinson's and palsies.
- Strengthens the medulla, thus used for vertigo and dizziness.
- Spinal cord injuries.

- Used for drug and alcohol withdrawal symptoms.
- As an aromatic, it calms the emotions.

Scientific name: *Scutellaria lateriflora*

Parts used: Herb, aerial portions.

Actions: Antispasmodic, nervine, sedative.

Senna

- Helps tone and strengthen the GI tract.
- Increases peristaltic action of the GI tract.
- Used as a strong laxative, so not recommended for prolonged usage by itself. (Can irritate in high dosages and prolonged use.)
- Helps clean the intestinal walls.

Scientific name: *Cassia acutifolia*

Parts used: Pods and leaves.

Actions: Purgative that also inhibits reabsorption in the intestines.

Shiitake Mushroom

- Strengthens the immune system by increasing T-cell function.
- Effective in the treatment of cancer, as reported in a joint study by the Medical Department of Japan.

Scientific name: *Lentinus edodes*

Parts used: Cap and stems. Sold dry.

Actions: Immune stimulating, nutritive, hypotensive, anti-cholesterol.

Siberian Ginseng (Eleuthero)

- One of the great endocrine gland herbs, especially great for the adrenal glands.
- Increases neurotransmitter and steroid production.
- Strengthens cells (cellular proliferator).
- Improves vitality and stamina.
- Used for chronic fatigue or loss of energy.
- Helps strengthen the immune system.
- Increases circulation by helping to reduce cholesterol.

- Strengthens the pancreas and helps control blood sugar issues.
- Helps relieve emotional, mental and physical stress.
- Helps lower blood pressure and strengthens the heartbeat.
- Used in cases of asthma, emphysema and C.O.P.D., where an adrenal gland relationship exists.
- A tonic for the whole body.

Scientific name: *Eleutherococcus senticosus*

Parts used: Root.

Actions: Demulcent, stimulant, rejuvenative.

Slippery Elm

- One of nature's great healers of the body.
- Pulls toxicity out of tissues.
- Soothes irritated and inflamed mucous membranes.
- Soothes the mucosa of the GI tract (stomach and intestines).
- Excellent for the urinary tract (strengthens and cleans).
- Well known for its beneficial effect upon the respiratory system.
- Soothes sore and inflamed throat tissues.
- Helps pull (expectorant) mucus from the respiratory tract.
- High in nutrition.
- Used in prostatitis.
- Ulcerated conditions of the body.
- Lesions of the GI tract.
- Used in gastritis, enteritis, colitis and diverticulitis.
- Great for abscesses and gangrene.
- Used in gout and arthritis.
- Helps remove acids from the tissues.

Scientific name: *Ulmus fulva*

Parts used: Inner bark.

Actions: Astringent, demulcent, emollient, expectorant, nutritive, vulnerary, yin tonic and soothing to the alimentary canal.

Turmeric

- An ancient herb used for liver and blood conditions.
- Stimulates bile flow and production.
- Helps dissolve and remove sediment in the liver.
- Has some antiparasitic actions, especially for protozoa infestations.
- Helps increase circulation.
- Has a beneficial effect upon the whole GI tract.
- Has strong anti-inflammatory properties, therefore very beneficial for arthritis, bursitis, tendonitis, etc.
- Aids in digestion.
- Promotes healing.

Scientific name: *Curcuma longa*

Parts used: Rhizome.

Actions: Aromatic stimulant, alliterative, analgesic, antiseptic, astringent, cholagogue, emmenagogue.

Uva Ursi or Bearberry

- A powerful antiseptic and cleanser of the urinary tract system.
- Has a strong influence upon the pancreas and used to help regulate blood sugars.
- Has a healthy effect upon the liver and spleen.
- Aids with the elimination of kidney stones.
- A great herb for the prostate gland (especially in prostatitis and prostate cancer).
- Great in congestive conditions of the body (especially the bladder, kidneys, liver, gallbladder, pancreas and spleen).
- A diuretic.
- Strengthens the liver, kidneys, bladder, uterus, prostate and spleen.
- Useful in correcting bedwetting issues.
- Useful as a douche for vaginal infections and disorders.
- Soothes, strengthens and tones the mucous membranes of the genitourinary (urinary organs, c.a. kidneys, urinary bladder) passages.
- Used in urethritis, cystitis, nephritis, incontinence, and urinary tract ulcerations.
- Used for CHF (congestive heart failure), cardiac edema.
- Used for piles and hemorrhoids.

Scientific name: *Arctostaphylos uva-ursi*

Parts used: Leaves.

Actions: Antiseptic, astringent, diuretic.

Valerian

- Valerian has soothed a lot of nerves through the years.
- A strong nervine and non-narcotic sedative.
- Aids in anxiety (adrenals), nervous tension, muscle spasms, epileptic seizures and depression (thyroid).
- Said to be somewhat of a cardiac tonic—helps regulate heart palpitations.
- Helps in hyperactivity.
- Helps reduce high blood pressure from stress and tension.
- Helps strengthen brain and nerve tissues.
- Aids in colic conditions, gas and indigestion from nervous stomach.

Scientific name: *Valeriana officinalis*

Parts used: Root, rhizome and also the herb.

Actions: Anodyne, antispasmodic, anti-thermic, aromatic, carminative, cathartic, diaphoretic, diuretic (lithotriptic), nervine (sedative), stimulant, tonic.

White Pond Lily

- This is another one of God's great cleansing herbs.
- Similar to white oak bark, but more for lower body cleansing.
- Helps remove toxicity from the tissues of the body.
- Has a healthy and toning effect upon tissues.
- Especially used to cleanse and strengthen the reproductive tissues in both male and female.
- It has pain-relieving properties.
- Use in cancerous conditions.

- Useful for abscesses, boils and tumors.
- Makes a great mouthwash to clean and heal swollen or ulcerated gums.
- Makes an excellent douche for cleansing the vaginal wall (infections, inflammation, A-typical cells, ulcerations, etc.).
- Strengthens prolapsed conditions and re-laxed vagina.
- Use for prostate conditions, especially prosta-titis and prostate cancer.
- Excellent for urinary tract system (kidneys and bladder).
- Use to heal wounds, sores, and the like.
- Helps remove congestion out of tissues.

Scientific name: *Nymphaea; Nymphaea Odorata* or *Castalia Odorata*

Parts used: Fresh root and leaves, rhizome.

Actions: Alterative, anodyne, anti-scrofulous, antiseptic, astringent, demulcent, deob-struent, discutient, tonic, vulnerary.

White Oak Bark

- Another tremendous herb of God.
- White oak bark is a great cleanser of the body.
- Has very strong astringent properties.
- Increases lymphatic flow and helps reduce swollen lymph nodes.
- A powerful cleanser of tissue, used for mouth-washes, poultices, douches, enemas and ab-scesses.
- Use as a douche for infections and A-typical cell formation.
- Strengthens cells (cellular proliferator).
- Superb for internal or external hemorrhages.
- Has diuretic properties, thus increases urine flow.
- Kills and expels small worms (pin worms, etc.).
- Used to eliminate gallstones and especially kidney stones.
- Helps clean and strengthen the GI tract.
- Excellent for prolapsed conditions, including intestinal, uterus, bladder, vascular system, etc.
- Used in all mouth and gum conditions.

- Has a powerful effect upon tooth enamel and bone growth.
- Used with plantain for snakebites.
- Ulcers, boils, gangrene, tumors, and the like.
- Use in all skin conditions including eczema, dermatitis and psoriasis.
- Hemorrhoids, piles and lesions.
- Used to strengthen the arteries, veins and capillaries; especially great for varicose veins and spider veins.

Scientific name: *Quercus alba: fagaceae*

Parts used: Inner bark, gall, acorn.

Actions: Anthelmintic (vermifuge), anti-emetic, antiphlogistic, astringent (strong), antiseptic, antivenomous, diuretic (litho-triptic), febrifuge, hemostatic, stimulant (mild), tonic.

Wood Betony

- Wood Betony is considered a top nerve tonic.
- It especially effects the nerves of the head and face.
- It acts like a tonic to the digestive system.
- A great blood and liver cleanser.
- Use in liver congestive issues like jaundice.
- A great spleen cleanser and strengthener.
- Known to expel worms.
- Used for headaches, convulsions, spasms and cramping.
- Use for nerve disorders like multiple sclerosis, Parkinson's, and palsies.
- Use in cases of neuralgia.
- Use in times of stress and nervous tension.

Scientific name: *Betonica officinalis*

Parts used: Whole herb, aerial portions.

Actions: Alterative, analgesic, anthelmintic, antiscorbutic, antispasmodic, antivenom-ous, aperient, aromatic, astringent, bitter tonic, carminative, febrifuge, nervine, seda-tive, stomachic.

Wormwood

- One of nature's top herbs for parasites.

- Wormwood is especially great for larger parasites, including worms of all types and flukes.
- Promotes digestion and liver function.
- Great for stomach paralysis and disorders.
- A strong herb for debilitated conditions.
- An excellent nerve tonic.
- Has antiseptic properties.
- Has been used to counteract the toxic effects of various poisonous plants.
- Use for nausea, morning sickness and upset stomach.
- Use in nervous conditions and nerve injuries.
- Great for jaundice and liver conditions and congestive issues.
- Shown to be beneficial in cases of gout and rheumatism.

Scientific name: *Artemisia absinthium*

Parts used: Whole herb and leaves, oil (external only).

Actions: Anti-bilious, antiseptic, anti-venomous, aromatic, astringent, carminative, febrifuge, hepatic, nervine, stimulant, stomachic (vermifuge), tonic, anthelmintic.

Yellow Dock

- One of the great liver and blood herbs.
- Strengthens the liver and promotes liver function.
- Promotes bile formation.
- Increases the oxygen-carrying capacity of the red blood cells.
- High in iron, thus used for anemia and low hemoglobin counts.
- A top blood builder.
- A great lymphatic cleanser.

- Used in all types of skin conditions.
- Strengthens the spleen and helps clean the blood.
- Has a strengthening effect upon the entire body.
- Excellent for swollen lymph nodes and tumors as well as abscesses and toxic conditions of the body.
- Use in all cases of cancer and HIV.
- Helpful in cases of fatigue and lack of energy.
- Helps increase red blood cell count.
- Helps to promote bile formation and secretion.

Scientific name: *Rumex crispus*

Parts used: Root.

Actions: Alterative, antiscorbutic, anti-scrofulous, anti-syphilitic, aperient, astringent, cathartic, cholagogue, detergent, nutritive (leaves).

Yucca

- A great anti-inflammatory (has steroid type compounds).
- Excellent for gout, rheumatism and arthritis.
- Excellent for prostatitis and cystitis.
- Helps relieve pain in inflammatory conditions.
- Used to help break up inorganic compounds stored in tissues and the vascular system, especially calcium.
- Alkalizes and increases the healing potential of the body.

Scientific name: *Yucca glauca spp.*

Parts used: Roots and leaves of non-flowering plants.

Actions: Alterative, anti-inflammatory, anti-rheumatic, laxative.

☀ Power Herbal Formulas

The formulas recommended in this section, or close facsimiles thereof, can be found in some health food stores, and by contacting the herb supply companies listed in the Resource Guide, Appendix C of this book.

The only true path to healing and tissue regeneration depends upon proper diet and the use of botanical formulas. When this realization occurs for more people, you will begin to see an explosion of interest in herbal products.

Single herbs are strong and work well in helping your body detoxify and rebuild itself. However, herbal formulas, with the combined synergistic action of several herbs, are many times stronger in their effect. In my experience over the last twenty-seven years, working with and creating herbal formulas, the "power" that a specific formula has to effect a cure lies in the unique blend of the herbs used.

I have used herbal formulas that I have created on thousands of clients with tremendous results. However, I am experimenting with new formulas all the time, especially those that will move the lymph system and break up masses and tumors. There's nothing that can come close to a great herbal formula for promoting body detoxification, and especially for the enhancement and regeneration of your organs and glands.

When detoxifying your body with herbal formulas it is prudent to work on your kidneys, GI tract, liver/pancreas, lymphatic system and endocrine glands **all at the same time**. In my opinion, you can safely take **six or seven herbal formulas at one time**. You will get far better results if you get a little aggressive with yourself. Many of my friends have consumed ten to twelve different formulas at one time. When you realize that most herbs simply enhance your body's organs and glandular functions, build your immune system, and increase detoxification, you will lose your fear of consuming them.

To increase filtration and elimination through your kidneys, as well as through your intestines and skin, use kidney and intestinal restorative formulas. To improve elimination through your skin, use a lymphatic and thyroid (endocrine) formula. Use a liver formula on top of this, to detoxify and increase digestion and improve metabolism.

Your lymphatic system is your "sewer system," of which your immune system is a part. This area of your body becomes the most congested and obstructed. This is where most of our problems and conditions begin. Masses, boils, tumors, and the like, are all side effects of a congested lymph system. A parasite formula is also advisable in the beginning of your detoxification.

Detoxification is an art and science, but easy to learn. Always consult an experienced detoxification specialist and herbalist for guidance. Once again, consult the Resource Guide, Appendix C, at the back of this book for recommendations of herbal companies that supply high-quality formulas.

ADRENAL GLANDS

An ideal herbal tincture for aid in the regeneration of the adrenal glands would contain all or most of the following herbs:

Astragalus Root (*Astragalus membranaceus*)
Licorice Root (*Glycyrrhiza glabra*)
Parsley Root (*Petroselinum crispum*)
Bayberry Root Bark (*Myrica cerifera*)
Jamaican Sarsaparilla Root (*Smilax ornata*)
Juniper Berries (*Juniperus communis*)
Kelp Fronds (*Nereocystis leutkeana*)

Alfalfa Leaf (*Medicago sativa*)
Prickly Ash Bark (*Zanthoxylum clava-Herculis*)
Parsley Leaf (*Petroselinum crispum*)
Siberian Ginseng Root (*Eleutherococcus senticosus*)

INDICATIONS

Adrenal insufficiency, arthritis, fatigue and chronic fatigue (not from Epstein-Barr virus), a specific for low blood pressure, high blood pressure (occasionally), weak pulse, systemic inflammation, female reproductive problems—especially estrogen dominance (ovarian cysts, sore breasts, uterine fibroids, etc), prostatitis, exhaustion, low endurance, neurotransmitting issues—e.g., multiple sclerosis, Parkinson's, palsys, tremors, Lou Gehrig's, etc. Post strokes, spinal cord injuries, all types of cancers, HIV (AIDS), skin conditions, heart arrhythmias, anxiety disorders.

SUGGESTED USAGE

Add to a little water or juice.
General: 1 full dropper 3 to 6 times a day.
Acute: 1 full dropper every 4 hours.

CAUTIONS AND CONTRAINDICATIONS

May elevate the blood pressure temporarily, please monitor in high blood pressure cases.

NOTES

1. The medulla of the adrenal glands produces neurotransmitters (epinephrine, norepinephrine and dopamine hydrochloride). These regulate the action of the heart and nerve response. Low blood pressure is always a sign of adrenal insufficiency.

2. The cortex of the adrenal glands produces the cortical steroids that act in the body as anti-inflammatory compounds. Adrenal weaknesses, in most cases, affect the production of these lipid (cholesterol) type steroids causing inflammation to go unchecked. A diet of mainly acid foods (a typical diet) causes inflammation within the tissues of the body. Long-term inflammation deteriorates tissue, eventually leading to ulceration, leading to deterioration or cancer.

BLOOD

An ideal herbal formula for the blood would cleanse impurities, alkalize the blood and tissues, and reduce vascular inflammation. Such a formula would help remove mineral deposits, lipid deposits, and metals as it strengthened the blood system overall. It would contain:

Red Clover Herb and Flowers (Frifolium pratense)
Yellow Dock Root (Rumex spp.)
Burdock Root (Arctium lappa)
Plantain Herb (Plantago lanceolata)
White Oak Bark (Quercus alba)
Prickly Ash Bark (Zanthoxylum clava-Herculis)

INDICATIONS

Detoxification, toxic blood conditions, septicemia, leukocytosis, all cancers (especially leukemia), AIDS, anemia, syphilis, leprosy, elevated cholesterol, fatigue, low iron levels, gangrene, exhaustion, parasitic invasion of weakened blood cells, blood disorders, chronic fatigue syndrome (except when caused from thyroid and adrenal weaknesses), toxic liver and spleen conditions. Low iron levels, low O_2 saturation, malabsorption.

SUGGESTED USAGE

Add to a little water or juice.
General: 1 full dropper 3 to 6 times a day.
Acute: 1 full dropper every 2 to 4 hours.

CAUTIONS AND CONTRAINDICATIONS
None known.

NOTE

In cancer cases, use with a parasite formula for microorganisms and a lymphatic formula.

BRAIN AND NERVOUS SYSTEM

And ideal herbal formula to strengthen and rebuild the brain and nerve tissues of the body would contain all or most of the following:

Gotu Kola Herb (Centella asiatica)
Siberian Ginseng Root (Eleutheroccocus sent.)
Ginkgo Leaf (Ginkgo biloba)

Schizandra Berries (Schisandra chinensis)
Skullcap Herb (Scutellaria lateriflora)
Prickly Ash Bark (Zanthoxylum clava-Herculis)
Calamus Root (Acorus calamus)

INDICATIONS
Weakened nervous system, marked by nerve rings in the iris (autonomic, sympathetic and parasympathetic), poor memory (short and long term), Alzheimer's (or Mad Cow Disease, as several doctors have reported), senile dementia, multiple sclerosis, Parkinson's, Bell's palsy, post strokes, headaches, migraines, spinal cord injuries, depression, jittery nerves, pituitary and pineal gland weakness, shingles (also use a general parasite formula and a parasite formula for microorganisms), spasms, epilepsy, twitching, electrical weaknesses of the heart (arrhythmias, depolarization and repolarization issues, etc.), dizziness, equilibrium issues and mental disorders.

SUGGESTED USAGE
Add to a little water or juice.
General: 1 full dropper 3 to 6 times a day.
Acute: 1 full dropper every 2 to 4 hours.

CAUTIONS AND CONTRAINDICATIONS
None known.

NOTES
1. I have seen tremendous nerve regeneration in quadriplegics and paraplegics with this type of formula, and a 100 percent raw food diet.
2. Deeper results can be attained using this type of formula together with a circulation (upper) formula plus a lymphatic system formula.
3. Alkalization of the body is essential for brain and nerve regeneration. Acidity causes inflammation, which leads to tissue weakness and deterioration.

CIRCULATION AND BLOOD PRESSURE

A cayenne/garlic combo would be an ideal herbal formula to lower blood pressure and increase circulation throughout the body. It would also strengthen the heart and vascular system. Such a cayenne/garlic formula in capsule form would consist of all or most of the following:

Cayenne Pepper Fruit (*Capsicum annum*)(40,000 HU maximum)
Garlic Bulb (*Allium sativum*)
Alfalfa Leaf (*Medicago sativa*)
Butcher's Broom Root (*Iuscus aculeatus*)
Licorice Root (*Glycyrrhiza glabra*)
Hawthorn Berries (*Crataegus spp.*)
Aloe (100:1)

INDICATIONS
High blood pressure, poor circulation, general body weaknesses, especially in the heart and vascular system. Nervous tension, headaches, internal bleeding, depression, sinus congestion, fatigue, poor memory, cold conditions of the body, especially hypo-activity of tissues.

SUGGESTED USAGE
General: 2 capsules, 3 times a day.
Acute: 2 to 3 capsules, every 2 to 4 hours.

CAUTIONS AND CONTRAINDICATIONS
Caution with low blood pressure. Low blood pressure is adrenal and/or pituitary weakness. In high blood pressure cases you should use an adrenal formula (without Licorice), especially if the iris shows adrenal weakness. However, monitor your own or your patient's blood pressure.

FEMALE REPRODUCTIVE SYSTEM

An ideal herbal tincture to help clean, strengthen, and regenerate the female reproductive system would consist of all or most of the following:

Chaste Tree Berries (*Vitex agnus-castus*)
Alteris Root (*True Unicorn Root*)
False Unicorn Root (*Chamaelirium luteum*) (*Aletris farinosa*)
Saw Palmetto Berries (*Serenoa repens*)
Wild Yam Root (*Dioscorea spp.*)
Red Raspberry Leaf (*Rubus idaeus*)
Black Haw Bark (*Viburnum prunifolium*)

Prickly Ash Bark (*Zanthoxylum clava-Herculis*)

INDICATIONS

All female reproductive issues including dysmenorrhea (painful menstruation), amenorrhea (lack of proper menstruation), PMS, and ovulation disorders. Discharges (use a lymphatic formula, a general parasite formula and a parasite formula for microorganisms), endometriosis, ovarian cysts and uterine fibroids (adrenal weakness), prolapsed uterus, menorrhagia (excessive bleeding, which is estrogen dominance), hot flashes and cramping (low thyroid function), edema, under-developed or sagging breasts, dry vaginal walls (low estrogen levels), premature births (estrogen dominance), lack of tone in the female body, cancers of the female reproductive organs (see notes), low sex drive (also underactive thyroid).

SUGGESTED USAGE

Add to a little water or juice.
General: 1 full dropper 3 to 6 times a day.
Acute:1 full dropper every 4 hours.

CAUTIONS AND CONTRAINDICATIONS

Be cautious during early pregnancy. May cut suggested usage in half.

NOTES

1. This formula may be used as a douche. Use 2 to 3 full droppers in skin-temperature water.
2. Females produce estrogen in primarily three places: the liver, fat cells, and ovaries (very acidic).
3. In cancers of the cervix, uterus, ovaries or vaginal wall, a heavy detoxification program is essential. Douching 2 to 4 times a day is also beneficial. Use with a lymphatic system and a general parasite formula, plus a parasite formula for microorganisms.
4. Seventy-five percent of females are considered estrogen dominant. Low blood pressure, excessive bleeding, ovarian cysts, uterine fibroids, premature births, sore breasts, osteoporosis, inability to conceive, etc. are just a few of the indicators of low progesterone levels. Low progesterone production occurs mainly from adrenal insufficiency. Use an adrenal formula to enhance and regenerate the adrenals. Low blood pressure is just one indicator of adrenal weakness.
5. Hot flashes and cramping can be an indicator of thyroid weakness. Add a thyroid formula to your program if this is the case.

GENERAL NUTRITION AND ENERGY

A daily nutritional supplement of the highest quality super-food blend would contain some of God's most energetic and nutritive foods known. These would include:

Royal Jelly
Wheat Grass
Alfalfa
Siberian Ginseng Root
Beet Root
Cinnamon Bark
Dandelion Leaf
Saw Palmetto Berries
Lemon Peel
Norwegian Kelp
Black Walnut Hull
Pau d'Arco
Chaste Tree Berries
Chickweed
Gotu Kola
Hawthorn Berries
Milk Thistle Seed
Barley Grass
Licorice Root
Ginger Root
Rye Grass
Astragalus Root
Flax Seed
Aloe 100:1
Ginkgo Biloba

INDICATIONS

The ideal super-food formula should be one that is designed for all ages and all walks of life. The formula suggested above is mega-nutritional, and fits in all situations, especially for highly depleted individuals. Even animals can benefit tremendously with this formula.

SUGGESTED USAGE BY WEIGHT
10 lbs. – 50 lbs. – 1/4 of a heaping teaspoon
50 lbs. – 100 lbs. – 1/2 of a heaping teaspoon
100 lbs. – 200 lbs. – 1 heaping teaspoon
200 lbs. – 300 lbs. – 1 tablespoon

SUGGESTED USAGE
Take 2 to 3 times a day. This super-food formula can be mixed in water or juice, or sprinkled over a salad.

CAUTIONS AND CONTRAINDICATIONS
Do not take before bedtime if you want to sleep as this formula is an energizer.

NOTE
Super-food complexes far exceed orthomolecular supplementation (separate vitamins and minerals). The whole far exceeds its parts.

HEART

An ideal herbal formula to strengthen and regenerate the heart tissue, and increase circulation and nerve response within the heart would contain all or most of the following:

Hawthorn Berries (*Crataegus spp.*)
Butchers Broom Root (*Iuscus aculeatus*)
Black Walnut Hull (*Juglans nigra*)
Dandelion Leaf (*Taraxacum spp.*)
Kelp Granules (*Nereocystis luetkeana*)
Motherwort Herb (*Leonurus cardiaca*)
Lily of the Valley Herb (*Convallaria majalis*)
Cayenne Pepper (*Capsicum annuum*)
Night Blooming Cereus Stem (*Selenicereus grandiflorus*)

INDICATIONS
Myocardial infarction (heart attack), mitral valve prolapse, pericarditis, bradycardia, tachycardia, angina pectoris (chest pains), palpitations, dyspnea, varicose and spider veins, arrhythmias, including atrial fibrillation and flutter, junctional rhythms, PACs, PVCs, heart blocks, heart or chamber hypertrophy (enlargement), weak heart (check adrenals), congestive heart failure, edema and aneurysms.

SUGGESTED USAGE
Add to a little water or juice.
General: 1 full dropper 3 to 6 times a day.
Acute: 1 full dropper every 2 to 4 hours.

CAUTIONS AND CONTRAINDICATIONS
Do not take during pregnancy. Monitor if you or your patients are on beta-blockers or calcium channel blockers. Heart medications can become too strong and drop blood pressure too low.

NOTE
For optimum results, use with circulatory, thyroid, kidney, adrenal glands and/or brain and nervous system formulas.

KIDNEY AND BLADDER

An ideal herbal formula would alkalize (remove inflammation), clean, strengthen, and regenerate the kidneys and bladder tissues. It should contain all or most of the following:

Couch Grass Root (*Agropyron repens*)
Corn Silk (*Zea mays*)
Pipsissewa Leaves (*Chimaphilla umbellata*)
Nettle Herb (*Urtica dioica*)
Coriander Seed (*Coriandrum sativum*)
Dandelion Leaf (*Taraxacum spp.*)
Lespedeza Herb (*Lespedeza capitata*)
Gravel Root (*Eupatorium purpureum*)

INDICATIONS
Kidney weakness or failure, bladder weakness, cystitis, nephritis, urethritis, urinary tract infections (use a parasite formula for microorganisms as well), lower back pain, prostatitis, edema (dropsy), eye weakness, bags under the eyes, blindness, gout, kidney and bladder stones, dialysis.

SUGGESTED USAGE
Add to a little water or juice.
General: 1 full dropper 3 to 6 times a day.

Acute: 1 full dropper every 2 to 4 hours.

CAUTIONS AND CONTRAINDICATIONS

This type of formula coupled with a raw fruit diet will considerably increase the need to eliminate through the kidneys. If your patient is on dialysis, you may need to increase their dialysis from three times a week to four times a week until self-urination has been achieved. Dialysis patients should eat 90 to 100 percent raw, living foods. Eliminate all meats and grains as these are acidic and irritating to the tissues of the urinary tract.

NOTES

1. Alkalization is essential to the regeneration of the kidneys.
2. Do not drink cranberry juice, as this is too acidic. Fresh watermelon is far better. Fresh fruits and fresh fruit juices are excellent kidney cleansers and regenerators.

LUNGS

An ideal herbal formula would assist the body in removing mucus and toxicity, interstitially and intracellularly within the lung tissues, promoting tissue repair and rejuvenation. It would include all or most of the following:

Platycodon Root (*Platycodon grandiflorum*)
Cayenne Pepper Fruit (*Capsicum annuum*)
Mullein Leaf (*Verbascum thaspus*)
Fenugreek Seed (*Trigonella foenum-graecum*)
Pleurisy Root (*Asclepias tuberosa*)
Horehound Herb (*Marrubium vulgare*)
Comfrey Root and Leaf (*Symphytum officinalis*)
Lobelia Herb (*Lobelia inflata*)

INDICATIONS

Congestive and degenerative lung issues including: bronchitis, pneumonia, emphysema, asthma, C.O.P.D. (Chronic Obstructive Pulmonary Disease), colds, sore throats, tonsillitis, lung cancer, lung tumors, TB, sinus congestion, dyspnea, pleurisy, influenza, coughs, bleeding of the lungs, hearing loss, loss of taste and smell, thyroid congestion (causing hyperthyroidism or hypothyroidism).

SUGGESTED USAGE

Add to a little water or juice.
General: 1 full dropper 3 to 6 times a day.
Acute: 1 full dropper every 1 to 2 hours.

CAUTIONS AND CONTRAINDICATIONS

Avoid during early pregnancy.

NOTES

1. Best when used with a parasite formula for microorganisms and a lymphatic system formula.
2. Gastrointestinal cleaning and rebuilding is a must.

MALE REPRODUCTIVE SYSTEM

An ideal herbal formula to enhance and strengthen the male system would include:

Damiana Leaf (Turnera diffusa)
False Unicorn Root (Chamaelirium luteum)
Chaste Tree Berries (Vitex agnus-castus)
Saw Palmetto Berries (Serenoa repens)
Siberian Ginseng Root (Eleutherococcus senticosus)

INDICATIONS

A weakened male system with symptoms including, but not limited to: impotence, premature ejaculation, low or excessive sex drive, general body weakness or fatigue, low ambition, low energy, pituitary weakness, adrenal weakness, anemia, depression, hormone imbalance, lack of endurance. Use when you desire a daily formula for longevity.

SUGGESTED USAGE

Add to a little water or juice.
General: 1 full dropper 3 to 4 times a day.

CAUTIONS AND CONTRAINDICATIONS

Do not take with prostate cancer.

NOTE

With prostate cancer, use a prostate formula together with lymphatic system formula, parasite for microorganisms formula, adrenal formula and blood formula.

PARASITES—MICROORGANISMS

An ideal herbal formula for microorganism infestations (viruses, bacterium, fungi, protozoas etc.) would contain all or most of the following:

Pau d' Arco Inner Bark (*Tabebuia impetiginosa*)
Thyme Leaf (*Thymus vulgaris*)
Black Walnut Hulls (*juglans nigra*)
Butternut Bark (*Juglans cinerea*)
Echinacea Angustifolia Root (*Echinacea angustifolia*)
Usnea Lichen (*Usnea spp.*)
Grapefruit Seed Extract (*Citrus paradisi*)
Lomatium Root (*Lomatium dissectum*)

INDICATIONS

Microbial infestations including viruses, bacterium, protozoas, fungi, molds, warts, etc., (specifically, but not limited to: streptococcus, staphylococcus, pneumococcus, pseudomonas, M.R.S.A., E-coli, and herpes), yeast infections (Candida albicans), hepatitis A, B, and C, pneumonia, whooping cough, food poisoning, dysentery, cholera, typhoid, syphilis, TB, colds, flu, urinary tract infections, ringworm, poison oak, insect bites, wounds, toxic skin conditions (psoriasis, eczema, dermatitis), itching, tonsillitis, bronchitis, gangrene, AIDS, cancer, tumors, abscesses, cysts, infections of all types.

SUGGESTED USAGE

Add to a little water or juice.
General: 1 full dropper 3 to 6 times a day.
Acute: 1 full dropper every 2 to 4 hours.

CAUTIONS AND CONTRAINDICATIONS

Do not use during early pregnancy.

NOTES

1. For heavy infestations especially with Candida albicans (fungi) this type of formula may be used for 4 to 6 months, if needed.
2. In spinal cord injuries (in quadriplegics, paraplegics, etc.) this formula will help eliminate urinary tract infections. This formula may be used on a regular basis to achieve this. Should be used with a lymphatic system formula.

3. In chronic conditions or heavy infestations, use a general parasite formula.

PARASITES—GENERAL USE

An ideal herbal formula especially for larger parasites, such as flukes and worms of all types would contain the following:

Wormwood Herb (*Artemesia absinthium*)
Betel Nut (*Piper betle*)
Male Fern Root (*Aspidium filix-mas*)
Wormseed (*Chenopodium anthelmin.*)
Parsley Root and Leaf (*Petroselinium crispum*)
Cloves (*Syzygium aromatic*)
Pau d'Arco Bark (*Tabebuia impetiginosa*)
Pink Root (*Spigelia marilandica*)
Tansy Herb and Flower (*Tanacetum vulgare*)
Casara Sagrada Bark (*Rhamnus purshiana*)

INDICATIONS

Parasites, especially larger ones such as worms (pin, hook, round, all types of tapeworm) and flukes (in the liver, pancreas), microorganisms including, but not limited to: viruses, bacterium, protozoa, fungi, molds, warts; chronic yeast infections (Candida albicans), hepatitis A, B, and C, chronic UTIs (use with a parasite tincture for microorganisms), ringworm, toxic skin conditions (like psoriasis, eczema, dermatitis), gangrene, AIDS, cancer, tumors, abscesses.

SUGGESTED USAGE

Add to a little water or juice.
General: 1 full dropper 3 to 6 times a day.

CAUTIONS AND CONTRAINDICATIONS

Do not use during pregnancy.

NOTE

In chronic conditions or with heavy infestations also use a parasite formula for microorganisms.

STOMACH AND BOWELS

An ideal herbal formula that acts like a gentle laxative, as it rebuilds, restores, and rejuvenates the gastrointestinal tract would contain the following powdered herbs:

Cascara Sagrada Bark (*Rhamnus pursh.*)
Slippery Elm Bark (*Ulmus fulva*)
White Oak Bark (*Quercus alba*)
Wild Yam Root (*Dioscorea spp.*)
Plantain Leaf (*Plantago spp.*)
Licorice Root (*Glycyrrhiza glabra*)
Barberry Root (*Berberis spp.*)
Gentian Root (*Gentiana lutea*)
False Unicorn Root (*Chamaelirium luteum*)
Ginger Root (*Zingiber officinale*)

INDICATIONS

Inflammation (gastritis, enteritis and colitis), ulceration, degeneration and cancer of the GI tract, constipation, chronic diarrhea, acid dyspepsia, acid reflux, mucoid plaque build-up, prolapsus, IBS (irritable bowel syndrome), diverticulitis (detoxification is a must), polyps (internal and external), Crohn's disease.

SUGGESTED USAGE

General: 1 to 6 capsules, 3 times a day.

CAUTIONS AND CONTRAINDICATIONS

None known. However, avoid during early pregnancy.

NOTES

1. This type of bowel formula is a bowel regenerator, not a laxative. The goal is to keep herbs working in the gastrointestinal tract, cleaning and rebuilding.

2. The goal is not to have loose stools, but nice soft stools. If diarrhea occurs, cut back on the number of capsules that you are taking. Bowels work on 12-hour cycles. Start with two to three capsules in the morning and two to three in the evening. With the above in mind, I always prefer three capsules, two times a day, A.M. and P.M. It is better to have more restorative intestinal herbs in your GI tract than less. You want the herbs to do their cleaning and strengthening actions there. At the same time, you don't want to use laxatives or produce loose stools. Pushing your food through too fast will void their proper digestion.

If you want to be more aggressive in your GI tract, you may wish to take a stomach and bowel formula three times a day. However, the formula you use then should have less stimulating herbs (like Cascara sagrada, Senna, and Aloe) and more cleaning and healing herbs (like Plaintain, Marshmallow, and Comfrey).

3. A liver/gallbladder flush is very important for everyone, especially those who have small intestinal ulcers, constipation, diarrhea and high blood pressure. (*See* instructions for Liver Flush in Chapter 9.)

THYROID

An ideal herbal formula to help clean, enhance, strengthen and regenerate the thyroid gland would contain all or most of the following in a tincture:

Bladderwrack (*Fucus vesiculosus*)
Fritillary Bulb (*Fritillaria cirrhosa*)
Poke Root (*Phytolacca americana*)
Mullein Leaf (*Verbascum thapsus*)
Bugleweed Herb (*Lycopus virginicus*)
Bayberry Root Bark (*Myrica cerif*)
Black Walnut Hull (*Juglans nigra*)
Irish Moss (*Chondrus crispus*)
Cayenne Pepper Fruit (*Capsicum annuum*)
Saw Palmetto Berries (*Serenoa repens*)

INDICATIONS

Hypothyroidism, fatigue (also check adrenals), chronic fatigue (not from Epstein-Barr; use a general parasite formula and a parasite formula for microorganisms for Epstein-Barr virus), heart arrhythmias, osteoporosis, cramps, rigid or brittle fingernails, hair loss, menstrual disorders (especially when pain is present), arthritis, bursitis, headaches, migraines, obesity (weight that is hard to eliminate).

SUGGESTED USAGE

Add to a little water or juice.
General: 1 full dropper 3 to 6 times a day.
Acute: 1 full dropper every 4 hours.

CAUTIONS AND CONTRAINDICATIONS

None known.

NOTES

1. Where inflammation and bone deterioration is present (as in arthritis, etc.), the thyroid and adrenal glands are always underactive.

2. Most thyroid medications (especially Synthroid®) do not affect T4 to T3 conversion well. This means that the thyroid is always hypoactive even when blood serum levels of TSHs, T4s and T3s appear to be normal (*see* Wilson's Syndrome).

3. Use the Basal Temperature Test (see Appendix A) for a more accurate indicator of thyroid function.

4. Also see Glandular System, p. 265.

MODULE 8.4

☀ Herbal Rejuvenation for Each Body System

This section contains a recommended diet, plus specific herbs or herbal formulas for each body system. Some of the Herbal Formulas (Detoxifiers and Strengtheners) recommended here have already been discussed and specified in Module 8.3: *Power Herbal Formulas*. For example, "Adrenal Glands," "Blood" or "Lungs." Other Herbal Formulas listed in this section are simply described by their generic application, such as "Spleen" or Liver-Gallbladder." Both the single herbs and the herbal formulas recommended can be found in many health food stores, or by contacting the herbal companies suggested in Appendix C: *Resource Guide* at the back of this book. While different herbal companies may call their herbal formulas by various names, the point is to find one designed for the particular body system or organ that needs rejuvenation.

CARDIOVASCULAR SYSTEM

STRUCTURES — Heart, vascular system (arteries, capillaries and veins), and the blood (also part of the digestive system).

DIET — A living, raw food diet consisting mainly of fruits will alkalize (create an anti-inflammatory effect) the vascular system, which creates an ionic reaction. This means that lipid (cholesterol) plaque and mineral deposits will dissolve, and red blood cells that have bonded will break free. This will increase circulation, blood biodynamics, "thin" the blood, and lower blood pressure. This reduces or eliminates the risk of strokes or heart attacks and increases oxygenation of your body.

SINGLE HERBS—DETOXIFIERS

    Butcher's Broom

    Horse Chestnut

    White Oak Bark

    Witch Hazel

    Red Clover

SINGLE HERBS—STRENGTHENERS

    Hawthorn Berries

    Ginkgo Biloba

    Bilberry Leaf

    Black Walnut Hull

HERBAL FORMULAS—DETOXIFIERS

    Circulation Formulas

    Cayenne/Garlic Combo

    Blood

Lymphatic System

HERBAL FORMULAS—STRENGTHENERS
Circulation Formulas
Adrenal Glands
Blood
Inflammation/Joints
Endocrine Glands

DIGESTIVE SYSTEM

STRUCTURES — Mouth and salivary glands, stomach, small intestines (duodenum, jejunum and ileum), pancreas, liver, gallbladder.

DIET — A living, raw food diet is full of enzymes, nutrition and fiber, all of which promote better digestion, bile flow and bowel function.

SINGLE HERBS—DETOXIFIERS
Chickweed
Marshmallow
Bitters
Dandelion Root
Dock Family (Yellow Dock, Burdock, Oregon Grape Root)
Ginger
Mint Family

SINGLE HERBS—STRENGTHENERS
Gentian
Dandelion Root
Milk Thistle

HERBAL FORMULAS—DETOXIFIERS
Stomach and Bowel
Circulation (a Cayenne/Garlic Combo)
Pancreas
Liver/Gallbladder
Lymphatic System

HERBAL FORMULAS—STRENGTHENERS
Stomach and Bowel
Circulation (a Cayenne/Garlic Combo)
Pancreas
Liver/Gallbladder
Adrenal Glands
Endocrine Glands

OTHER — A Liver/Gallbladder Flush is also recommended (see Chapter 9 for instructions in applying this.)

ELIMINATIVE SYSTEMS

See Lymphatic System, Immune System, Intestinal System, Integumentary System, Urinary System.

GLANDULAR SYSTEM

STRUCTURES — The pituitary gland, pineal gland, thyroid and parathyroid glands, thymus, adrenal glands, pancreas (Islets of Langerhans), glands within the intestinal mucosa, ovaries and testes.

DIET — A living, raw food diet promotes glandular function. It also helps balance hormone and steroid responses, which in turn increases utilization of nutrients. Creates a homeostasis of body chemistry.

SINGLE HERBS—DETOXIFIERS
Bugleweed Leaf
Dandelion Leaf
Parsley Leaf
Poke Root
Kelp
Saw Palmetto Berries

SINGLE HERBS—STRENGTHENERS
Licorice Root
Astragalus Root
Panax Ginseng Root
Siberian Ginseng Root
Kelp
Saw Palmetto Berries
Chaste Tree Berry
Hawthorn Berries
Bugleweed
Dandelion Leaf
Parsley Leaf
False Unicorn Root

HERBAL FORMULAS—DETOXIFIERS
  Lymphatic System
  Prostate
  Liver/Gallbladder
  Circulation Formulas
  Blood

HERBAL FORMULAS—STRENGTHENERS
  Endocrine Glands
  Adrenal Glands
  Thyroid Gland
  Pancreas
  Male Reproductive
  Prostate
  Liver/Gallbladder
  Circulation Formula
  Blood

LYMPHATIC SYSTEM

STRUCTURES — Spleen, thymus, appendix, tonsils, lymph nodes, lymph vessels, and lymph fluid.

DIET — A living, raw food diet consisting mainly of fruits which are full of antioxidants and astringents. They clean, enhance, rebuild and restore the health of your cells. The "kings" of these fruits are grapes and lemons.

SINGLE HERBS—DETOXIFIERS
  Poke Root
  Blood Root
  Fenugreek
  Mild Cayenne Pepper
  Cascara Sagrada
  White Oak Bark
  Cleavers
  Red Clover
  Blue Flag
  Plantain
  Red Root
  Yellow Dock

SINGLE HERBS—STRENGTHENERS
  Yellow Dock
  Poke Root
  Blue Flag

White Oak Bark
Reishi Mushroom
Maitake Mushroom
Shiitake Mushroom

HERBAL FORMULAS—DETOXIFIERS
  Lymphatic System
  Kidneys and Bladder
  Stomach and Bowel
  Liver/Gallbladder
  Blood Formula

HERBAL FORMULAS—STRENGTHENERS
  Kidneys and Bladder
  Stomach and Bowel
  Liver/Gallbladder
  Immune System
  Blood Formula

NOTE — The organs of your eliminative system are tied to your lymphatic system. Work with both systems. Your lymph and blood send their wastes into your eliminative channels (this includes your kidneys and colon) to be excreted.

IMMUNE SYSTEM

STRUCTURES — Lymphatic system, which includes the thymus and spleen, bone marrow, immune cells (lymphocytes, monocytes, basophils, macrophages, T-lymphocytes, B-cells, helper T and B cells, etc.), liver and beneficial parasites.

DIET — A living, raw food diet alkalizes and helps remove acids, foreign proteins and substances from the tissues that cause inflammatory immune responses. This enhances and eases the function of your immune system.

SINGLE HERBS—DETOXIFIERS
  Poke Root
  Blood Root
  Blue Flag
  Bugleweed
  Red Clover Flower
  Fenugreek Seed
  Plantain Leaf

Oregon Grape Root

SINGLE HERBS—STRENGTHENERS

Reishi Mushroom

Shiitake Mushroom

Astragalus Root

Kelp/Bladderwrack

Antler (Elk or Deer)

Panax Ginseng

Echinacea (all types: Purpurea, Angustifolia and Pallida)

Siberian Ginseng

Maitake Mushroom

Schizandra Berries

HERBAL FORMULAS—DETOXIFIERS

Lymphatic System formula

Lymph Nodesformula

HERBAL FORMULAS—STRENGTHENERS

Immune Formula #1, for general use

Immune Formula #2, (Super-Immune) for general use, bone marrow strengthening and improved B-cell production.

Adrenal Glands

Thyroid Gland

Spleen

Liver/Gallbladder

INTEGUMENTARY SYSTEM

STRUCTURES — Skin, nails, hair, oil and sweat glands.

DIET — A living, raw food diet is highly cleansing and strengthening to the liver and skin. Raw fruits and vegetables alkalize and dissolve fatty deposits in the skin and liver (stones). These foods also enhance the function of your thyroid gland and increase body heat and elimination through your skin.

SINGLE HERBS—DETOXIFIERS

Dock Family (Yellow Dock and Oregon Grape Root)

Milk Thistle

Poke Root

Chaparral

White Oak Bark

SINGLE HERBS—STRENGTHENERS

Dock Family (Yellow Dock and Oregon Grape Root)

Milk Thistle

Horsetail

Comfrey Root and Leaf

HERBAL FORMULAS—DETOXIFIERS

Lymphatic System

Liver/Gallbladder

Stomach and Bowel

Blood

Circulation Formulas

HERBAL FORMULAS—STRENGTHENERS

Liver/Gallbladder

Stomach and Bowel

Blood

Circulation Formulas

OTHER — A Liver/Gallbladder Flush (Chapter 9) and skin brushing (Chapter 9) are also recommended.

INTESTINAL SYSTEM

STRUCTURES — Colon, lymphatic system, urinary system, immune system and the skin.

DIET — A living, raw food diet is rich in "electrical" fiber and nutrition for optimal elimination.

SINGLE HERBS—DETOXIFIERS

Cascara Sagrada

Psyllium Seed

Flax Seed

Dock Family

Marshmallow

Slippery Elm

White Oak Bark

SINGLE HERBS—STRENGTHENERS

Cascara Sagrada

Mullein

Chickweed

Dock Family

Marshmallow

Slippery Elm
Gentian

HERBAL FORMULAS—DETOXIFIERS
Stomach and Bowel
Liver/Gallbladder
Lymphatic
Kidneys and Bladder
Parasite—for microorganisms
Parasite—a general formula
Strengtheners
Stomach and Bowel
Liver/Gallbladder
Kidneys and Bladder
Parasite—for microorganisms

OTHER — A Liver/Gallbladder Flush is also recommended (see Chapter 10).

MUSCULAR SYSTEM

STRUCTURES — Muscles, tendons, and connective tissue.

DIET — A fresh, raw food diet consisting of lots of green leafy vegetables and vegetable juices helps to rebuild strong muscle tissue. These foods are high in superior amino acids and minerals, especially usable calcium.

SINGLE HERBS—DETOXIFIERS
Poke Root
Plantain
Blood Root
Fenugreek Seed
Chaparral
White Oak Bark
Blue Flag
Red Clover
Burdock Root
Dandelion Root

SINGLE HERBS—STRENGTHENERS
Alfalfa
Kelp
Panax Ginseng
Comfrey Root and Leaf
Horsetail

HERBAL FORMULAS—DETOXIFIERS
Lymphatic System
Circulation Formulas
Lymph Nodes

HERBAL FORMULAS—STRENGTHENERS
Bones
Thyroid Gland
Adrenal Glands

NERVOUS SYSTEM

STRUCTURES — The brain, spinal cord (Central Nervous System), the Autonomic Nervous System, sensory organs (eyes, ears, nose, olfactory nerves, etc.).

DIET — A living, raw food diet consisting primarily of fruits. These foods hold the highest electromagnetic energy of all foods (alkalizing) and promote nerve and brain regeneration.

SINGLE HERBS—STRENGTHENERS
Gotu Kola
Ginkgo Biloba
Skullcap
Kelp
Saw Palmetto Berries
Chaste Tree Berries
Panax Ginseng
Siberian Ginseng
Parsley Root and Leaf
Hawthorn Berries
Astragalus Root
Licorice Root

SINGLE HERBS—ANTISPASMODICS
Lobelia
St. John's Wort
California Poppy
Passion Flower
Skullcap

SINGLE HERBS—RELAXANTS
Valerian
St. John's Wort
Passion Flower
California Poppy

HERBAL FORMULAS—DETOXIFIERS
Lymphatic System
Lymph Nodes
Stomach and Bowel Formulas

HERBAL FORMULAS—STRENGTHENERS
Brain and Nervous System
Adrenal Glands
Thyroid Gland
Kidneys and Bladder
Neuromuscular Spasms

NOTE — Many of the herbs listed strengthen the adrenal glands, which in turn increases low neurotransmitter production. By increasing low neurotransmitter production (adrenal insufficiency), you will strengthen your nervous system.

REPRODUCTIVE SYSTEM

STRUCTURES — Testes, ovaries, sperm, ova, mammary glands and prostate gland. The reproductive system works hand-in-hand with your glandular system.

DIET — A living, raw food diet energizes the gonads and the glandular system. A raw food diet is also an anti-inflammatory to these tissues (prostate, uterus, etc.).

SINGLE HERBS—DETOXIFIERS
Saw Palmetto Berries
White Pond Lily
Poke Root
White Oak Bark

SINGLE HERBS—STRENGTHENERS
Kelp
Chaste Tree Berries
False Unicorn
Saw Palmetto Berries
Panax Ginseng Root
Siberian Ginseng Root
Damiana Leaf
Astragalus Root
Licorice Root
Black Cohosh
Red Raspberry Leaf

Pumpkin Seed
Black Haw Root

HERBAL FORMULAS—DETOXIFIERS
Lymphatic System
Prostate
Female Reproductive

HERBAL FORMULAS—STRENGTHENERS
Adrenal Glands
Thyroid Gland
Male Reproductive
Female Reproductive
Prostate

NOTE — It is not advisable to use Panax-type Ginseng in the presence of inflammation or cancer. Panax-type Ginseng may promote estrogen and testosterone, which can stimulate or feed these processes.

RESPIRATORY SYSTEM

STRUCTURES — Lungs, trachea, bronchi, bronchial tubes and alveoli.

DIET — A diet of raw foods is not mucus-forming or congesting. The effects of these foods is the opposite; they help clean the lungs, throat, bronchi, etc. Fruits are especially good!

SINGLE HERBS—DETOXIFIERS
Mullein
Fenugreek
Pleurisy Root
Lobelia
Elecampane
Comfrey Leaf
Horehound

SINGLE HERBS—STRENGTHENERS
Mullein
Lobelia
Elecampane
Comfrey Leaf
Horehound

HERBAL FORMULAS—DETOXIFIERS
Lungs

Lymphatic System
Strengtheners
Lungs
Neuromuscular Spasms
Adrenal Glands

SKELETAL SYSTEM

STRUCTURE — Bones, cartilage and connective tissue.

DIET — A living, raw food diet, which includes dark-green leafy vegetables, alkalizes and nourishes the whole system, especially the skeletal/muscular system. These vegetables have a high content of electrolytes (alkaline minerals: calcium, magnesium, sodium and potassium). Raw vegetables are high in calcium and magnesium with the proper balance of phosphorus. This is vital for bone regeneration.

SINGLE HERBS—DETOXIFIERS
Black Walnut Hull
White Oak Bark

SINGLE HERBS—STRENGTHENERS
Oat Straw
Horsetail
Kelp
Comfrey Root and Leaf
Black Walnut Hull
Alfalfa
White Oak Bark
Chickweed

HERBAL FORMULAS—DETOXIFIERS
Lymphatic System
Lymph Nodes
Blood

HERBAL FORMULAS—STRENGTHENERS
Bones
Adrenal Glands
Blood
Kidney and Bladder
Pancreas
Thyroid Gland

URINARY SYSTEM

STRUCTURES — Kidneys, bladder, ureter and urethra.

DIET — A raw food diet is essential because of its high alkalizing effect upon the urinary system. Acidosis, especially from high protein diets, deteriorates this system rapidly.

SINGLE HERBS—DETOXIFIERS
Corn Silk
Juniper Berries
Saw Palmetto Berries
Pipsissewa
Uva Ursi
Couch Grass Root
Parsley
Dandelion Leaf

SINGLE HERBS—STRENGTHENERS
Juniper Berries
Saw Palmetto Berries
Pipsissewa
Uva Ursi
Lespedeza
Couch Grass Root
Parsley
Dandelion Leaf

HERBAL FORMULAS—DETOXIFIERS
Kidneys and Bladder
Lymphatic System
Prostate
Blood

HERBAL FORMULAS—STRENGTHENERS
Kidneys and Bladder
Adrenal Glands
Blood
Prostate

ALL SYSTEMS

SINGLE HERBS—TONICS
Panax Ginseng
Astragalus
Gotu Kola
Siberian Ginseng

Antler
Alfalfa
Fo Ti
Pau d'Arco
Chaste Tree Berries

SINGLE HERBS—PARASITE ELIMINATION
Black Walnut Hull
Pau d'Arco
Wormwood
Male Fern
Cloves
Garlic

Grapefruit Seed extract

HERBAL FORMULAS—TONICS
Immune #2 (or Super-Immune)
Male Reproductive
Female Reproductive
Endocrine Glands
Thyroid Gland
Adrenal Glands

HERBAL FORMULAS—PARASITE ELIMINATION
Parasite—a general formula
Parasite—for microorganisms
Lymphatic System

MODULE 8. 5

☀ Pharmaceutical Antibiotics vs. Nature's Anti-Parasitics

Throughout this book I've touched upon parasites (including bacteria, funguses, and worms) and their role in nature. Now as we consider chemical medications versus herbs, I think it's important to understand two things. First, there are no such "things" as diseases—there are only varying degrees of acidosis and toxicity. Secondly, you can't "treat" acidosis and toxicity with more acidosis and toxicity (e.g., chemical medications). Treatment of "disease" symptoms by chemical medications is ludicrous, toxic, damaging to cells, and many times deadlier. In my opinion, among the many chemical forms of treatment, antibiotics stand out as being some of the worst, especially in the side effects they create in your body.

One of the main tenets of the allopathic medical philosophy is the "germ theory"—perpetuated by Louis Pasteur, who believed that because microorganisms were present in most disease processes, that they must certainly be the "cause." He did not consider the idea that they were only secondary to the cause.

The naturopathic view has always considered parasites to be secondary to the real causes of disease—toxicity and acidosis. (We have covered most of this in Chapter 5 when we considered parasites and the causes of disease.)

Especially in the last four generations, humans have weakened their organs and glands considerably. We have weakened our cellular structures and functions through our lifestyle and diet, and passed these weaknesses along to our children. With each generation, cells are becoming weaker while the body's inflammatory responses to toxicity are greater than ever before, and the lymphatic highway (lymph system) has become highly obstructed. This has greatly affected the immune response. Our ability to digest and absorb our foods has dramatically decreased. Add all the above factors together and you can begin to see why your cells succumb to parasites.

Remember, parasites are God's way of keeping your body clean. They consume by-products of metabolism and digestion, as well as other toxins. They also eliminate your weak or dying cells. Because this can be life-threatening in many toxic, weakened and congested people, modern medical science has sought to fight back. Thus, the world of antibiotics was born.

Humans themselves have created a great many strains of microorganisms, especially bacteria. These include M.R.S.A. (methicillin-resistant staphylococcus aureus), Sinorhizobium meliloti bacterium and the Rhizobia (RMBPC) bacterium, just to name a few. From these and many others we see conditions like "hoof and mouth" disease, M.R.S.A. infections, and "Mad Cow Disease." Many of these conditions lead to death.

Viruses are a whole different subject. Many deadly and debilitating viruses have been created due to contamination; in the search for weapons of biological warfare; and even as forms of simple population control. For a frightening look into the subject of viruses and their use by the scientific community, refer to *Emerging Viruses* by Leonard G. Horowitz.

Now let's look at antibiotics, both the pharmaceutically-manufactured and the natural.

PHARMACEUTICAL ANTIBIOTICS

Pharmaceutical antibiotics are also known as sulfa drugs. Most contain primarily a sulfur derivative with additional highly toxic chemical compounds. This type of sulfur is inorganic and has a cumulative effect within your body. If you consume too many sulfa drugs, you will eventually become allergic and/or immune to them.

Sulfur is an inhibitor with affinity to intestinal and lymphatic tissues. This creates hypoactivity in these areas. Typically, when a person comes down with a simple cold and/or flu-like symptom because he/she has congested him/herself by consuming sugars, diary products, or other congesting foods, the following process takes place:

- A stimulus—like an overload of bacteria, fungi, cold winds or weather, or excessive weakness—trips the body into a healing or cleansing process. But the allopathic medical community sees this as a disease it must treat.
- Because this congestion or mucus is loaded with microorganisms, it is now labelled an "infection."
- Antibiotics are given for suppressing, and thus eliminating these types of symptoms.
- These sulfa drugs, however, inhibit the lymph system.
- The body's natural efforts to eliminate this congestion are stopped.

Congestion and toxicity must be eliminated not just suppressed. Otherwise, your body is forced to store this congestion. These toxins, plus any added sulfur and other chemicals that you may have consumed to treat your condition, are stored within your tissues (intestinal, lymph, lymph nodes, etc.). You can't just kill the microorganisms that feed and live in this toxic congestion. You must remove the toxic congestion too.

Over time, suppressing the body's natural cleansing processes creates a steady decline in cellular health and/or causes tumors to be formed. It also goes without saying that this creates a continuous inflammatory response by your immune system. The end result of this scenario in today's world is cancer, in one form or another.

Let's take a look at CIPRO, one popular antibiotic that is frequently being used. It was highly recommended for anthrax until people caught on to the devastating side effects to all the systems of the body. These include:

GI — Nausea, vomiting, diarrhea, oral candidiasis, dysphagia, intestinal perforation, dyspepsia, heartburn, anorexia, pseudo-membranous colitis, flatulence, abdominal discomfort, GI bleeding, oral mucosal pain, dry mouth, bad taste.

CNS — Headache, restlessness, insomnia, nightmares, hallucinations, tremor, lightheadedness, confusion, seizures, ataxia, mania, weakness, drowsiness, dizziness, psychotic reactions, malaise, depression, depersonalization, paresthesia.

GU — Nephritis, crystalluria, hematuria, cylindruria, renal failure, urinary retention, polyuria, vaginitis, urethral bleeding, acidosis, renal calculi, interstitial nephritis, vaginal candidiasis, glucosuria, pyuria, albuminuria, proteinuria.

SKIN — Rashes, urticaria, photosensitivity, flushing pruritus, erythema nodosum, cutaneous candidiasis, hyperpigmentation, edema (of lips, neck, face, conjunctivae, hands), angioedema, toxic epidermal necrolysis, exfoliative dermatitis, Stevens-Johnson syndrome.

OPHTHALMIC — Blurred or disturbed vision, double vision, eye pain.

CV — Hypertension, syncope, angina pectoris, palpitations, atrial flutter, myocardial infarction (heart attacks), cerebral thrombosis, ventricular ectopy, cardiopulmonary arrest, postural hypotension.

RESPIRATORY — Dyspnea, bronchospasm, pulmonary embolism, edema of larynx or lungs, hemoptysis, hiccoughs, epistaxis.

HEMATOLOGIC — Eosinophilia, pancytopenia, leukopenia, neutropenia, anemia, leukocytosis, agranulocytosis, bleeding diathesis.

MISCELLANEOUS — Super-infections; fever; chills; tinnitus; joint pain or stiffness; back, neck or chest pain; flare-up of gout; flushing; hyperpigmentation; worsening of myasthenia gravis; hepatic necrosis; cholestatic jaundice; hearing loss. After ophthalmic use: Irritation, burning, itching, angioneurotic edema, urticaria, maculopapular and vesicular dermatitis, crusting of lid margins, conjunctival hyperemia, bad taste in mouth, corneal staining, keratitis keratopathy, allergic reactions, photophobia, decreased vision, tearing, lid edema. Also, a white, crystalline precipitate in the superficial part of corneal defect (onset within 1-7 days after initiating therapy; lasts about 2 weeks and does not affect continued use of the medication). Contraindications include: never use in children and lactating mothers.

This information is taken from the *RN's NDR-93 (Nurse's Drug Reference)* by George R. Spratto and Adrienne L. Woods.

As you can see, the side effects of CIPRO are shocking, and the FDA allows this! It makes you question the FDA and who really controls it. (The FDA is supposed to be a consumer protection agency.) I learned of CIPRO's devastating side effects from one of my clients who developed a urinary tract infection and went to his medical doctor, instead of asking me first. His wife called me from the Emergency Room when he developed three blood clots and had a heart attack as a probable result of consuming CIPRO, which he had just started taking three days earlier.

Each antibiotic, depending upon its chemical composition, has its own set of side effects. Not only do they kill your overgrowth bacteria, they also kill your beneficial digestive bacteria, and at the same time increase the growth of fungi and yeasts. They also inhibit your immune system and lymphatic system, making it very difficult for your body to clean and properly protect itself. As previously stated, this eventually leads to cellular death and the degeneration of your body.

NATURE'S (GOD'S) ANTIBIOTICS

Now let's examine nature's remedies to toxic human lifestyles. When nature creates anything, it has multifaceted purposes and responses. An excellent example of this is nature's botanical kingdom. Herbs are non-hybrid vegetables . . . with a twist. This twist is the herb's active principles that give it its unique action within your body. Take Black Walnut Hull, for example. It is a powerful antibiotic, antifungal, anti-worm, anti-protozoa, anti-fluke, as well as a cellular proliferator (strengthener). It is also an immune enhancer, has astringent properties for cleansing, and is lymphatic enhancing. It's high in calcium and known to strengthen bones and connective tissues. I can go on and on about just this one herb.

Even more amazing, Black Walnut Hull does not kill all the beneficial bacteria like chemical antibiotics do, and it has no harmful side effects. God never ceases to amaze me!

The above is true of the effects of almost all herbs. There are some toxic ones, but we don't use those. All non-toxic herbs are also nutritive. In other words, they are full of vitamins, minerals, and a whole host of other nutritive factors.

One case out of literally thousands that I have worked with will show you the difference between manufactured antibiotics and nature's botanical gifts. A female client of mine contracted E-coli. Where she got it we were not sure. It could have been in a restaurant, or at home using uncleaned vegetables, or in the fish that she had eaten on the day she became ill.

She became deathly sick and went to the Emergency Room. Consequently, they admitted her to the hospital and put her on strong antibiotics. Because she had been on a healthy program for a year or so, her body was very sensitive to toxins. The antibiotics were making her even sicker. She felt a multitude of side effects, which were ignored by the staff.

Her husband became very alarmed and finally pulled her out of the hospital, after a lengthy battle with her M.D. This doctor finally told my client that she would be dead within two days if she left the hospital. Within three days, however, I had her up and around and feeling great, all because of dietary interventions and herbal formulas that left her with no side effects or damaged tissue.

As you learn about the true causes of disease and the nature of parasites, this truth will set you free. As you learn the ways of nature, you will save yourself a lot of needless suffering.

And God said, "Behold, I have given you every herb-bearing seed which is upon the face of all the earth."
— Genesis 1:20

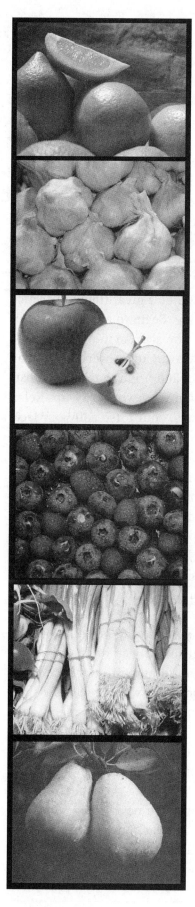

CHAPTER NINE

Tools for Healthy Living

This chapter will introduce you to or reacquaint you with other health modalities besides diet that can assist you on your journey. As you turn these pages you will be entering through a golden door into a vast and incredible world, full of truths, information, new hobbies and ways to enhance your ultimate growth potential.

In the first section you will learn about Nine Healthy Habits that can be used on a daily or regular basis to up-level your health. Some of these, like exercise and deep breathing, you may already be doing. Others, like dry skin brushing and foot reflexology, may be new for you.

In Module 9.2 you will receive instructions for many of the adjunct tools that we have suggested throughout this book, including the Liver and Gallbladder Flush.

Have fun and be happy as you enter here. Remember, this is your life, your body and your choice. Nature is endless. Enjoy the many tools God has created for you.

☼ Nine Healthy Habits

HABIT #1
BE GOOD TO YOURSELF

It is said you are born alone, you live alone (within yourself), and you die alone. So, love the one you're with! Make every moment count. Most people do not know themselves very well and many do not even like themselves. One day in meditation a voice said to me, "You are my creation." I realized that all life is God's expression. We are all divine, no matter what we look like, how smart we are, or how "good" or "bad" we are. We are only *using* our physical bodies. Who we are as soul is much greater than the bodies we use.

Love yourself, but not egotistically. Be like the sun, which shines its light and warmth on all life, without judgement or separation. Love everything, as all things are made of God. You are divine and owe it to yourself and all life to get yourself healthy and happy. Be good to yourself and all life.

HABIT #2
MEDITATION: RELAX! RELAX! RELAX!

Stress constricts the circulation, the bowels, the organs and the glandular functions. This constriction leads to discomfort and tissue weakness, including constipation, lower back pain, adrenal gland and kidney weakness, anxieties, heart problems and poor food digestion, just to name a few possible conditions.

Meditation is one of your greatest tools for relaxation. It allows you to relax every muscle and cell in your body. As the body relaxes, this also relaxes the mind and emotions, which are the main cause of stress in the first place. Meditation is simple, fun, and with practice can be done anywhere, at any time.

It is best to start a meditation practice by finding a quiet place where no one will bother you. Give yourself thirty minutes or so. It is also best if you can set up a routine, starting at the same time each day if possible. You will want to sit or lie down in a position that is comfortable for you, and where you will not be disturbed.

Close your eyes and take about ten deep breaths. This would be a great time to practice abdominal breathing. Begin to relax all over, allowing your mind a break from thinking. You are now going to just relax and observe. You may start with your toes and begin to relax each part of your body as you work your way up. Relax your legs, your arms, your torso and your face. Allow yourself to relax to the point of feeling like air, where you are like a floating feather, with no direction or desire for anything. Observe and listen, but do this totally relaxed, as if you're a watcher of a movie. Once fully relaxed you may wish to purposely move your attention anywhere. (If you hear a "pop," and find yourself "out of your physical body," do not be alarmed. You've just had an O.B.E., out-of-body experience. Relax.)

Meditation is your time to be with yourself, without external influences or the constant demands of the mind and emotions. Meditation will open doors that were previously shut, and will allow true healing to take place. Your knowingness of, and relationship with, God will expand greatly. By opening yourself in the above manner, spirit can flow through you unobstructed. This can bring great healing, and if you're "listening," you never know what you might experience. It is far better to listen to God than to speak to God.

Remember, just *be*.

HABIT #3
EXERCISE

If we lived in much earlier times we might have been wanderers and gatherers, walking far and collecting foods for survival. Of necessity we would have moved about a great deal more than we do today. Movement plays a vital role in our health issues. Much of your blood and lymph flow, especially in your lower extremities, moves by muscle activity. Notice when you are inactive for a while, either sitting or lying down, you tend to become stiff until you start moving around. The less toxic a person is, the less stiff he or she will be after periods of inactivity.

Many great forms of exercise are available. I recommend walking, swimming, rebounding, tai chi, stretching, yoga, passive aerobic exercise, to name a few, as anyone in almost any condition can do these forms, in part or whole.

Keep yourself active. If you are in a weakened state, build up slowly, but increase your activity level as much as you can every day. Exercise is essential to becoming healthy.

HABIT #4
DEEP BREATHING

The air we breathe is the life force for our physical body. Without it we would die. God created a natural cycle whereby we breathe in oxygen, carbon, hydrogen and nitrogen from plants, and we exhale carbon dioxide, which is the essential breath or physical life force for plant life. Oxygen, of course, is vital to your life. It is a great energizer, alkalizer and oxidizer. The air we breathe (which is created by plants and trees) is alkaline, while the carbon dioxide by-products we exhale are acidic. Being a predominately alkaline species, it is vital that we learn to breathe properly and spend some time deep breathing. This charges the system with negative ions creating a cationic condition in the body, whereas shallow breathing creates over-acidity and an anionic situation in the body. Oxygen and simple sugars are the main fuels for our cells, as carbon dioxide is one of the main fuels for plants.

Most humans were never taught to breathe properly, so we have become what are called "shallow breathers." If our breath becomes shallow, so does our life. Human beings and nature are not separate, but work together as one. It is when the human's ego separates him or her from nature that disease sets in.

Deep breathing energizes the system, increasing circulation and lymph flow. Deep breathing also clears the mind and settles the emotions, allowing us to feel more at peace with ourselves and with nature.

The breath, in spiritual traditions, has been called the *prana, chi, ki,* life force, spirit, *mana,* the *ECK,* and many other names. There are a few individuals who consume mainly air as their food. I read about a Catholic nun who supposedly lived only on snow, high in the Himalayan mountains. I was personally moving in the direction of trying to live solely on air back in the early seventies. I lived as a hermit in the national forests and state parks around Florida. I lived on oranges only, for six months, hoping to eventually eliminate those. However, my energy was so high that I kept having out-of-body experiences and I became unbalanced with respect to this world. It was hard for me to communicate with others. (Human awareness, on earth and in this physical realm, is very low when it comes to understanding true reality and the ability to interact with all life.) Eventually, I balanced out my eating habits with raw fruits and vegetables.

Try the following deep-breathing exercise to increase the oxygen content within your body. The more you work with it the more you will develop a better breathing pattern. Lie on your back on a couch, floor or bed. RELAX, RELAX, and RELAX! Place your right hand on your abdomen just above your navel. Breathe in through your nose without moving your shoulders. Watch as your hand moves up and down with your breathing. This requires breathing into the lower lobes of your lungs. Each time you breathe in, make your abdomen expand, or move up (raising your hand with it), then exhale from your mouth. Your abdomen will naturally contract as the air is released. Your hand will move as your abdomen lowers.

After you have done this for several breaths, try increasing your intake of oxygen by breathing first from the abdomen—that means, as if filling the abdomen. It expands. Then fill the top lobes of your lungs by inhaling more air in the upper thoracic cavities. This will raise your shoulders. Then, exhale gently.

Now let's look at this again. First fill the lower lobes of your lungs by breathing to expand your abdomen. Keep inhaling and fill your upper lobes, elevating your chest and shoulder areas to allow for complete filling. Once full, exhale gently.

You can practice deep breathing in any position. Work with this until it becomes second nature to take deeper and more filling breaths. Deep breathing will help alkalize and increase cellular respiration as well as increase elimination of acid gases. This is a great exercise to do before you meditate or just as a calming technique. Open yourself to nature in every way and vitality, youthfulness, and a sense of connection will be yours.

HABIT #5
DRY SKIN BRUSHING

In previous chapters we covered the skin and its disorders (for example, see Chapter 5, Module 5.9). Remember that you eliminate up to two pounds of metabolic wastes and toxins per day through your skin. It is your largest eliminating organ. When the layers of your skin become full of acids and toxins you develop rashes, pimples, boils, and other conditions. Skin care should be one of your top priorities. It is important to clean the skin every day with a bath or prefer-

ably a shower. It would be valuable to put a water softener or reverse osmosis (R/O) system in your house, as inorganic minerals clog and block the pores of the skin. You will notice the difference in your skin and the softness of your hair when using pure, soft water over hard, mineralized water.

Another great way to enhance skin health is through dry skin brushing. This removes old and dead skin cells and promotes circulation and lymph flow, allowing the skin to "breathe" much better. All you need is a long-handled vegetable-fiber brush, which is generally available at your local health food store. Do not use a nylon-bristle brush for the skin. Brush your feet, legs and hands first. It does not matter which direction you brush in, however brushing toward the center of your body is beneficial. Since there are nerve endings in your hands and feet, you will experience a tingling sensation as you stimulate your nervous system. Cleaning the skin in this manner is of great benefit to gain vibrant, healthy skin. Over the years, people who attended Dr. Jensen's seminars learned what healthy skin should look like. Even up to his death at ninety-three, Dr. Jensen's skin was always as soft and healthy as a baby's.

Try to spend some time in the fresh air with as few clothes on as possible. Let your skin breathe.

HABIT #6
SAUNAS AND STEAM BATHS

Sweating plays an essential role in daily detoxification. The skin, called the third kidney, eliminates as much waste (by-products and toxins) as your lungs, kidneys and bowels. The skin is your largest eliminative organ. When thyroid function is low, or when one leads a sedentary life, the body does not sweat well. The subcutaneous layers of the skin become clogged or stagnant with toxicity. This causes dry skin, rashes, pimples, rosacea, dandruff, dermatitis and the like. Sweating is an essential mechanism for getting healthy.

Saunas and steam baths are extremely beneficial, especially when using various essential oils. Public facilities may be less desirable, so know the owners and their awareness about cleanliness (the environment should be as sterile as possible) both physically and psychically. If saunas are not available in your area, they can be built or purchased. You can create a steam bath in your own bathtub. Use mustard, cayenne pepper or other herbs added to the water for additional cleansing effects. (Also see instructions for cold sheet treatments in Module 9.2.)

HABIT #7
SLANT BOARDING

A slant board is simply a board or table that is fixed at a 45° angle. By lying down with your head lower than your feet you can improve cerebral circulation and increase lymphatic flow in the lower extremities. After years of living upright, gravity can take its toll on your body. We develop poor cerebral circulation and edema in our legs and feet. Our skin and organs begin to sag and prolapse, restricting proper functions. The slant board is a great way to return good blood flow to the brain. This can also help our internal organs, relieving some of the pressure that gravity puts on them.

HABIT #8
COLOR THERAPY (SUNLIGHT)

All life in one way or another looks to the sun for its energy and healing. Sunlight offers us full-spectrum color healing, and each individual ray of color presents a unique energy for healing the body. Each color has its own special effect upon tissue. Added together, all these individual color rays provide a powerful healing energy that flows through all the cells of the body, uplifting, healing and giving succor to each cell.

Remember to maintain balance in using the sun, however. The sun is acidic in nature, and too much is just as bad as not enough. Most people are far too acidic as it is. This is why many do not like the sun, or burn too easily. The more alkaline you become, the more you will enjoy the sun and its healing power. Enjoy God and nature; bathe in its energies; they're all around and flowing through us.

There are many great books on color healing (see the Bibliography for a few suggestions), and we will deal with more about this subject later in this chapter where you will learn about the different colors and their individual powers to heal. It's fun to study about color, and the observation of colors in one's daily life brings more awareness about the colors in your dreams. The heavens have more colors than one can even imagine. Open yourself to the higher energies of God. It's an exciting trip.

HABIT #9
FOOT AND HAND REFLEXOLOGY

Acid crystals (uric, phosphoric, carbonic, lactic, etc.) and cellular wastes build up under the nerve endings in your feet. Since these nerve endings reflex all through your body, these acids and toxins can have a devastating effect in related areas. The nerve that feeds the heart, for example, ends in your hands and feet. If acid crystals or a toxic build-up affect the ending of this nerve, it can lead to heart palpitations, high blood pressure (when standing or walking), chest pain, etc. This is true with all your organs and glands as the nerves that feed them also end in your hands and feet. Rubbing the bottoms of your feet and the palms of your hands on a daily basis will break-up these crystals and toxic accumulations, relieving the symptoms.

Reflexology is an incredible science. I have saved three individuals in cardiac arrest with the techniques of reflexology. This is another simple science that can save much suffering. Study and learn this health-enhancing system.

☀ Four Healthy Tools to Assist Your Detoxification . . . and Your Life

TOOL #1
LIVER AND GALLBLADDER FLUSH

This process helps to remove liver stones and gallbladder stones.

Items Needed

- 8-ounces of pure, cold-pressed, extra virgin organic olive oil.
- 6- to 8-ounces of freshly squeezed (if possible) pink grapefruit juice or the juice of 2 lemons.
- Freshly squeezed apple juice (enzymes assist with reducing nausea).
- Optional: a preparation to aid in the softening of possible stones, such as Phosfood Liquid®, produced by Standard Process Laboratories. (See Resource Guide for ordering.)
- Optional: Intestinal cleansing formula.

Suggested Preparation

- Three days of eating mainly raw fruits and vegetables (organic preferred).
- One 8-ounce glass of freshly juiced apple juice in the morning and one in the evening, for three days.
- Three days of bowel detoxification. Use an intestinal cleansing formula, with formula strength depending upon your bowel regularity. Use a gentle formula if bowels move at least one time daily; a moderate-strength formula if bowels move at least once in a two-day period; and a strong formula for bowels that resist regular movement.
- In lieu of herbal detoxification, an individual may choose to take an enema one-day prior to the flush. It is important that your bowels are moving well.

- Optional: You can add 45 drops of Phosfood Liquid to your apple juice, two times a day (A.M. + P.M.). This will help loosen and soften any stones you might have.

NOTE: No solid foods should be consumed after noontime on the day of the flush (fresh fruit juices or distilled water are acceptable).

Directions

- Stop all fluid intake at 6:30 P.M., or thirty minutes before the flush is started.
- Begin the flush between 7:00 P.M. and 9:00 P.M., or as you wish.
- Mix or blend 8-ounces of olive oil with 6 to 8 ounces of pink grapefruit juice or the juice of two lemons.
- Consume at a rate that best suits you. You may wish to consume it all at one time, or you may consume 1/4 cup every 15 minutes, or you may drink it even more slowly. After the olive oil is consumed you should retire for the evening, lying on your right side.

Considerations

- If nausea and/or vomiting sensations are experienced, the olive oil/citrus juice mixture can be chased with small amounts of freshly-made apple juice. Resume consumption of the mixture as soon as possible. If the feeling of nausea continues, consume only as much of the mixture as you possibly can, then go right to bed, lying on your right side.
- Watch stools for stones. Stones are usually green, but may be yellow, red or black. Stones range from a pea-size to that of a quarter, or larger. Most liver or gallbladder stones are soft in nature, as they are lipid/bile stones.

- With degenerative problems, the liver and gallbladder flush should be supervised by a health care professional.

TOOL #2
DISTILLED WATER

Natural water from springs, wells, rivers, lakes, and the water that comes through your faucet is full of mineral elements that have been collected from contact with soil and rocks. Most water sources are full of impurities including chemicals from fallout, boats, raw sewage, and pesticides.

The minerals from these water sources are inorganic. There is a vast difference between the minerals in the human body and those in the earth. Earth minerals (which are inorganic) do not have the same electrical frequency as those found in the human body and within the botanical kingdom. Elemental (earth) minerals are basically inert. They are low in electromagnetic charges.

As rain (distilled water) falls from the sky and saturates the soil, it becomes electrified with the energies of the minerals and other properties of the soil. The water is then absorbed into plant root systems and drawn up into the plant. This energy, mixed with the energy of the sun, transmutes these inorganic minerals into tissue salts, which build and maintain the plant.

As plants develop from the seed through enzyme action, the constituents establish themselves in compounds. The minerals in plants are called "cell salts," because many have bonded together creating more of a synergistic response. They need each other and other compounds synergistically to be properly absorbed and utilized by the cells of the animal or human. Animals and especially humans need to live upon a higher-frequency food source than elemental minerals.

Inorganic minerals, if allowed through the bowel wall, act only as stimulants. Their electrical charge is low and they cannot pass through a cell membrane wall. An example of this is iodine. Inorganic iodine is used in hospitals for dyes and thyroid work. This type of iodine only stimulates the thyroid and can deposit and accumulate in the thyroid tissues, causing inflammation and additional thyroid problems. Just as a water pipe in your house becomes clogged from an accumulation of inorganic minerals and debris, our veins, arteries and tissues become clogged with inorganic minerals as well.

Distilled water is said to be the greatest solvent on earth. It is the only true water that can be taken into the body without damage to the tissues. It assists by dissolving nutrients so they can be assimilated and taken into every cell. It dissolves the wastes of cell life so the toxins can be removed. Distilled water is also great at dissolving inorganic mineral substances lodged in the tissues of the body so that such substances can be eliminated in the process of purifying the body. It does not leach out body minerals. There have been many blood tests conducted during distilled water fasts showing improved and more homeostatic electrolyte percentages. Distilled water does collect and remove minerals that have been rejected by the cells of the body and are therefore nothing more than debris, obstructing normal functioning of the system.

It is important to keep ourselves hydrated. We should receive the majority of our water from raw and ripe fruits and vegetables. In their raw state, these foods are composed of 60 to 95 percent water.

Always brew your herbal teas with distilled water. Being void, distilled water pulls the nutrients from the herbs into the water. Water that is full of inorganic minerals and other matter cannot leach all the compounds of the herb into it, which causes a much weaker tea.

If you cannot get distilled water, I recommend R/O (reverse osmosis) water. You can put an R/O filter under your sink, which makes it very convenient to use. Remember that water is one of nature's greatest catalysts. Drink plenty of fresh, pure, distilled or R/O water, but don't overdo it. Follow your natural instincts. Many people try to drown themselves with too much water. Remember, a raw food diet gives you plenty.

NOTE: Never drink with your meals. This dilutes your digestive enzymes and affects proper food digestion.

TOOL #3
CASTOR OIL PACKS

Castor oil, also known as Palma Christi (the Palm of Christ), has been used for healing for hundreds of years, and is a treatment that medical intuitive Edgar Cayce often prescribed for many different conditions. Preliminary studies on castor oil packs performed at the George Washington School of Medicine indicate that they improve immune system functioning, aid with dilation, and soften tissues and muscles.

Castor oil packs used on the abdomen are detoxifying to the system. They may also be used for pain syndromes, slipped discs, tumors, tinnitus, nausea, inflammation, hard or swollen organs (such as the spleen, liver, kidneys, lymph nodes, and bowels), and a variety of other problems. Applied topically, they may help loosen or dissolve cancerous masses. They are especially beneficial for lung problems, such as asthma.

Lung clients are difficult to detoxify as many of them use inhalers which block or hold the toxicity in the lung tissue itself instead of allowing this congestion to come forth or expectorate. The chambers of the lungs may be clear, but the tissues (interstitially) can be saturated. This can, and often does, affect the nervous system, causing spasms. It is imperative to detoxify the lungs if you want to completely eliminate problems like asthma.

Castor oil packs can assist greatly during the spasmodic time when the client needs air. One may also ingest 1 teaspoon of a tincture of Lobelia every ten minutes as an antispasmodic. This herbal remedy is used in place of an inhaler. Be aware that some clients are so locked into using inhalers that they may need to use them somewhat during this process. Push to eliminate, not suppress.

Castor oil packs are useful for female indications such as abdominal pain and distention, ovarian and uterine fibroids and cysts, endometriosis, and menstrual discomfort.

Castor oil packs are easy to use.

Items Needed

- Soft, flannel cloth (cotton or wool).
- Cut flannel to the appropriate size (example 10 inches to 12 inches for abdomen).
- Cold-pressed castor oil (available at most health food stores).
- Wax paper or plastic wrap.
- Heat source (a non-electric source is preferable such as a hot water bottle. However, you can use an electric blanket or heating pad, if necessary).

Directions

- Fold the cloth into a two-to-four-inch thickness.
- Saturate the cloth with the cold-pressed castor oil.
- Apply the cloth directly to the skin in the area that needs the treatment.
- Place a piece of wax paper or plastic wrap over the soaked flannel cloth.
- Apply heat over the wax paper or plastic wrap (if the temperature of the heat source is too hot, wrap in a towel).
- Maintain in place for at least an hour.
- Leave on overnight, if necessary.
- The recommended frequency for use of castor oil pack is three to seven times per week.
- The flannel pack does not need to be discarded after one application. It may be kept in a glass container in the refrigerator for future use.

During this treatment, be aware of the thoughts and feelings that may arise. It is common during a detoxification process to experience toxic thoughts and feelings from the past. Don't worry, these are being released along with the physical toxins.

TOOL #4
COLD SHEET TREATMENT

The cold sheet treatment is a powerful hydrotherapy procedure that was enhanced and brought to the public's attention by the late Dr. John Christopher, and popularized by Dr. Richard Schulze. The cold sheet treatment can be a vital tool in assisting the detoxification process. This is a very strong procedure that pushes and draws body toxins from the skin.

Because it is such a strong and oftentimes enervating procedure, I do not recommend it in highly debilitated conditions, such as advanced cancer. The value of this treatment at this level goes without saying; however, the risk of too much enervation to an individual who has very little energy to begin with is too risky.

NOTE: If you or your patient is very weak, I prefer to build the energy in these clients before I purge them with this cold sheet procedure. You *can* detoxify too fast. When you go on a 100 percent raw food diet and take high quality herbal formulas, this can be a very powerful process by itself.

The following is a basic cold sheet treatment that anyone can do at home with the assistance of a mate or friend.

Step 1

I suggest a raw food diet for a few days before you start this procedure. This will clean the putrefying animal matter from the bowels. You may wish to give yourself an enema the night you start your treatment. Dr. Richard Schulze recommends a garlic implant after this. This would have to be done with a rectal syringe.

Dr Schulze recommends "putting eight to ten large cloves of Garlic in a blender with 50 percent apple cider vinegar and 50 percent distilled water." I find this very strong on raw food eaters, but it certainly can be used by many toxic individuals. The healthier you are, the more sensitive you get toward pungent foods.

Step 2

Start drawing yourself an extremely hot bath—as hot as you can stand it without burning or hurting the skin. Place 1 ounce of Dry Mustard herb inside a small cotton sack or bag. In another clean cotton bag place one ounce of ground Ginger Root. If you want to "kick it up another notch," fill and add another cotton bag with Cayenne Pepper. I recommend you try the cold sheet treatment without the pepper first.

Place these cotton sacks of herbs into the water and allow them to filter throughout the hot water. You must place petroleum jelly (like Vaseline®) on all your sensitive body parts, including genitals and nipples. You will want to stay in the hot water at least 10 to 15 minutes. You are stimulating sweating by creating a fever through heat.

I suggest drinking a hot herbal tea made from Yarrow or Ginger Root to increase this heat-inducing process and to maintain hydration. As the heat begins to dilate or open the skin, coupled with the diaphoretic properties of the herbs, especially Yarrow, you will begin to sweat. This also stimulates the blood and lymphatic systems, increasing circulation and elimination through the skin.

Drink as much tea as possible. If you feel faint, have your assistant put a cool washcloth over your forehead or over the back of your neck. It is advisable to have tincture of lobelia on hand in case of body spasms. I personally suggest not letting it go that far.

Prior to starting this treatment, place an all-white, double-bed size cotton sheet in the freezer of your refrigerator or in a bucket of ice water. You will need this sheet as soon as you step out of the bath.

Step 3

Enter the tub and try to cover your whole body, except your head, with water. This is very stimulating and dilating, especially if the Cayenne Pepper is added. Stay in the water as long as you can possibly stand it. Push it somewhat. As you exit the water, have your assistant wrap the frozen cotton sheet from the freezer or ice water around you. Believe me you will not feel the cold. You're so hot you will enjoy the sensation. The mixture of the hot body and the cold sheet creates a further drawing action on the skin pulling out more toxins.

Step 4

You are now going directly to bed, wrapped in the cold sheet. This is a time to rest and sleep the night away. You will want to put some plastic or waterproof material on your bed so it won't get wet. Put a cotton sheet over that. Have your assistant place another cotton sheet over you as well as a cotton or wool blanket.

Wrap yourself like a cocoon. A "garlic paste" may be applied to the bottom of the feet for further stimulation, immune response, and anti-parasitic properties.

In the morning examine the sheet that was wrapped around you. You will see some of the toxicity that is stored within you. You will want to shower and clean your skin well. Dry skin brushing would be beneficial at this time. You should continue on a raw food diet eating mainly fresh fruits, juices, and distilled or R/O water. Make sure your bowels are moving well.

There are many natural therapies you can use to assist in the detoxification process. Be patient, the body loves to respond, but has a mind of its own. The single most important issue is what you eat. Have fun with your journey into vibrant health. It's your journey alone. You know your body better than anyone. Listen to it. Be intuitive and don't push yourself too far. Health will come if you're persistent. You will be amazed at how deeply and how quickly you can achieve good health. From there, vitality is just around the corner. Take it a day at a time until healthy living is your new lifestyle.

The natural force within each of us is the greatest healer of disease.
— Hippocrates

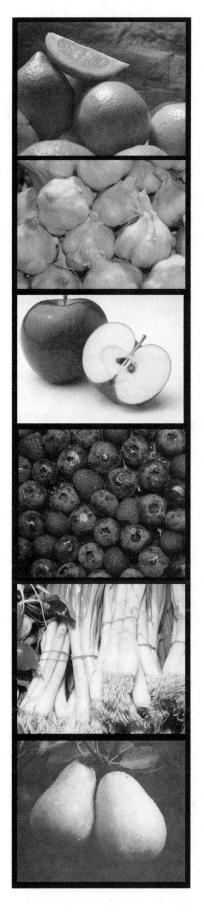

CHAPTER TEN

Health and Spirituality

We are much more than our physical bodies. We have different "bodies," many levels to ourselves, that few people understand. However, the unity and simplicity of life is seen when one appreciates the meaning of consciousness or awareness.

At your core, you are pure awareness, without thought or emotion. This is the "true you" that always abides no matter what your experience is in the outer world. You cannot hide from your true self—this awareness—which is always observing what your mind and emotions create. This "you" is the observer of the observed. Even though many people use drugs or alcohol in an attempt to hide from themselves, this is impossible. Your awareness is the one thing that you cannot kill or get rid of. It does not die. It is the part of you that can expand without limit.

Contrary to popular belief, one does *not* need to think to exist. You *become* awareness itself when you stop thinking, planning and desiring. Presently, however, you are chained to your thoughts, feelings and desires by the attention you give these energies. This wasn't always the case. Remember when you were a child? Time as we know it did not exist for you. You simply played until suddenly your mother called you in for dinner.

Consciousness or awareness is the life force that experiences and radiates in everything. True health is a result of wholeness, wherein the body, mind, and emotions are kept in harmony with this soul awareness and with God. The toxic conditions we experience are essentially self-created. Since we create them by our lifestyles, including our diets and our thoughts, we can turn them around. We can renew and revitalize body and mind.

The Physical Body

Although the physical body is necessary for you to experience and enjoy the journey in this physical world, who you are is not

Anatomy of Creation

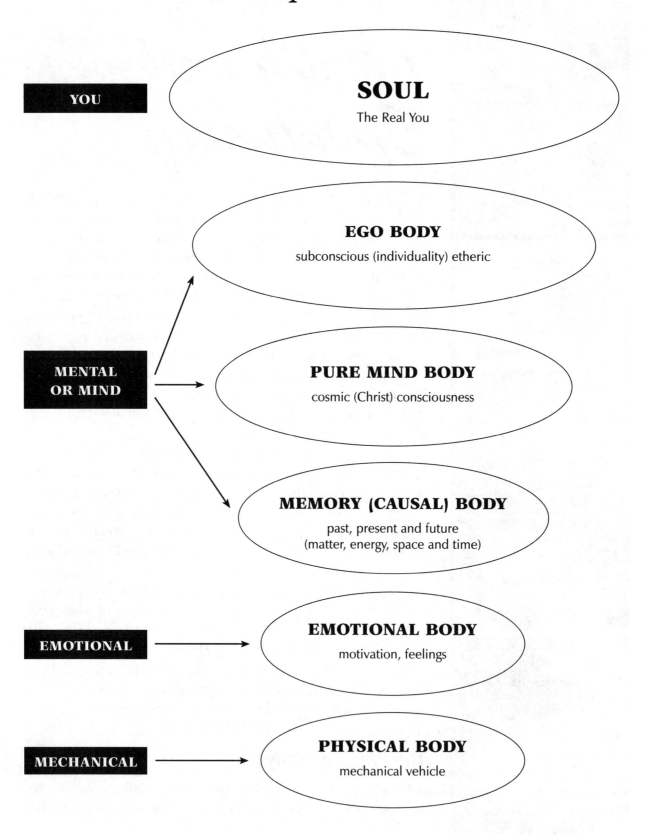

limited to your body. The physical body is a vehicle, like your car, that carries you around and takes you wherever you wish. It is a self-regulating machine. Its basic need is only survival. Its awareness is cellular. This body is your protection. It is very dense; made up of mainly water, cells, toxins and minerals. The nervous system and brain are its messenger/communication service, without which one cell would not know what and how to respond to external stimuli or to any other cell. For all its amazing abilities and strengths, however, the physical body has a very short life span when you compare it with eternity.

Now let's stop and think for a minute. If our physical body is only made up of matter, where do we get our awareness from? And where do thoughts and emotions come from? It becomes much easier to understand these questions if you have had an out-of-body experience. Many people today have come to know that they are not limited to the body, based on having a near-death experience for one reason or another. Many practice "out-of-body" travel on a daily basis. I spent years working in emergency medicine, and I was honored to have been close to those who had such experiences, as well as those who passed into the next adventure. I also spent many years experimenting as a traveler "out of body," learning and experiencing the many levels or heavens that exist. (Remember that Jesus said, "In my Father's house, there are many mansions.") We only *use* the physical body, however, giving it life with our consciousness . . . our awareness. When it is time for us to leave our bodies, we will simply withdraw our attention from them and move on.

Through an expanded awareness comes the God-realization that we are all one. Once you have experienced this level of awareness and understanding, you will find absolute love, and you will discover that you are God's expression. The healthier you are in all your bodies, the greater and happier your life is, and the more love and God you will experience as an active part of every moment of your life.

Our awareness, our consciousness, comes from our union with God, our inseparability from the One. I think most people who believe in God will agree that God is omnipotent, omniscient, and omnipresent. This means that God is infinite. There is no place in which God is not. God has no boundaries, and thus cannot be a limited being in any way. Therefore, God cannot have form or substance, as we know it, or God would be limited. God cannot be limited to a body, or to emotions, or even to thoughts, as all of these are limiting and based upon conditioning and experiences, not truth.

The Emotional Body

The existence of your emotional body, called by many the "astral body," has been well documented by many travelers. This astral or emotional body is a distinct body from your physical body, but looks very much like it. This is the body of feelings and emotions. This body drives thought and gives motivation to the physical body. Without desire, your ability to create in the physical world would not exist.

Your emotions or your emotional body are not you; they are only used by you to further experience creation. However, the health of your physical body can be greatly affected by your emotional body. Anger, hate and rage will destroy your liver. Jealousy, anxiety and negative emotions will affect kidneys and adrenals. Fear, gossip and ego will shut down the heart. You can see how important it is to gain control of this body that you use to express emotion.

The Mental Body

This consideration of the emotional body leads us to the mind, or mental body. God created this mental body to actually form creation. This body or level is where thought manifests. This is where true duality exists. This is where male/female, up/down, black/white, small/large, etc., is created. To experience anything you must first think about it. You must have an image or create an image out of what you already know or have experienced in the past. Then, with this data you create your future. Thought is totally limited to past experiences or conditioned responses. The best example I can give you is that the mind is like a computer; it can only function as it has been programmed.

Your emotional body and physical body only respond to thought. Thought is the creator and the emotions are the driving force or manifester, so to speak, of these images. All thoughts and emotions are like your physical body—they go through birth, life and death. The mind is just another "body" that you use to experience and "create experience" with.

The Ego

The ego is the "body of separation." It says, "I am separate and different from the rest." This is the first body that you as soul must use to begin your journey into creation. This is the first separation that you have from God, and the last you must drop to be free again from creation. When you go beyond your ego, which is a limited and limiting "little" self, you can then experience the truth of the *real* you, the unlimited you, again. You will find that you have "always been there" or "here" all along. What hides your true self is your bodies and their functions. All this is necessary in the scheme of things so that God and you can experience endlessly. God being omnipotent, omniscient and omnipresent needs this separation in order to experience.

All Together

The reason I have concluded with this chapter in *The Detox Miracle Sourcebook* is to help you connect to your true self and to give you some

understanding of why we use the terminology "body, emotions, mind and soul." All of your bodies must become healthy if you wish to have longevity and true vitality. Each of the "bodies" you use affects all the others. They fit and interact so closely that you and most scientists are fooled into thinking they are one body. They are not. They exist to give color, aroma, form and texture to creation. Each of these bodies you use is created from the atoms of its respective dimension of heaven. Each of these bodies creates an electrical reaction in the physical body, which is their mechanism of response. One must look beyond the veil of the physical, emotional and mental worlds (bodies) if one wishes to experience and know truth.

The Bottom Line

Break free of the chains that bind you to this world. "Become like little children," free to enjoy the present moment. The present moment is eternal, and pure awareness (which is what you are) only lives in the present moment. Remember, it is thought that is based in time. Past and future are only concepts of the mind, as memory and desire weave your future.

Use the natural laws of God to create a vibrant state of health. Look to the power and expansion of the infinite, not the limitation and confinement of the finite. Realize that you are God's expression and that what you experience, God experiences. Why else would God create?

See every moment as a spiritual experience. Feel and see the divine in all things. The future is unimportant; it doesn't matter what changes the earth will make to cleanse itself. What is important is you and your survival. One day it will be time for you to leave your body, so spend time alone with yourself and get to know who you truly are.

Years ago, a very old master told me "that alone exists." Everything is born alone, lives separate from everything else, and passes (dies)

When It's Your Time to Move On

In extreme cases, and in some advanced cancer cases, failure to get well may indicate that it is a person's turn to leave this planet. Our physical, emotional, and mental bodies are only our vehicles while we're on a journey in this creation. They can't and won't last forever.

One should never fear God or the journey that one takes. "You" can never die—only your bodies die. You, as soul, live forever. This physical world is one of the hardest of God's worlds to function and live in. If it is your time, it can be experienced as a blessing and a great joy to move on to the next world. When I have journeyed out of my physical body I have found nothing but joy, awareness, ecstasy and pure love.

Always fill yourself full of love and God. If everyone did this at all times, this world would be a much different place. Live in every moment for the moment and forget the past. Live in the "Now" and the future never comes. Learn to enjoy every moment, regardless of what medical condition you have or how chronic and hopeless it seems. Make your life what you want it to be. If you want your body to be healthy, then so be it – make it healthy. It is up to you, and you alone, to make it healthy. You choose.

---

alone. Get to know who you are in this alone state. Most people cannot live without a TV or radio. They fear this aloneness. At the physical and emotional levels, souls have become codependent because of this fear and this longing for God. Use prayer, meditation or contemplation; not to petition God, but to listen to and experience God. God is omnipresent; there is no place God is not. If you are constantly talking, thinking or desiring, how will you experience or be able to recognize this eternal presence of God?

Open the doors of exploration and allow yourself to grow and expand. This will remove the stress out of all your bodies and will allow healing to take place. True healing is integrated; treatment is specific, separate. Healing is expansive; treatment is constricted or limited. See everything and everyone as God's expression and give divine love to all. When you experience the beauty of total love and God, then true vitality will be yours. Keep your heart opened at all times.

Learn to step back from thought and emotions and observe. "Be" your true self. This is what true prayer and meditation is all about—separating yourself from your bodies so you can have true communion with God. Clean and strengthen yourself in every way.

May the blessings be!

Appendixes

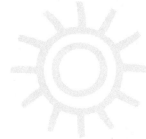

Basal Temperature Study for Thyroid Function

The basal temperature test is quite accurate when the temperature is tested in the axilla (armpit) each morning for a period of four days. If the temperature is consistently low, then there is a hypo- or under-functioning of the thyroid gland in spite of what any other laboratory analyses indicate.

How to Take Your Own Basal Temperatures

At night, before retiring, shake down a thermometer and lay it beside your bed, on your night table, or chair. BE SURE IT IS SHAKEN DOWN.

Next morning, on awakening, don't get up or move around. Place the thermometer under your armpit pressing your arm against your bare body. Relax and LEAVE THE THERMOMETER THERE FOR TEN MINUTES BY THE CLOCK. Take it out, read it, and write down your results.

This record of your early morning basal temperature is a great aid in determining hypothyroidism. The most important issues of hypothyroidism are metabolism and calcium utilization.

Normal reading is between 97.8° to 98.2°

When your basal temperature is below 97.8, this shows varying degrees of hypothyroidism. When your temperature is above 98.2, this may indicate hyperthyroidism.

Basal temperatures between 97.0 and 97.8 are much easier to cure than temperatures in the 96s or 95s. These temperatures are chronically low, requiring much more aggressive detoxification and herbal therapy. Raw thyroid glandulars

and organic iodine may be needed with low basal temperatures. Most underactive thyroid conditions are congestive in nature, coming from mucus, acids, and foreign proteins that literally clog the tissues of the thyroid. Hyperthyroidism, especially, is also a congested condition. Detoxification is the main key to eliminating these thyroid conditions.

Today, many people have genetically weak thyroids. The answer is always the same: detoxify and strengthen these tissues and the body. Give it time. It could take you a year or more to change these chronic levels.

Date_____ Temperature _____

Date_____ Temperature _____

Date_____ Temperature _____

Date_____ Temperature _____

For menstruating females, also do temperatures on the second and third days of your period.

Date_____ Temperature _____

Date_____ Temperature _____

Date_____ Temperature _____

Date_____ Temperature _____

ADDITIONAL READINGS

Date_____ Temperature _____

Date_____ Temperature _____

Date_____ Temperature _____

Date_____ Temperature _____

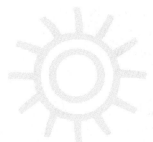

The Family of the Natural Sciences

God offers a wide range of natural healing modalities, some of which have not yet been discovered. The beauty of natural therapies is how they make you feel. Some can be painful at first, as they dig deep into your tissues to release toxins. Others are soft and gentle, enhancing your energy flow and elevating your consciousness. Natural therapies affect not only the physical body, but also your mental and emotional bodies.

Curing the cause is much different from simply treating the symptom. Nature's healing therapies can basically be divided into two categories: treatment systems or detoxification systems. Some treatment systems, like massage, actually promote detoxification. Both treatment and detoxification systems are needed in today's world because of the depth of our tissue weakness and toxicity. However, I personally prefer the detoxification modalities because the results will be permanent. Vitality and the restoration of weakened or degenerative tissue to vibrancy should be your goals. Have fun using nature's therapies as you clean and reshape your physical and spiritual bodies.

ACUPUNCTURE & ACUPRESSURE

Acupuncture and Acupressure are systems that use either needles or pressure to move stagnant energy, especially through areas of weakness or congestion.

The body naturally focuses its energy where irritation or congestion exists. This can cause pain and discomfort. By moving stagnant energy, we increase circulation (blood and lymph flow) through these areas as well. This increases

the immune, nutritional, antioxidant and electrolyte responses, and helps to remove the inflammation and toxicity in these stagnant areas.

Acupuncture and Acupressure have helped millions of people to enjoy a higher quality of life. Detoxification mixed with either of these two arts makes an unbeatable pair.

BIOELECTROMAGNETICS

Emerging out of the current spiritual renaissance is the science of Bioelectromagnetics or Energy Medicine. This science is closely related to quantum physics and encompasses electricity and electromagnetic energies and their effects on your cells, tissues, organs and glands. The study of electrical currents will always lead you to God and God's creations because we are simply talking about energy.

All matter is condensed energy. Without energy nothing exists, including consciousness. Consciousness is pure energy in its most static yet active form. This is another paradox. That is to say, God, the creator, is pure energy without limit, while its creation is this pure energy condensed and confined into forms. As pure energy moves out into creation, it creates electrical currents. The energy that these electrical currents give off is called electromagnetic energy.

Every single atom gives off electromagnetic energy from its movement. When it "clusters" with other atoms, thus creating compounds and structures, these energies combine, giving off a rainbow of hues. The true beauty of creation is its unlimited rainbow of colors emanating from its expressions. This energy flows from your consciousness, or soul, down through the mental worlds of your mind, into the emotional worlds (the astral level), and into this physical world. This electromagnetic energy gives off many different colors depending upon the frequencies or types of structure that soul takes on—be it animal, human, flower, or mineral. One's awareness and lifestyle affects and defines the way this energy is experienced, since all life in creation is defined energy. The state or level of consciousness or individual expression (whether human, flower, animal, etc.) determines the level and color of energy involved. When there are obstructions to this energy flow, there is dis-ease.

Creation is energy in movement. One must consume and live with energies that are in harmony with one's level of awareness. These energies are contained in foods, thoughts, emotions, external influences, etc. One's level of awareness can change as one grows spiritually. Any discord in these energies and dis-ease begins to settle in. When an element or form of energy is internal to your physical body, it is called an "endogenous field of energy." When it's external to your physical body, it is called an "exogenous field of energy."

There are, of course, endless bands and frequencies of energies. There are simple, low-frequency bands of DC currents; mid-level currents of radio, microwave, radar and infrared currents; and high-level X-rays and gamma rays.

In Chapter 4, dealing with alkaline (cationic) and acid (anionic), we discussed ionization. Simply put, ionization is the breaking down of structures into other structures. Ionization is vital to life, as life is ever changing. This includes everything from our awareness, to our structure, to the world we live in. Creation is in a constant state of flux or change; ever growing and expanding.

Electro-pollution is a word given to the toxic effects of electrical currents and their electromagnetic energies that damage tissue. X-rays and gamma rays are strong ionizers that can destroy biological tissue. Ultraviolet and some of the visible light bands are somewhat ionizing. Even though your radio, microwave, radar and infrared bands are considered non-ionizing, it is my opinion that these bands can affect brain and nerve tissue in a destructive way, especially with prolonged exposure. These "non-ionizing" bands are divided into two categories: the thermal or heat-producing type, and the non-thermal or non-heat producing type. The thermal or heat-producing currents are, of course, the more destructive of the two, to biological tissue.

We use non-thermal, non-ionizing energy bands in the medical field as a way of observing and diagnosing tissue weakness. The EKG and the EEG instruments are two examples of this.

Humans are coming closer and closer to an understanding of the life force and how it works. You must always seek truth and remain open minded, allowing yourself to grow and explore the endless worlds of God within and without.

NOTE — When you are acidic, this condition changes the electromagnetic energy of the body, which causes increased thermal energy and ionization. This damages the tissues throughout your body.

AROMATHERAPY— USING ESSENTIAL OILS

I've always said that if you breathe it, you eat it. Aromatherapy is based upon the power of the essential oils from plants to enhance, heal, stimulate and revitalize tissue. These oils can be administered either by breathing, ingesting or by absorbing them into the skin. The FDA does not recommend ingesting essential oils, but millions of people worldwide do ingest them, especially when you consider that if you put them on your skin, you ingest them.

Essential oils are extremely potent. They are said to be one of the strongest compounds of a plant. They have deep-reaching effects upon tissue and, when used wisely, the results are tremendously valuable. Try using essential oils as an adjunct to getting healthy. Different oils, like different herbs, will have specific effects on various organs or processes of the body. Consult the Bibliography for additional resources in this field.

Essential Oils and Their Benefits

BASIL OIL — Anti-spasmodic. Use for migraines, mental clarity, nervous system support (due to anxieties, etc.), thyroid support (due to depression), adrenal gland support.

BERGAMOT OIL — For skin conditions, congestive conditions of the respiratory tract, sinuses, lymphatic system, inflammation, urinary tract system, parasites, endocrine glands. This oil is said to affect the hypothalamus of the brain.

BIRCH OIL — For arthritis, pain, detoxifying, lymphatic congestion and skin conditions.

CHAMOMILE OIL — A smooth muscle relaxant; use for allergies, bladder, anxieties, and digestion.

CINNAMON OIL — For digestion, parasites (cinnamon has anti-bacterial properties), cardiac issues, increasing circulation, support for the kidneys, toothaches.

CLARY SAGE OIL — This hormone balancer provides glandular support to the lymphatic system. Also use to support the nervous system, as a tonic, and for headaches.

CLOVE OIL — For respiratory congestion, rheumatism, allergies (clove provides lymphatic support), stress, toothaches, and tuberculosis. Strong anti-parasitic.

CORIANDER OIL — For the pancreas (helps digestion), for cardiac support, for circulation, and for pain.

CYPRESS OIL — Lymphatic. Use for arthritis, hot flashes, pancreatic support, and circulation.

EUCALYPTUS OIL — For any lung congestion or condition, diabetes, headaches, sinus congestion, lymph congestion, or kidney inflammation.

FENNEL OIL — Respiratory conditions, especially asthma; constipation; digestion; liver support.

FRANKINCENSE OIL — Immune system support, lymphatic system support, for enhancing red blood cells, for tumors, inflammation, and urinary tract support.

GALBAUNUM OIL — Said to enhance spirituality. An anti-parasitic due to its anti-bacterial properties. Use for lymphatic support, for stress, and for circulation.

GERANIUM OIL — For the pancreas (particularly in cases of diabetes, or for digestion), for liver/gallbladder; a detoxifier; urinary system support; for skin; for the lymphatic system.

GINGER OIL — A digestant. Use for the pancreas, for circulation, arthritis, cramps, tooth-aches, as a laxative, and for hangovers.

GRAPEFRUIT OIL — Lymphatic support. Use for skin, liver, glandular support. An anti-parasitic.

HYSSOP OIL — Anti-parasitic (anti-bacterial, viral, anti-fungal). An expectorant for the respiratory system. Also supports the lymphatic, urinary and digestive systems. This is a strong oil. Use with caution!

JASMINE OIL — For inflammation (itis's), for adrenal support (in cases of anxiety), liver conditions, respiratory issues, nervous system support, and for muscles.

JUNIPER OIL — Urinary tract, especially kidneys; for diabetes (because this oil supports the pancreas); for endocrine glands; "ego" issues; adrenal glands; gout; lymphatic system support. (Strong oil—use with caution!)

LAVENDER OIL — Great for kidneys and bladder, headaches, earaches, and as a relaxant for the nervous system. This oil slowly feeds the nerves. Use as a liver and gallbladder detoxifier.

Also works well for all skin conditions, including burns.

LEMON OIL — For the pancreas (in cases of diabetes, and for digestion, among other uses). Provides lymphatic support; helps the urinary tract (kidneys and bladder); heals scar tissues; helpful in cases of bleeding.

LEMON GRASS OIL — For conditions involving connective tissue; also used as a digestant (helps the pancreas, liver, etc.); great for the lymphatic system, urinary tract, respiratory system, nervous system; and help for the muscles.

MARJORAM OIL — Supports the adrenal glands (for anxiety, nervous system issues, stress). Great for the thyroid (for depression, headaches, or in cases of bruising). An anti-fungal. Supports the respiratory tract and the muscles. Helps in removal of ticks. Relieves inflammation.

MOUNTAIN SAVORY OIL — Anti-microbial, including bacterial, fungal, and viral properties. Said to be somewhat of a tonic.

MYRRH OIL — Helps inflammation, respiration congestion, and hyperthyroidism. Use for its anti-fungal, anti-bacterial, and sedative properties.

NUTMEG OIL — A digestant (helps the pancreas), and a laxative. Helps relieve vomiting. Support for the heart.

ORANGE OIL — Helps the spleen, adrenal glands (anxiety, stress, shock, etc.), heart, liver and blood. Also used for anti-fungal properties and as a laxative.

OREGANO OIL — An anti-parasitic (due to its anti-fungal, bacterial, viral components); good for immune system support.

PATCHOULY OIL — Helps the nervous system, the lymphatic system, and the glandular system especially the adrenals in conditions of anxiety and stress, and the thyroid in cases of depression, headaches, fever. Good for the skin; use as a diuretic; use for mental clarity, and for allergies where lymphatic support is needed.

PEPPERMINT OIL — Ideal for respiratory congestion; for use as an anti-spasmodic; a great digestant (helps the pancreas, liver, etc.). Use for skin conditions; for inflammation; for urinary tract support; and mental clarity. Helps relieve morning sickness, shock, nausea, dizziness and fatigue. Use for gallstones, and for toothache.

ROSE OIL — Supports the endocrine glands; good for issues involving the emotions; useful for lung congestion, TB, impotency, ulcers, skin conditions, depression (due to its thyroid supporting properties.) Contains hemostatic properties (useful in stopping both internal and external bleeding).

ROSEMARY OIL — Use for inflammation, liver conditions, skin conditions, endocrine glandular support, pancreas support (for diabetes), epilepsy, gout, cardiovascular conditions (heart and circulation), mental confusion and conditions, respiratory and sinus congestion, stress. Also useful in childbirth.

ROSEWOOD OIL — Anti-parasitic properties (bacterial, fungal, etc.). Useful to the skin, liver, nervous system, adrenals (to ease stress, anxiety, worry).

SAGE OIL — Another great detoxifier, which aids in lung, lymphatic, sinus, liver, skin, and circulatory congestion and obstructions. Sage is also a good diuretic and aids digestion. Useful for inducing sweating, which encourages skin elimination. Also said to be anti-bacterial, anti-fungal, and anti-viral.

SANDALWOOD OIL — Believed to have positive effects on the DNA and RNA. Useful as a digestant by supporting the pancreas and liver. Good for the bladder, thyroid support (especially with depression, calcium issues), skin conditions, stress, and vomiting. Contains anti-fungal properties.

SPEARMINT OIL — Similar to Peppermint, Spearmint supports the liver, urinary tract, and lymphatic system. Good for respiratory conditions, and as a relaxant to the nervous system. Contains anti-fungal properties.

SPRUCE OIL — Use for inflammation (various itis's), urinary tract support, anti-fungal properties, and hypothyroidism in conditions relative to the bones, skin, sweating.

TARRAGON OIL — A digestant (which supports the pancreas, liver). Use for inflammation (various itis's), as a laxative, and as an anti-parasitic. Valuable in cases of anorexia, and for support of the nervous system.

TEA TREE OIL (MELALENCA) — A great oil for support of the immune and lymphatic systems. Useful for shingles, as an anti-fungal, or anti-viral. Good for burns, shock, and eliminating warts.

THYME OIL — Anti-parasitic for all types of parasites: fungal, bacterial, viral, or worms. Use in cases of lung congestion, stress, anxiety and tension (when adrenal glands need support), skin disorders, thyroid-related problems (like depression or skin conditions), lymphatic/congestive conditions, tumors, nausea, gout, cardiac problems, circulation, and throat congestion.

WILD TANSY OIL — Provides support for the immune system, lymphatic system, adrenal glands (especially emotional issues).

WHITE LOTUS OIL — Useful as tonic. Uplifting, said to bring euphoria. Spiritual properties. Immune system enhancing. Anti-cancer properties.

In my sister's herb shop we have a sauna in which we use essential oils. This offers a great benefit to the body, especially in assisting elimination through the skin, lungs, kidneys and even the bowels. Using oils in this way can literally pull the toxins from your skin. I recommend using Eucalyptus, Birch, Sage or Lavender oil (see their properties and uses above).

Essential oils can also be burned in oil lamps or special essential-oil burners. They can be used in the bag of your vacuum cleaner, which allows the essential oils to neutralize many toxic particles that escape from your sweeper. This method also spreads the oil throughout the area that you are vacuuming.

Let the aroma of the oils invigorate you and enhance your life in endless ways.

CHIROPRACTIC AND KINESIOLOGY

Chiropractic is a therapeutic system based upon the interaction of the spine and the nervous system. A trained chiropractor can use a variety of methods to manipulate the spinal column, making adjustments to specific vertebrae, and thereby opening energy pathways and releasing energy blockages to various parts of the body.

Kinesiology is a feedback system of diagnosis that involves testing the strength of particular muscles. The theory is that the muscles are weakened when any part of the body is threatened or weak. By "asking" the body specific questions, and then testing the strength of the muscles, the trained kinesiologist can pinpoint which system is in need of attention, and determine how best to strengthen it.

When used together, chiropractic and kinesiology have saved many suffering souls. The combination is important, as spinal vertebrae oftentimes move out of place from toxic, weak muscles. Muscles hold the skeletal system in place. The body naturally stores toxins in muscles first, in order to save the vital organs. Dairy products, refined sugars, and starches all cause lymphatic congestion, which eventually lead to muscle and tissue weakness. This can leave some muscles weaker than others. The stronger muscles then begin to pull bones out of place.

Of course, we can also displace our skeletal system through injuries. When your skeletal system is out of place, you can suffer severe pain and discomfort. I have seen convulsions occur from spinal misalignments. If you add detoxification to chiropractic you could truly heal the muscular/skeletal system.

COLON THERAPY

See section 6. 9 on "Healthy Bowel Management," in Chapter 6.

COLOR THERAPY

Without color, life would not exist. The energies that make up the millions of colors create, support and sustain the untold dimensions that exist beyond our sight. The power of colors to enhance tissue is phenomenal. I developed a color therapy machine years ago and had great fun experimenting with colors and their effects upon the body. The sun is the ultimate provider of color therapy. Full-spectrum rays surround and flow through us, healing and embracing our cells. All life looks to the "light," one way or another.

As we have discussed, energy creates, supports, sustains and changes the universe. This energy manifests from consciousness, and extends out into creation. As it moves, it gives off colors (light) and music (sounds). These energies, their colors and music, are both dramatic and subtle. Duality dictates that colors or energies move between hot (acid) and cold (alkaline), or light (acid) and dark (alkaline).

Everything that exists has a main energy or energies that support or sustain it, whether this is a human, animal, plant, planet or universe. An example of this would be a planet, like Mother Earth, where gemstones play a major role in channeling these energies that sustain her. There are also lay lines or electromagnetic energy lines that crisscross the earth. Where they meet is said to be a place of very high energy—a place where more spiritually-minded people tend to congregate and live. Sedona, Arizona is an example of such a place.

Another example of energy centers is found within the bodies of animals and humans. There are basically seven main energy centers within each of us. These main energy centers correspond to different aspects or different bodies that we use. Most people cannot see these types of energies. Those who can we call psychic; however, anyone can train himself or herself to see these. Your ability to achieve anything depends upon the degree of your desire for it. These centers of energy are "seen" as follows:

First Center

Dimension: physical (survival)
Location: base of spine (fourth sacral)
Color: red

Second Center

Dimension: physical (social, healing)
Location: 2 inches below the naval
Color: orange

Third Center

Dimension: emotional (astral, survival)
Location: solar plexus
Color: yellow/pink

Fourth Center

Dimension: emotional (healing, astral)
Location: center of chest (heart) first, second, third thoracic
Color: green

Fifth Center

Dimension: mind (survival)
Location: throat first through third cervical
Color: sky blue

Sixth Center

Dimension: mind (healing)
Location: third eye, pineal gland
Color: indigo

Seventh Center

Dimension: ego (crown)
Location: crown of head, pituitary gland
Color: purple/violet

Eighth Center

Dimension: soul itself
Color: yellow/white

The above main centers are expressed through your physical body and are called chakras (pronounced: sha'-crahhz).

When one has physical, emotional or mental disease, these centers will begin to shut down respectively. These energies emanate from and through your physical body. Your aura, or the electromagnetic energies emanating from you, can be read and analyzed to determine weaknesses or strengths.

In the aura, white or yellow are the colors of Consciousness. The main creative and sustaining energies of Earth, divided into five basic influences or elements, are seen in the aura in the following colors:

Air element = violet

Fire element = red

Ether element = blue

Water element = orange

Ground element = green

The following are examples of colors and the specific tissues that they affect.

Color Energies and Tissues They Affect

RED	ORANGE	YELLOW	GREEN	BLUE	VIOLET
Prostate gland	Repiratory stimulant	Overall vitality	Pituitary	Liver	Individuality
Colon	Stomach	Spinal cord	Cell activation	Pelvic area	Sexual organs (females)
Muscles	Solar plexus	Growth	Cleansing	Cerebral (brain tissue)	Lymphatic system
Red blood cells	Parathyroid/ Thyroid	Immune system	Healing	Blood	Stomach
Excretory		Heart	Muscle builder	Small intestines	Menstruation
Organs (general)		Lymphatic activator	Tissue builder	Oxygenation of tissues	Digestive system (pancreas)
Liver (energizer)		Cerebral stimulant		Adrenal glands	Pregnancy
Adrenal glands		Bones			Lower extremities
		Nervous system			Parathyroid
		Brain			Spleen Immune
					Blood

By using different colors, or electromagnetic frequencies, therapeutically, we can affect tissue in a positive way. It will respond or function in a greater capacity. Today, we need all the healing power we can get because of the severe hypo-conditions that most of us have in our cells, tissues, organs and glands as a result of our diets and genetics.

If you truly wish to become healthy physically, emotionally, mentally and spiritually, then you must reconnect with God. In this world we are interconnected with nature, without which life could not exist as we know it. Nature offers us an abundance of tools to assist us in the quality of our expression while we live on this planet. Take control. Use all of these tools available to you, to obtain your goals.

Below is a list of foods and their specific colors. Eat more of the foods that fit the area of your body you wish to work on.

In creation there is always duality or opposites. Without opposites there would be only one thing – God! Opposites give us matter, energy, time and space. There are always two processes or forces at work in nature: anabolism and catabolism. Anabolism is the process of growth, repair, building, enhancement and dynamic energy. The essential opposite to this is catabolism, which is the destructive or the "tearing down" side. This side affects change; balances out over-growth; maintains the shape and size of forms; and destroys the weak, to make room for the strong. Catabolism creates the wastes from metabolism, while anabolism moves these out through the lymphatic system. Life in these material worlds requires duality for its existence. We need to understand both sides of life's essential processes.

Colors add beauty and elevate the consciousness in one's life. Surround yourself in color,

Foods and Their Specific Colors

RED	ORANGE	YELLOW	GREEN	BLUE	VIOLET
cherry	carrot	carrot	romaine	blueberry	pear
watermelon	orange	cataloupe	lettuce	blackberry	asparagus
strawberry	tangerine	corn	spinach	plum	celery
tomato	pumpkin	lemon	celery	grape	parsnip
yams	rutabaga	grapefruit	parsley	all blue-skinned fruits and vegetables	potato
watercress	melon, some	mango			
radish	yam	onion			
cabbage	garlic	papaya			
onion	nuts, some	persimmon			
garlic	all orange-skinned fruits and vegetables	squash			
peppers		orange			
ginger		tangerine			
eggplant		turnip			
beet		peach			
parsley					

harmonious music, and the energy of God. You will then know what true vitality really is.

FLOWER ESSENCES

Nature is so beautiful and powerful. One of its most beautiful creations is the flower. I love to go to flower gardens and embrace the loving energies of these most precious gifts. Without these "balancing" gifts of royal beauty, life on this planet would truly be dull.

Have you noticed the multitude of aromas found in the flower kingdom? Each aroma affects your physical, emotional, mental and soul bodies in an uplifting and healing way. Each flower is designed, like each herb, to enhance and expand the consciousness of your cells, your emotions, and your thoughts. Edward Bach was the modern day founder of a healing modality that uses flowers to enhance each facet of your life. Kathren Woodlyn Bateman has created a fantastic selection of flower essences (Flower Essences of Running Fox Farms™ in Worthington, Massachusetts). I have used these formulas to balance the emotional trauma that people have experienced in hospital Emergency Rooms, in the Oklahoma City bombing, and in mental health clinics. I have seen these subtle energies work with amazingly positive results.

In physics you learn that all things exist as energy fluctuating between two poles. These energies can be disruptive to the emotional and mental parts of ourselves, or they can be harmonious, yielding balance and upliftment. This is important to know because what you think and what you feel affects your health as much as what you eat.

Many flower essence formulas have been created. They are similar to herbal formulas in that the quality of the formula depends upon the quality of the flower and the ability of the practitioner who made it. Of all the formulas created, "Emergency Relief" by Bach Flower Essences is the most famous. Many companies have copied this one to some extent. "Emergency Relief" can be used in almost any traumatic experience, especially when shock is involved. "Moonshine Yarrow" (by Fox Mountain) is another great formula for shock, anxiety attacks, and especially for depression.

Most men typically do not think or dream in color. One night I was meditating on this subject and had a vivid out-of-body experience in a heaven that was crystalline, where all the trees and plants flashed an endless variety of colors and hues. This experience changed the way I looked at, and dreamt about, life. Flower therapy is very much a part of color therapy and aromatherapy. We just need more of it.

Flowers can also be eaten for their nutritional and energetic values. Nasturtiums, daisies, and dandelion flowers are just some of these edible beauties. Enjoy the "Power of the Flower." You will be surprised as God's rainbow foods enhance, calm, expand and revitalize you. Add plenty of flowers and flower essences into your life and it will help you open your heart and bring forth the music of God.

GEM STONE THERAPY

Gem stone therapy has been practiced for thousands of years. Many gemstones, such as rubies, were ground to a fine powder and given internally for sickness and disease. The vibration and stimulation of the inorganic compounds had a beneficial effect upon biological tissue. Other gemstones were worn as jewelry around the neck, on the arms, or over the infected area. Crystal therapy is widely used today to absorb disease and to focus healing energy to weakened areas of the body. This is done by placing a crystal over an infected area of the body and allowing the energy of the crystal to do its magic. Gem stones carry a great deal of power that humans generally do not yet understand. It is an exciting science to explore. To learn more about this subject I recommend *Love is in the Earth* by

Melody (Earth-Love Publishing House, 1995); *Crystal Enlightenment* by Katrina Raphaell (Aurora Press, 1985); and *Cunningham's Encyclopedia of Crystal, Gem and Metal Magic* by Scott Cunningham, (Llewellyn Publications, 1987).

HERBOLOGY

Whether you call it phytotherapy, botanical medicine, or herbology, God's non-hybrid plants hold the power of nature to heal, clean and revitalize tissue. Science likes to extract, separate, and mega-dose constituents found in plants to treat bodily symptoms. Plants were never intended for this. The whole plant is powerful enough, when you learn how to use botanicals correctly. I have used herbal formulas for over twenty-five years, well before they were fashionable. That's because my desire has always been to help others heal themselves, not treat their symptoms. I have used gallons of herbs on just one patient. Herbs can be very powerful and strong. There are only a few that I do not recommend due to their toxic nature. However, these are exotic herbs, not used in mainstream herbology.

Besides all the different properties of herbs, including anti-inflammatory, astringents, bitters, stimulants, antispasmodics, etc., they have nutritional value. Herbs are full of vitamins, minerals, tissue salts, flavins, amino acids and sugars, not to mention their electromagnetic energies. Study and experiment with botanicals. Without them, humans will not survive the many damaging effects they have created on this planet.

HOMEOPATHY

Homeopathy is a treatment-based system using remedies from animal parts, plants, and minerals. The strengths and dosages of these formulas are very mild. Homeopathy is founded on a philosophy of "like treats like." If you had a case of poison ivy, for example, the treatment would be to consume poison ivy internally in minute amounts. This modality works more with building immune response than actual tissue healing. Homeopathic remedies are based upon the essence of their constituents rather than potency, realizing that electromagnetic energy, not the potency, is the key. Homeopathy is not a deep detoxification and regenerating modality, but gets tremendous results in relieving symptoms.

HYDROTHERAPY (KNEIPP THERAPY, AND OTHER FORMS)

Hydrotherapy, or water therapy, has been used for thousands of years. In modern times we credit the late Sebastian Kneipp, a Catholic priest in Bavaria, with refining and publicizing hydrotherapy to the world.

Water can be used to stimulate both blood and lymphatic circulation. Water also is a transporter of elements and toxins to and from the cells via the GI tract or skin. We know the benefit of heat, as it dilates and increases circulation. The body uses this method internally by diaphoresis (sweating and fevers) and histamine response, to increase blood and lymph flow. As we increase circulation to the tissues, we increase nutrition, oxygen, immune and electrolyte (alkalization) response. These are all important to tissue circulation. On the opposite side, cold is a constrictor and can block energy circulation to tissue. Adding both of these aspects of stimulation together, water therapy using a hot application followed by a cold application can get tremendous response in disease situations.

One could consider the consumption of water as a form of hydrotherapy. The average person does not consume nearly enough of it as a beverage or from cooked foods. Water is vital to the oxidation and ionization processes of the body. Water is essential to proper movement of the bowels, proper hydration and proper renal (kidney/bladder) function.

Mineral baths, another type of hydrotherapy, are great in stimulating tissue. However, over-exposure to heavy mineral water can clog the skin making it dry and crusty. It can make the hair coarse, and can slow down hair growth by blocking the hair follicles. Over-stimulation is not the key to vitality; dynamic energy is.

IRIDOLOGY

Iridology is the science and study of the iris of the eye and its relationship to the tissues in your body. It is a highly detailed road map to all your cells, their functions, and their failures.

My old friend, the late Dr. Bernard Jensen, calls Iridology the "Master Science." The iris of the eye shows us in detail the genetics, tissue weaknesses or strengths, and the congestive (or toxic) conditions of the body. It shows us obstructions, prolapsed conditions and chemical accumulations. Not only does it show us our tissue weaknesses and congestion, the eyes show us the degree of these issues. You do not truly know your physical body until you've had a neuro-optic analysis.

For the practitioner, iridology not only gives a picture of all the cells, but of the structures and systems of the body. This is essential to seeing reflex conditions, particularly the importance of the GI tract (gut tissue) and its relationship to all the cells in the body. In the allopathic medical world, many times a symptom has no known origin, and no known reflex or contributing areas of toxicity or weakness. Iridology gives us this information.

Iridology is soft tissue analysis. It provides a type of information that is so badly needed in today's diagnostic and analytical world. Your eyes are not only the windows of your soul, but also the windows into your physical body. Iridology is an easy science for all to learn and highly recommended. It will help you unveil the mystery of your genetics and the weaknesses within your body.

MASSAGE (ALL TYPES) AND REFLEXOLOGY

The golden hands of a good massage therapist are truly magical as they reshape and restore the tissues of your body. There are so many forms of massage—from light stimulation and relaxing massage, to deep tissue and sacral cranial massage. Massage work is an important field in many ways, from assisting the body to heal itself from injuries, to promoting lymphatic drainage and detoxification. The body stores toxins in muscles, sparing as long as possible the major organs. But, in storing these toxins the body becomes stiff and sore, driving us to exercise to stimulate lymph flow. When we have the inability to exercise or we become too toxic, massage is extremely vital.

Foot Reflexology, noted under Healthy Habits in Chapter 9, is a special form of massage and a most valuable tool. I have saved several people from cardiac arrest with my thumb and their left foot. The power of stimulating the nervous system and lymphatic system by pressure to points on the hands and feet cannot be underestimated. Toxicity and acid crystals build up under the nerve endings in the hands and feet. This toxicity can cause a multitude of symptoms from high blood pressure to gallbladder weakness.

NAPRAPATHY AND POLARITY THERAPY

Naprapathy encompasses Dr. Randolph Stone's Polarity Therapy combined with manipulation. "Polarity" refers to a type of energy balancing. Naprapathy is a combination of chiropractics (structural realigning), kinesiology, polarity therapy and nutrition. Its goal is to remove energy obstructions by manipulating the muscles and skeletal system. My old friend Dr. Rudy Splavic was taught by Dr. Stone, and was a naprapath for fifty years. When he was age eighty-six I saw him work miracles on people, completely changing their posture and structure after thirty years of deformity. He could tell you the year of your injury or when the disease began; and could feel a hair under seven sheets of paper. However, some modern naprapaths swing toward conventional medicine.

Always seek to know your practitioner. It is important to keep your body, and its injuries, in balance. It is equally important to learn why they get out of balance.

NATUROPATHY

The name "naturopathy" was coined by Benedict Lust, but can be traced back to Hippocrates and before. The science of naturopathy is based upon a 100 percent natural, organic system of detoxification and nutrition, which leads to tissue regeneration. This establishes true vitality and longevity.

A naturopath will use only nature and nature's remedies to accomplish this. Naturopathy is one of the greatest sciences on the planet. It encompasses chemistry, physics, hydrotherapy, vibrational therapy, color therapy, phytotherapy (herbs), massage therapy, thermotherapy, electrotherapy, bioelectromagnetic therapy, emotional therapy, reflexology, raw food therapy, fasting therapy, proper food-combining, and the like. Detoxification and alkalization is at the core of naturopathy.

Naturopathy is based upon the premise that disease is a natural process. When your body is acidic and full of such things as mucus, pus, parasites, chemicals, preservatives, antibiotics, pesticides, and carbon by-products, you can't expect to be healthy.

Naturopathy is truly holistic—it covers body, emotions, mind and soul. Since we are highly integrated beings, disease can and is experienced on many levels, mostly unknown to the patient. Naturopathy opens all of these doors and allows the individual to reconnect to life spiritually. I consider naturopathy to be the highest healing modality on this planet. Naturopathy is concerned with causes not effects.

Naturopathic Medicine

Naturopathic medicine is a system or modality similar to naturopathy. However, it is more treatment-minded than naturopathy. Naturopathic physicians use orthomolecular science (vitamins and minerals), tissue salts, glandular supplements and other separated constituents to treat symptoms in an effort to correct the cause of the problem. Naturopathic medicine uses some detoxification principles and stresses diets consisting mainly of fresh fruit, vegetables and grains.

VIBRATIONAL THERAPIES (ENERGY HEALING)

This is a large category and could include Therapeutic Touch™, magnet therapy, crystal therapy (gem stone therapy), radionics, qi gong (Chinese energy healing), spiritual healing, psychic healing, feng shui, biofeedback, and the like. Even though each of the above modalities is uniquely different, they all use "spirit" in one way or another to affect tissues, increasing circulation and elimination. These therapies change the vibrational energy of cells, thus improving cellular respiration and vitality. Our magnetic energies become out of balance by toxicity, acidic foods, negative thoughts, negative derogatory emotions and unhappiness.

Vibrational therapies move stagnant or restricted energies and allow this energy to circulate through cells and tissues better. This reduces or eliminates pain, increases overall circulation, and stimulates elimination. This increases tissue function and repair.

We are only at the first stage of new discoveries in this area. Vibrational therapies will dominate the future, in one form or another.

ALLOPATHIC MEDICINE

Allopathic medicine, in my opinion, should be limited to emergency medicine, diagnostic procedures and surgeries. Emergency medicine has saved hundreds of thousands of lives, and many surgeries are essential to life, as humans have literally destroyed their health and the tissues in their bodies.

I spent many years involved in emergency medicine, and especially enjoyed anything that dealt with the heart. However, there are a lot of hospital Emergency Rooms that could learn about nature and how to apply more non-invasive techniques that could save even more lives and increase the quality of life for many, many more. There are far too many tissue-damaging techniques used in Emergency Rooms today, including chest compressions, which crack or break the sternum.

Many surgeries are unnecessary, however. They often cause the patient great distress, and in many cases, a dismal future. Open-heart surgery, for example, can mostly be avoided. Nature can clean out the vascular system in short order if the patient is willing to change his/her lifestyle. In fact, eighty to ninety percent of all dis-eases can be cured without chemical medicine or invasive procedures. Naturopaths are non-invasive and seek a cure for the cause of the problem.

Conclusion

Avoid a future of immobility, despair, sexual impotence and massive diseases. Don't wait until it is too late. Become healthy now. Health, vitality and fun can give you a new life of freedom, tranquility, vibrancy and longevity.

It is beyond the scope of this book to cover all the natural therapies that currently exist, for which I send out my deepest apologies. I have tried to give you an overview of the most well-known and important ones. Each one deserves much more recognition. Each natural modality is a science within itself, offering you a magnificent journey to restoration of the self. Read, study, and learn all you can about each one and enjoy what they have to offer you. The Bibliography at the end of this book will suggest many fine books that will help you in your study.

It is time that each individual takes responsibility for his/her own health issues. Empower yourself. You will enjoy how your body feels as it becomes more vital and dynamic. If you seek anything, seek to be vibrantly healthy: physically, emotionally, mentally and spiritually.

NOTE: The sciences described above are the greatest tools that nature offers you in restoring your vitality. However, they are only as good as the practitioner who uses them. A director of the American Medical Association was once interviewed on the news program 60 Minutes and asked about how people could protect themselves from poor M.D.s. His response was to quote the old adage, "Let the buyer beware [*Caveat Emptor*]."

I challenge you to make your life a masterpiece. I challenge you to join the ranks of those people who live what they teach, who walk their talk. Live with passion!

— Anthony Robbins

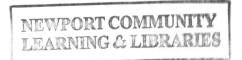

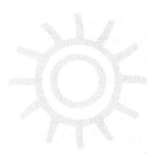

APPENDIX C

Resource Guide

BOOK AND VIDEO SOURCES

Sunfood
(888) RAW-FOOD (Toll Free)
(888) 729-3663
www.rawfood.com

Carries a great line of natural products and hard-to-find books by the old raw-food masters.

Nutri-Books
A Division of Royal Publications
P.O. Box 5793
Denver, CO 80217
(303) 788-8383
www.nutribooks.com

Carries an extensive line of natural health books.

Health Research
P.O. Box 850
Pomeroy, WA 99347
(888) 844-2386 (Toll Free)
www.healthresearchbooks.com

Carries an extensive line of old and hard-to-find health and spiritual books.

CHILDREN'S PRODUCTS

The Natural Baby
www.naturalbabyhome.com

FLOWER ESSENCES

Flower Essences of Fox Mountain
P.O. Box 383
Chester, MA 01011
(413) 667-8820
www.foxmountain.net

Supplies high quality flower essences, including two of our favorites—"Emergency Relief" and "Moonshine Yarrow."

FOODS, SEEDS, NUTS, GRAINS, SPROUTING SEEDS—ORGANIC

Bautista Family Organic Date Ranch
P.O. Box 726
Mecca, CA 92254
(760) 396-2337
www.7hotdates.com
kissme@7hotdates.com

Earth Source Tropicals
19901 SW 264th Street
Homestead, FL 33031
(305) 792-8882
www.earthsource.us
Service@earthsource.us

Carries wonderful organic tropical fruits sourced from local, small farms.

Pavich Family Farms
P.O. Box 10420
Terra Bella, CA 93279
(925) 202-8020
www.terrabellafamilyfarm.com

Carries some of the finest organic raisins, dates, and other natural foods available.

Eco Organics
P.O. Box 202191
Austin, TX 78720
(877) 596-2727 (Toll Free)
http://www.ecoorganics.com/

Distributes organic fruits, vegetables, etc.

Johnny Selected Seeds
P.O. Box 299
Waterville, Maine 04903
(877) 564-6697 (Toll Free)
Fax (US Only): (800) 738-6314
www.johnnyseeds.com

Organically grown seeds, herbs and other products

Oskri
528 E. Tyranena Park Road,
Lake Mills, WI 53551
(920) 648 8300
www.oskri.com

Dried fruits, nuts and wonderful sesame bars

Sun Organic Farm
(888) 269-9888 (Toll Free)
www.sunorganic.com

Distributes organic raw seeds, nuts, grains, sprouting seeds, low-temperature dried fruits, virgin oils, herbs and spices.

The Raw Food World
406 Bryant Circle, Unit E
Ojai, CA 93023
(866) 729-3438
http://www.therawfoodworld.com/

Resource for raw foods, snacks and supplies

Sunfood
(888) RAW-FOOD (Toll Free)
(888) 729-3663
www.rawfood.com

Raw organic olives, coconut butter, stone-crushed olive oil, dried fruits and nuts, etc.

Mountain Valley Growers
38325 Pepperweed Road
Squaw Valley, CA 93675
(559) 338-2775
(559) 338-0075 (Fax)
www.mountainvalleygrowers.com

Live plants and seeds

Territorial Seed Company
P.O. Box 158
Cottage Grove, OR 97424
(800) 626-0866
(888) 657-3131 (Fax)
http://www.territorialseed.com/

Seeds

Horizon Herbs, LLC
The Cech Family
P.O. Box 69
Williams, OR 97544-0069
(541) 846-6704
(541) 846-6233 (Fax)
http://www.horizonherbs.com/

Richter's
357 Highway 47
Goodwood, Ontario
Canada L0C 1A0
(905) 640-6677
(905) 640-6641 (Fax)
www.richters.com

Seeds

Southern Exposure Seed Exchange
P.O. Box 460
Mineral, VA 23117
(540) 894-9480
(540) 894-9481 (Fax)
http://www.southernexposure.com/

Herb and vegetable heirloom and non-GMO seeds

GREEN PRODUCTS
God's Herbs
525 Tamiami Trail
Port Charlotte, FL 33953
(941) 766-8068
(941) 766-8067 (Fax)
www.naturesbotanicalpharmacy.com

God's Garden Superfood Blend (*25 of the most power-packed herbs on earth!*)

Sunfood
(888) RAW-FOOD (Toll Free)
(888) 729-3663
www.rawfood.com

Sun is Shining

Green Foods Corporation
2220 Camino Del Sol
Oxnard, CA 93030
(805) 983-7470
www.greenfoods.com

Green Magma

Christopher's Original Formulas
155 W. 2050 N.
Spanish Fork, Utah 84660
(800) 453-1406
(801) 794-6801 (Fax)
http://www.drchristopher.com/

Vitalerbs *and* Jurassic Green

HERBS AND HERB PRODUCTS
God's Herbs
525 Tamiami Trail
Port Charlotte, FL 33953
(941) 766-8068
(941) 766-8067 (Fax)
www.naturesbotanicalpharmacy.com

Offers the highest quality and most powerful herbal formulas known for detoxification and cellular regeneration.

Dr. Morse's Clinic
525 Tamiami Trail
Port Charlotte, FL 33953
(941) 255-1979
(941) 255-8067 (Fax)
www.naturesbotanicalpharmacy.com

High quality herbal pharmacy and Dr. Robert Morse's Clinic

Mountain Rose Herbs
P.O. Box 50220
Eugene, OR 97405
(800) 879-3337
Fax (510) 217-4012
International Calls (541) 741-7307
http://mountainroseherbs.com/

Herbal formulas, bulk herbs, supplies, etc.

Uncle Harrys Natural Products
6975 176th Ave. NE Ste. 360
Redmond WA, 98052
(425) 558-4251
http://www.uncleharrys.com/store/
Natural beauty supply products including dental care

A. C. Grace Company
1100 Quitman Road
P.O. Box 570
Big Sandy, Texas 75755
(903) 636-4368
(903) 636-4051 (Fax orders)
www.acgrace.com
Offers the finest vitamin E on the market.

V.E. Irons, Inc.
705 McGee Street
Kansas City, MO 64106
(816) 221-3719
(800) 544-8147
(816) 221-1272 (Fax)
http://veirons.com/
Quality detoxification products, especially for colon regeneration

Kroeger Herb Products Co., Inc.
805 Walnut Street
Boulder, CO 80302
(303) 433-0261
(800) 516-0690
(303) 443-0108 (Fax)
www.kroegerherb.com
Carries high quality herbal products, and an especially good parasite program.

Dr. Hulda Clark
www.naturalhealthsupply.com
www.huldaclark.com
These web sites carry Dr. Hulda Clark's detoxifying herbs, etc.

Dr. Christopher's Original Formulas
Provo, Utah 84601
(800) 453-1406
www.drchristopher.com
High quality herbal formulas

Blessed Herbs
109 Barre Plains Road
Oakham, MA 01068
(800) 489-4372
(508) 882-3755 (Fax)
www.blessedherbs.com
High quality herbal products

**Sage Mountain Herbal Products—
Rosemary Gladstar**
P.O. Box 420
East Barre, Vermont 05649
(802) 479-9825
(802) 476-3722 (Fax)
http://sagemountain.com/
Herbal information, classes and information

Frontier Natural Brands
3021 78th Street
P.O. Box 299
Norway, WI 52318
(800) 669-3275
www.frontiercoop.com/
Large, natural-products co-op

Starwest Botanicals, Inc.
161 Main Ave.
Sacramento, CA 95838
(800) 800-4372
(916) 853-9673 (Fax)
www.starwest-botanicals.com/
Products for natural healing

American Botanical Pharmacy
P.O. Box 9699
Marina Del Rey, CA 90292
www.DrRichardSchulze.com
Dr. Richard Schulze's herbal formulas

The Heritage Store, Inc.
984 Laskin Road
Virginia Beach, VA 23458
(800) 862-2923
www.caycecures.com/
Dr. Edgar Cayce's formulas

Health Concerns / K'an Herb Company
380 Encinal St., Suite 100
Santa Cruz, CA 95060
(800) 543-5233
(831) 438-9457 (Fax)
www.kanherb.com
High quality, traditional Chinese herbal formulas

Motherlove Herbal Company
P.O. Box 101
LaPorte, CO 80535
(970) 493-2892
(970) 224-4844 (Fax)
Email: mother@motherlove.com
www.motherlove.com

Specializes in products for pregnancy, childbirth and breastfeeding, both wholesale and retail.

Pacific Botanicals
4840 Fish Hatchery Road
Grant's Pass, OR 97527
(541) 479-7777
(541) 479-7780 (Fax)
www.pacificbotanicals.com

This is the most experienced and diversified medicinal herb farm in North America; sells wholesale only.

HERBS — CHINESE BULK

East Earth Herbs
P.O. Box 2808
Eugene, OR 97402
Reishi extracts and products; bulk herbs

East Earth Trade Winds
144 Hartnell Avenue
Redding, CA 96002
(530) 223-4849
(800) 258-6878
(530) 223-0944 (Fax)
www.eastearthtrade.com/
Bulk Chinese herbs, patent medicinals, books and supplies

Mayway Corporation
1338 Mandela Parkway
Oakland, CA 94607
(510) 208-3113
www.mayway.com
Chinese herbs and ready-made products

Shen Nong
(877) 252-5436
(866) 526-8359 (Fax)
www.chineseherbsdirect.com/
Bulk Chinese herbs

Spring Wind
2325 4th Street #6
Berkeley, CA 94710
(510) 849-1820
https://springwind.com/
Wholesale to practitioners

HERBAL ASSOCIATIONS

The Herb Growing & Marketing Network
also: **The Herbal Green Pages**
c/o Maureen Rogers
P.O. Box 245
Silver Spring, PA 17575
(717) 393-3295
(717) 393-9261 (Fax)
Email: herbworld@aol.com
www.herbworld.com

Herbworld is the largest trade association for the herb industry, with around 2000 members. They are an information service, covering over 3000 books and over 200 periodicals. They monitor twelve internet mailing lists and search the Web looking for resources and research on the herb industry to pass on to their members. They produce the Herbal Green Pages—*a must for anyone in the field!*

American Botanical Council (ABC)
P.O. Box 144345
Austin, TX 78714
(512) 926-4900
(800) 373-7105
www.herbalgram.org/

For over a decade, the ABC has educated the public, governmental agencies, research institutions and industries on solid scientific research on the safe and effective use of medicinal plants. They publish the well-respected peer-reviewed journal, Herbalgram.

American Herbal Products Association (AHPA)
8484 Georgia Avenue
Suite 370
Silver Springs, MD 20910
(301) 588-1171
(301) 588-1174 (Fax)
www.ahpa.org

AHPA exists to promote the responsible commerce of herbal products. Offers a searchable database and more.

The American Herbalists' Guild (AHG)
14 Waverly Court
Asheville, NC 28805
(617) 520-4372
www.americanherbalistsguild.com

The AHG is a non-profit, educational organization that represents the goals and voices of herbalists. It is the only peer-review organization for professional herbalists who specialize in the medicinal use of plants.

Herb Research Foundation (HRF)
4140 15th Street
Boulder, CO 80304
(303) 449-2265
www.herbs.org/

HRF is the world's first and foremost source of accurate, science-based information of the health benefits and safety of herbs, and expertise in sustainable botanical resource development.

American Herbal Pharmacopoeia (AHP)
P.O. Box 66809
Scotts Valley, CA 95067
(831) 461-6318
(831) 438-2196(Fax)
www.herbal-ahp.org/

The AHP's goal is to produce 300 qualitative monographs on therapeutic botanicals to serve as a primary reference in the U.S.

American Association of Oriental Medicine
9650 Rockville Pike
Bethesda, MD 20814
(866) 455-7999
(301) 634-7099 (Fax)
www.aaaomonline.org/

This group has a website with a searchable database that allows you to find a certified acupuncturist or expert in Chinese herbal medicine, as well as research, news, and political updates.

Herb Med
www.herbmed.org/

HerbMed is an interactive, electronic herbal database that provides hyperlinked access to the scientific data underlying the use of herbs for health. It is an evidence-based information resource for professionals, researchers, and the general public.

NATURAL SOAPS AND BODY CARE PRODUCTS

Thursday Plantation
548 Broadhollow Road
Melville, NY 11747
(800) 645-9500
www.thursdayplantation.com

Tea tree oil

Tom's of Maine
P.O. Box 710
Kennebunk, ME 04043
(800) 367-8667
www.tomsofmaine.com/

Natural toothpaste and body care products

Lotus Light Enterprises, Inc.
Box 1008, Lotus Drive
Silver Lake, WI 53170
(262) 889-8501
(800) 548-3824
http://www.lotuslight.com/

Health and wellness products including natural body brushes, loofahs, cosmetics, bath and skin care, pet care, etc.

Weleda Inc.
1 Bridge St
Suite 42
Irvington, NY 10533
(800) 241-1030
(914) 268-8574 (Fax)
www.weleda.com

Personal care products

Ginesis Natural Products
2143 Arlington Blvd., Suite 2
Florence, AL 35630
www.ginesis.com

Natural personal care products, including Kleen Kill, "Not Nice to Lice" laundry soap, for bug problems

OILS — ORGANIC

Omega Nutrition
1924 Franklin Street
Vancouver, BC Z5L IR2
(604) 253-4677
(800) 661-FLAX (3529)
(604) 253-4228 (Fax)
http://www.omeganutrition.com/

Organic oil products

PREMIUM SUPPLEMENTS AND GLANDULARS

Progressive Research Labs
9396 Richmond, Suite 514
Houston, TX 77963
(800) 877-0966
www.prlab.com/home.htm

Premium supplements and glandulars (for sale to practitioners only)

Standard Process
1200 West Royal Lee Drive
P.O. Box 904
Palmyra, WI 53156-0904
(800) 848-5061
www.standardprocess.com

Premium supplements and glandulars (for sale to practitioners only)

RAW FOOD RESOURCES

Listing of healthy foods and restaurants by area
www.happycow.net

Sunfood
(888) RAW-FOOD (Toll Free)
(888) 729-3663 (Toll Free)
www.rawfood.com

Raw food resources including organic raw olives, the best stone-pressed extra virgin olive oil, organic raw food bars, etc.

Creative Health Institute
112 West Union City Road
Union City, MI 49094
(517) 278-6260
www.creativehealthinstitute.com/

Health educators in Michigan

Gold Mine Natural Food
7805 Arjons Drive
San Diego, CA 92126-4368
(800) 475-3663
www.goldminenaturalfoods.com

Supplies all-natural and organically-grown foods, and more.

Herbal Answers, Inc.
P.O. Box 1110
Saratoga Springs, N.Y. 12866
(518) 581-1968
(518) 583-1825 (Fax)
www.herbalanswers.com

Fine quality raw, organic aloe

Jaffee Brothers Natural Foods
28560 Lilac Road
Valley Center, CA 92082
(877) 975-2333
(760) 749-1282 (Fax)
http://organicfruitsandnuts.com/

Organically grown fruits, nuts, nut butters, salad oils and foods

Rawganique.com
Box 81
Denman Island BC V0R1T0
(877) 729-4367

Food and clothing for a fragile planet

The Grain & Salt Society
4 Celtic Dr.
Arden, NC 28704
(800) 867-7258
(828) 654-0529 (Fax)
http://www.celticseasalt.com/

The finest quality sea salt, and more

Bobarosa's
22151 U.S. Highway 19 North
Clearwater, FL 33765
(727) 791-9339
(727) 791-6019 (Fax)
(800) 796-9339
www.bobarosa.com
Garden-fresh pickled garlic

Flora, Inc.
P.O. Box 73
Lynden, WA 98264
(800) 446-2110
(888) 354-8138 (Fax)
http://www.florahealth.com/home_usa.cfm
Organic, genuinely cold-pressed oils

Healthforce Nutritionals
1532 Encinitas Blvd.
Encinitas, CA 92024
(800) 357-2717 (Orders only)
(760) 479-0944 (Fax)
http://healthforce.com/
Carry an excellent selection of enzyme-active, whole-food-based vitamins, minerals, spirulina, etc.

Wakunaga of America Co., Ltd.
23501 Madero
Mission Viejo, CA 92691-2764
(800) 421-2998
http://www.kyolic.com/
Natural garlic products (Kyolic)

Maine Coast Sea Vegetables
3 George's Pond Road
Franklin, ME 04634
(207) 565-2907
(207) 565-2144 (Fax)
www.seaveg.com
Offers the finest organic kelp, dulse and sea vegetable products; natural minerals; iodine for thyroid; and great salt substitute.

Sun Organic Farm
(888) 269-9888 (Toll Free)
www.sunorganic.com
Distributes organic foods, nuts, grains, sprouting seeds, low-temperature dried fruits, virgin oils, herbs and spices.

The Spice Hunter
P.O. Box 8110
San Luis Obispo, CA 93403-8110
(800) 444-3061
(805) 544-3824 (Fax)
www.spicehunter.com
Carries organic herbs and spices. They do not purchase products grown from genetically altered seeds, and their products are not irradiated.

Urban Organic
240 Sixth Street
Brooklyn, NY 11215
(718) 499-4321
http://urbanorganic.com/
Home delivery service of organic produce. If you refer someone who registers with them, they will send you a free box! (N.Y.C. residents only)

World Organics
5242 Bolsa Ave
Huntington Beach, CA 92649
(714) 893-0017
Liquid chlorophyll, regular or with spearmint

Oskri Organics
1240 West Elmwood Avenue
Ixonia, WI 53036
(800) 628-1110
(800) 615-0765 (Fax)
www.oskri.com
Raw sesame tahini, date syrup, sesame spread, dates, etc.

Paws for Health
4588 Ashton Road
Sarasota, FL 34233
(941) 924-7297
(941) 924-7230 (Fax)
www.pawsforhealth.net
Raw and all natural pet food

Barleans
4936 Lake Terrell Road
Ferndale, WA 98248
(360) 384-0485
(800) 445-3529
http://www.barleans.com/
Provides flaxseed oil and borage oil that is processed at temperatures not exceeding 96°.

Bio International
215 East Orangethorpe Ave. #284
Fullerton, CA 92832
(800) 246-4685
(888) 808-8276 (Fax)
http://www.organicfoodbar.com/
Delicious organic raw food bars

Rejuvenative Foods
P.O. Box 8464
Santa Cruz, CA 95061
(800) 805-7957
(831) 457-0158 (Fax)
http://www.rejuvenative.com/
Provides raw nut and seed butters, and raw cultured vegetables.

Sunorganics
411 S. Las Posas Road
San Marcos, CA 92078
(888) 269-9888 (Toll Free)
(760) 510-9996 (Fax)
http://www.sunorganic.com/
Carries an extensive line of dried fruits, dehydrated vegetables, dates, maple sugar and syrup, date sugar, oils, raw butters and tahini, carob, bee pollen, herb teas and spices

Date People
P.O. Box 808
Niland, CA 92257
(760) 359-3211
http://datepeople.net/
Carries over 50 varieties of organic dates that are raw, fresh and non-hydrated.

RAW FOOD RESOURCE CENTERS

We invite all Resource Centers to contact us so that we can add them to our next revision or new edition.

Creative Health Institute (CHI)
918 Union City Road
Union City, MI 49094
(517) 278-6260
http://www.creativehealthinstitute.com/
Health educators in Michigan

True North Health
1551 Pacific Ave
Santa Rosa, CA 95404
(707) 586-5555
(707) 303-4377 (Fax)
http://www.healthpromoting.com/
Fasting center and healing center

Mothers for Natural Law
P.O. Box 1177
Fairfield, IA 52556
(515) 472-2809
(515) 472-2011 (Fax)
http://www.safe-food.org/-campaign/about.html

Provides information on bio-technology, and is working to get genetically-engineered products labeled.

Native Seeds/Search
3061 N. Campbell Avenue
Tucson, AZ 85719
(520) 622-5561
http://www.nativeseeds.org/

Dedicated to preserving ancient desert crops and heirloom farming practices. They offer both heirloom and wild seeds for gardens.

Price-Pottenger Nutrition Foundation
7890 Broadway
Lemon Grove, CA 91945
(619) 462-7600
(619) 574-1314 (Fax)
http://ppnf.org/

Collects and disseminates information on a variety of health-related topics. Offers books, reprints, videos and audio tapes.

Food & Water, Inc.
389 Vermont, Route 215
Walden, VT 05873
(800) EAT SAFE
(802) 563-3300
(802) 563-3310 (Fax)

A national non-profit dedicated to educating the public about various threats to the nutritional integrity of the food and water supply.

Rhio's Raw Energy Hotline
(212) 343-1152
http://rhiosrawenergy.com/hotline/main.html

Provides information about health-related issues, and raw food and living foods events.

SPROUTING AND SUPPLIES

Sprout House, Inc.
P.O. Box 180
Summertown, TN 38483
(800) 695-2241
www.sproutman.com/

The source for Steve Meyerowitz's sprouting supplies. Offers a wide variety of seeds, sprouting baskets, bags, mini-greenhouses, etc., and how-to books on sprouting.

The Sproutpeople
170 Mendell Street
San Francisco, CA 94124
(608) 735-4735
(877) 777-6887 (Toll Free)
(608) 735-4736 (Fax)
http://sproutpeople.org/

Carries a wide selection of organic seeds and sprouting supplies.

SCHOOLS (HERBAL)

We invite all Herbal Schools to write, email or call us with their information to be added to the next edition.

International School of Detoxification
(Dr. Robert Morse)
525 Tamiami Trail
Port Charlotte, FL 33953
(941) 255-1979
(941) 255-8067 (Fax)
http://www.drmorsesherbalhealthclub.com/

The Australasian College of Herbal Studies
5940 SW Hood Ave.
Portland, OR 97239
(800) 48STUDY / (800) 487-8839
https://www.achs.edu

Sage Mountain Herbal School
(Rosemary Gladstar)
P.O. Box 420
E. Barre, VT 05649
(802) 476-3722
www.sagemountain.com

East/West School of Herbalism
(Michael Tierra, L.Ac., O.M.D.)
P.O. Box 712
Santa Cruz, CA 95061
(800) 717-5010 (Toll Free)
(408) 336-4548 (Fax)
www.planetherbs.com

Natural Healing Institute
(800) 559-HEAL / (800) 559-4325
www.naturalhealinginst.com

The School of Natural Healing
(Dr. John Christopher's Teachings)
P.O. Box 412
Springville, UT 84663
(800) 372-
www.schoolofnaturalhealing.com

Blazing Star Herbal School
P.O. Box 6
Shelburne Falls, MA 01370
(413) 625-6875
(413) 625-6972 (Fax)
http://blazingstarherbalschool.typepad.com/

Dominion Herbal College
#271-5489 Bynre Road
Burnaby, B.C.
Canada V5J 3J1
(604) 433-1926
(604) 433-1925 (Fax)
http://dominionherbalcollege.com/

The California School of Herbal Studies*
P.O. Box 39
Forestville, CA 95436
(707) 887-7457
http://cshs.com/
*Started by Rosemary Gladstar in 1982 and now run by James Green.

Rose Kalajian Herbalist
26403 Chianina Drive
Wesley Chapel, FL 33544
(813) 991-5177
http://www.imherbalist.com/

SCHOOLS (NATUROPATHIC)

Academy of Oriental Medicine
2700 W. Anderson Lane
Suite 204
Austin, TX 78757
(512) 454-1188
www.aoma.edu

Bastyr College
14500 Juanita Dr. NE
Kenmore, WA 98028-4966
(425) 602-3000
(425) 602-3090 (Fax)
http://bastyr.edu

Boucher Institute of Naturopathic Medicine
4375 St. Catherine Street
Vancouver, British Columbia V5V 4M4
(604) 602-3330
http://binm.org

The Canadian College of Naturopathic Medicine*
60 Berl Avenue
Toronto, Ontario M8Y 3C7
Canada
http://www.ccnm.edu/
*Formerly The Ontario College of Naturopathic Medicine

Southwest College of Naturopathic Medicine & Health Sciences
2140 E. Broadway Road
Tempe, AZ 85282
(480) 858-9100
www.scnm.edu

University of Bridgeport College of Naturopathic Medicine
126 Park Avenue
Bridgeport, CT 06601-2449
(203) 576-4108
www.bridgeport.edu/naturopathy

Westbrook University
120 Llano Street
Aztec, NM 87410
(800) 447-6496
www.westbrooku.edu

Everglades University
(4 Florida branches)
(888) 854-8308
http://www.evergladesuniversity.edu/

TEAS — ORGANIC HERBAL

San Francisco Herb and Natural Food Co.
250 14th Street
San Francisco, CA 94103
(800) 227-4530
http://sfherb.com/
Wholesale herbs, spices and tea

Jason Winters International
P.O. Box 94075
Las Vegas, NV 89193
(702) 739-8277
(702) 739-0461 Fax
http://www.sirjasonwinters.com/
Jason Winter's Tea

God's Herbs
525 Tamiami Trail
Port Charlotte, FL 33953
(941) 766-8068
(941) 766-8067 (Fax)
http://www.drmorsesherbalhealthclub.com/
Heal-All *tea (anti-cancer and more)*

Pronatura, Inc.
2474 E. Oakton Street,
Arlington Heights, IL 60005
(800) 555-7580
(847) 718-0988 (Fax)
www.pronaturainc.com/
Kombucha tea, capsules and extracts

WATER SYSTEMS

Berkey Water Filtration (Fluoride filtering)
Berkey Filters
2648 Santa Fe Drive, Unit #18
Pueblo, CO 81006
(800) 350-4170
http://www.berkeyfilters.com/

Clean Water Revival, Inc.
85 Hazel Street
Glen Cove, NY 11542
(516) 674-2441
(800) 444-3563
Ceramic water filtration systems

En Garde Health Products
7702 Balboa Boulevard #10
Van Nuys, CA 91406
(818) 901-8505
www.oxymoxy.com
Dynam02

Global Water Tech.
c/o **Amvi Science Products**
P.O. Box 1101
Tacoma, WA 98401
(206) 922-9113
Pres-2-Pure *and* Pump-N-Pure—*reported to be far superior to R/O and less expensive.*

Multi-Pure Corp.
(800) 689-4199
http://www.multipure.com/
Large manufacturer of home water filters

Nutrition Coalition
P.O. Box 3001
Fargo, ND 58108
(218) 236-9783
(800) 447-4793
www.willardswater.com
For genuine Willard Water

Waterwise
Leesburg, FL
(352) 787-5008
(800) 874-9028
(352) 787-8123 (Fax)
www.waterwise.com
Large manufacturer of home water distillers

WATER THERAPY

Axel Kraft Int. USA Inc.
Fort Lauderdale, FL 33301
(800) 667-7864
www.axelkraft.com

Offers hydrotherapy products, soaps, aromatherapy, personal care, herbs, supplements and more.

Kneipp Corporation of America
105-107 Stonehurst Court
Northvale, NJ 07647
(800) 937-4372 (Info. Line)
http://kneippus.com/

The original hydrotherapy methods and related products

Weleda Inc.
1 Bridge St., Suite 42
Irvington, NY 10533
(800) 241-1030
(800) 280-4899 (Fax)
http://usa.weleda.com/

Personal care products

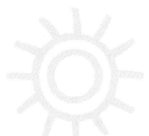

APPENDIX D

All About Blood Analysis

This Appendix will teach you a lot about blood chemistry and help you to interpret the results of any blood-work that your healthcare practitioner may suggest for you. This Appendix consists of four parts:

1. An overview of the most common types of blood analysis.

2. A sample Laboratory Report to familiarize you with how results are tabulated.

3. A detailed description of each blood test, explaining why it is used and what diseases or conditions its results may indicate.

4. The shortcomings of blood analysis.

PART I
OVERVIEW OF BLOOD ANALYSIS

Most Common Blood Analysis Ordered

The "Complete Blood Count and Differential Count," abbreviated as "CBC and diff." This analysis includes:

RBC
Red Blood Cell Count
Hemoglobin (HGB)
Hematocrit (HCT)
MCV (Mean Corpuscular Volume)
MCH (Mean Corpuscular Hemoglobin)
MCHC (Mean Corpuscular Hemoglobin
    Concentration)

WBC
White Blood Cell Count and Differential Count
Neutrophils
Lymphocytes

Monocytes
Eosinophils
Basophils
Platelet count

CANCER TUMOR MARKERS (ANTIGENS) CEA (CARCINOEMBRYONIC ANTIGEN) — A protein that normally appears in fetal gut tissue. However, it is also found in the bloodstream of adults with colorectal tumor and other carcinomas including breast, pancreatic, liver and gastric (stomach). It is also found in non-cancerous (benign) conditions including ulcerative colitis, diverticulitis and cirrhosis.

CA 19-9 — Useful tumor marker (antigen) for liver and pancreatic cancers. It is primarily used in the diagnosing of pancreatic carcinoma (70 percent). CA 19-9 markers can also indicate gastric cancers, colorectal cancer, pancreatitis, gallstones, cirrhosis and cystic fibrosis.

CA 15-3 — A tumor marker best used for metastatic breast cancer. It can also be elevated in ovarian disease, non-malignant breast masses and non-breast malignancies.

CA 125 — An epithelial cell tumor marker for ovarian cancer.

AFP (ALPHA-FETOPROTEIN) AND HCG (HUMAN CHORIONIC GONADOTROPHIN) — Germ cell tumor markers for the ovaries.

PSA (PROSTATE-SPECIFIC ANTIGEN) — A glycoprotein found in the cytoplasm of prostate epithelial cells. Elevated PSAs can indicate inflammation and/or cancer of the prostate. The higher the PSA levels, especially above 5, the more likely that this inflammation has become cancer.

Blood Typing

Human blood is categorized according to the presence or absence of blood antigens. These antigens are called **ABO** and **Rh Antigens**. The two major antigens that comprise **ABO** blood typing are the **A** and **B** antigen, which serve as the basis for the ABO system.

Type A blood contains type A antigens. Type B blood contains type B antigens. Type AB blood contains type AB antigens. Type O blood does not contain type A or B antigens.

The presence or absence of Rh antigens (factors) determines whether your blood is Rh-positive or Rh-negative.

Blood typing is important for transferring blood from one person to another. Antigens are the immunity of the individual and reflect one's ability to fight pathogenic invasions.

Other Common Terms and Tests Used

Electrolyte Panels: Show glucose and blood serum electrolytes.

Thyroid Panels: Show T4s (Thyroxin), T3s (Systemic converted Thyroxin), and TSHs (Thyroid stimulating hormone, from pituitary).

Lipid Profile Panels: Show cholesterol (LDLs and HDLs) and blood triglyceride levels.

PART II
HOW TO INTERPRET YOUR BLOOD TESTS

General Chemistry

GLUCOSE — In general, basic serum glucose levels may be an indicator of many conditions within the body. Elevated levels may indicate diabetes mellitus, hyper-parathyroidism, Cushing's disease, stress, pancreatitis, corticosteroid and diuretic therapy, pheochromocytoma, and cellular acidosis. Decreased levels may indicate hypoglycemia, hypothyroidism, liver disease and Addison's disease.

MINERALS — The minerals sodium, potassium, chloride and calcium are the main electrically-charged cations and anions, which constitute the body's electrolytes.

SODIUM — Sodium is the most abundant cation (positively charged) mineral in extracellular fluids. Therefore, it is the major salt in determining extracellular osmolality (transportation) of nutrients and constituents. Blood sodium is a direct result of the balance between dietary intake and kidney (renal) excretion and reabsorption.

Many hormones affect this balance of sodium by controlling the excretion through the kidneys (e.g., aldosterone, ADH, NH, etc.)

Low sodium levels create hyponatremia (low sodium), which can create weakness, confusion, coma and death. Too much sodium (hypernatremia) creates thirst, dry mucus membranes, convulsions, restlessness, etc. Many drugs can create both hypo- and hypernatremia, including antibiotics, steroids, laxatives, diuretics, sulfides, heart medications, etc.

Cancer will also decrease sodium levels. The body will use any alkaline component in it to fight acidosis. Sodium has a strong affinity for oxygen and is a vital inorganic metal in maintaining electrolyte balance.

POTASSIUM — Potassium is one of the major cations within the cell. There is almost forty times more potassium in a cell as opposed to the fluid that surrounds a cell. Potassium is affected by sodium reabsorption by the kidneys. Aldosterone lowers potassium by increasing kidney excretion. Your body always seeks to maintain the acid-based balance within it. Acidosis pulls potassium out of a cell, causing electromagnetic changes which affect cell wall permeability of nutrients and the electro-potentiality of a cell. Symptoms of elevated blood potassium (hyperkalemia) include nausea, vomiting, irritability, diarrhea, depressed electrical depolarization of the heart, muscle contractility, (S.O.B., chest pain, etc.) and acidosis. Low serum levels (hypokalemia) include a de-

Sample Blood Tests

	Result	Out of Range	Units	Reference Range
General Chemistry				
Glucose	103		mg/dL	70–115
Sodium	142		meg/L	133–145
Potassium	4.3		meg/L	3.3–5.3
Chloride	104		meg/L	96–110
Carbon Dioxide	33		meg/L	21–24
Bun	10		mg/dL	6–27
Creatinine	0.8		mg/L	0.5–1.5
Calcium	9.7		mg/dL	8.4–10.6
Total Protein	7.5		g/dL	5.9–8.4
Albumin	3.6		g/dL	3.4–4.8
Bilirubin Total	0.3		mg/dL	0.0–1.2
Alkaline Phosphatase	98		u/L	51–131
SGOT (AST)	19		u/L	0–50
SGPT (ALT)	23		u/L	0–50
Thyroid Testing				
T3 uptake	32.0		Percent	25.0-40.0
T4	10.7		ug/dL	4.9–11.7
T7	3.42		Calc.	1.25–4.55
TSH (ultrasensitive)		L <0.010	uiu/m/L	0.350–4.950
Miscellaneous Chemistry				
CEA	1.9		ng/mL	0.0–5.0
CBC, Platelet CT, and Diff				
White Blood Cell (WBC) Count	505		4.0–10.5	X 10-3/uL
Red Blood Cell (RBC) Count	4.42		4.10–5.60	X 10-6/uL
Hemoglobin		12.2 L	12.5–17.0	G/dL
Hematocrit	36.7		36.0–50.0	%
MCV	83		80–98	fL
MCH	27.6		27.0–34.0	pg
MCHC	33.2		32.0–36.0	G/dL
Platelets	183		140–415	X 10-3 uL
Polys	44		40–74	%
Lymphs	43		14–46	%
Monocytes	10		4–13	%
Eos	3		0–7	%
Basos	0		0–3	%
Polys (Absolute)	2.4		1.8–7.8	X 10–3/uL
Lymphs (Absolute)	2.4		0.7–4.5	X 10–3/uL
Monocytes (Absolute)	0.6		0.1–1.0	X 10–3/uL
Eos (Absolute Value)	0.2		0.0–0.4	X 10–3/uL
Baso (Absolute)			0.0–0.2	X 10–3/uL
Lipid Panel w/ LDL/HDL Ration				
LDL/HDL Ratio	2.5		0.0-3.6	Ratio units

crease in the contractility of smooth, skeletal and cardiac muscles, which can cause a host of symptoms including pain, paralysis, general weakness, and cardiac arrhythmias.

CHLORIDE — Chloride is an extracellular anion. It's considered one of the body's main electrolytes and serves to maintain electrical neutrality. Being a companion with sodium, its fluctuation mostly matches sodium, especially in fluid retention. However, chloride is not always affected by cancer like sodium is. In many cancers, the body will use its sodium to help alkalize this highly acidic condition. Chloride also helps maintain acid/alkaline balance. Chloride replaces intracellular bicarbonate in the neutralization of carbon dioxide, thus maintaining the alkaline balance of the cell and its fluids. Hypochloremia is low chloride levels and hyperchloremia is elevated chloride levels.

Hypochloremia

Hyperactivity of nerve and muscle tissue
Hypotension
Difficult and shallow breathing
Acidosis
CHF
Overhydration
Vomiting
Chronic respiratory

Hyperchloremia

Weakness
Fatigue
Dehydration
Cushing's Syndrome
Multiple myeloma
Kidney dysfuntion
Anemia

CALCIUM — Serum Calcium is used as an indicator of parathyroid function and calcium metabolism. This test is very inaccurate in determining calcium utilization. Blood calcium levels can rise or fall from cancer, chemical medication, detoxification, excessive milk drinking, high protein diets, vitamin-D supplementation, hyper-/hypo- or parathyroidism, renal failure, inflammation of the bones, malabsorption, pancreatitis, and other conditions.

CALCIUM-IONIZED — Ionized calcium does not bind with albumin, so is unaffected by albumin imbalances. Therefore it is seen as a more accurate picture for hyperparathyroidism.

CARBON DIOXIDE — Carbon dioxide levels are used to determine acidosis or alkalosis. It can also be an indicator of poor oxygenation, electrolyte imbalance (cellular), neutrality of extra and intracellular fluids, poor elimination (from kidneys and lungs), renal failure, salicylate toxicity, diabetic ketoacidiosis, starvation, shock, emphysema, and other conditions.

BUN (BLOOD UREA NITROGEN) — This test measures the amount of urea nitrogen in the blood. Urea is a substance formed in the liver as the end result of protein metabolism. As amino acids are catabolized (broken down or changed), ammonia is formed and then converted mostly to urea.

Urea is also formed in the lymphatic system. These ureas are transported to the kidneys for elimination. One can determine toxic levels of protein consumption, liver metabolism (of proteins) and kidney excretory functions by urea levels in the blood. Most kidney conditions create low levels of urea.

High levels can reflect over-consumption of proteins, GI bleeding, liver inflammation, and deterioration. Extracellular protein toxicity can also be a factor.

BUN and creatinine combo tests are used as renal function indicators. Dehydration or overhydration can affect blood ureas, as well as many drugs, including aspirin and diuretics.

Prostatitis and hypertrophy of the prostate gland can also cause abnormal urea levels. Malnutrition and lack of proper protein digestion and synthesis is also a big factor.

CREATININE — Creatinine is a product of catabolized creatine. Creatine is used for skeletal muscle contraction and strength. Creatinine is excreted entirely by the kidneys and can be an indicator of kidney or muscle breakdown (decreased levels). Increased levels can be an indicator of inflammation of the kidneys, urinary obstructions, dehydration, CHF, diabetes, shock or trauma.

TOTAL PROTEIN — Proteins are formed from building materials called amino acids. They are used in all structural and most functional aspects of the body. They are constituents of muscle, cell membrane walls, hormones, enzymes, neurotransmitters, and hemoglobin, and used as transport vehicles. Proteins significantly contribute to the osmotic pressure within the vascular system. This is significant to nutrient transport and metabolism.

ALBUMIN — Albumin is a protein formed within the liver. It constitutes almost 60 percent of the total protein of the body. Albumin has many responsibilities including maintenance of cellular osmotic pressure, and transportation of enzymes, hormones, etc. Albumin levels can give an insight into liver conditions, hepatitis, cirrhosis, cancer, malnutrition, wasting conditions including those of the vascular and intestinal (Crohn's) systems.

BILIRUBIN TOTAL — Bilirubin is one of the best indicators of liver function. It can become elevated during detoxification as the urine eliminates water-soluble toxins. There is indirect (unconjugated) or direct (conjugated) bilirubin depending upon the organ involved, (spleen or liver, respectively). Provides insight as to the proper functioning of these organs and the inflammation or damage therein. Obstructions of these organs, as well as the bile duct, such as with tumors or stones, will increase bilirubin levels. Other conditions that increase these levels include pernicious anemia, sickle cell anemia, hemolyte anemia, and damage from drug consumption.

ALP (ALKALINE PHOSPHATASE) — Alkaline phosphatase is a phosphatase enzyme that works in the presence of an alkaline environment. ALP is found mostly in the Kupffer's cells of the liver, bile tract epithelium (surface cells), and in the bones. When acidosis is present in these tissues, depending upon the degree (tumors, inflammation, cancer, etc.), the ALP will increase. The elevation of ALP can also be a result of healing fractures and normal bone growth, among other things. Many drugs and chemicals can play a major role in affecting ALP levels. These include antibiotics, heart medications, fluorides, oral contraceptives, oxalates, sulfates, and cyanides. Low levels can indicate hypothyroidism, pernicious anemia, excess vitamin-B ingestion. Some doctors give mega B-vitamin injections to drive ALP down when they are high. As previously stated, increased levels may indicate cancer (liver, gallbladder, bone, etc.), however, normal growth factors can also affect ALP levels.

AST (ASPARTATE AMINOTRANSFERASE) — Formerly SGOT (serum glutamic-oxaloacetic transaminase), AST is an enzyme found in liver cells, heart muscle cells, skeletal muscle cells, and to a smaller degree in kidney and pancreatic cells. The elevation of AST may suggest liver inflammation, as in hepatitis, cirrhosis and cancer, as well as myocardial infarction (heart attack), muscle conditions like myositis and myopathy, and renal disease and pancreatitis.

ALT (ALANINE AMINOTRANSFERASE) — Formerly SGPT (serum glutamic-pyrovic transaminase). ALT is an enzyme formed predominately in liver cells. However, it is found in heart muscle cells, skeletal muscular cells, and kidney cells, like AST. ALT enzyme is considered a specific in liver conditions such as hepatitis, cirrhosis, cancer, and necrosis.

Drugs and chemicals will affect both AST and ACT enzymes. These include antibiotics, aspirin-type drugs, heart medications, and many others. The list is a long one.

Immune Panel

For a complete explanation on immune function and its cells, see Chapter 2, Immune System, Module 2.7.

WBC (WHITE BLOOD CELLS) — Basically, white blood cells (leukocytes) are the body's armed forces, which protect it from foreign bodies—substances including proteins, chemicals and weakened or dying cells. When WBCs are elevated we know the body is fighting something. That something could be inflammation from foreign substances, tissue necrosis, or weakness and toxicity. This all leads to what is called infection. Trauma and stress also may affect WBCs.

When WBC count is low, ask yourself "Why are they low now?" "Why is my body under-producing them?" Or, "Why are they not getting into my bloodstream?" These questions may lead you to consider the presence of bone marrow weaknesses or disease, chemical and radiation therapies (which suppress and kill bone marrow cells), and/or a highly congested lymphatic system. All of these situations and more will affect the body's WBCs. Low WBC count is called **Leukopenia** ("penia" meaning "deficiency"). Elevated WBCs are called **leukocytosis**. An increase in total WBCs may indicate inflammation (acidosis), infection (acidosis), trauma, stress, and tissue neurosis. A decrease of WBCs may indicate drug toxicity, dietary deficiency, bone marrow failure or disease.

There are many types of white blood cells (leukocytes). They include:

Cell Types	% In Body
Neutrophils	55% – 70%
Lymphocytes	20% – 40%
Eosinophils	01% – 04%
Basophils	0.5% – 01%
Monocytes	02% – 08%

Most immune panels provide what is called a differential count. Each type of immune cell has its own function. When the percentage of any particular type of WBC changes, it will give insight into what condition the body is fighting. For example, **neutrophils** indicate inflammation, **lymphocytes** indicate anything from infection to cancer, **monocytes** indicate conditions from parasites to ulcerative issues (types of tissue destruction).

The following are some of the causes related to the increase or decrease of individual WBCs.

Neutrophils
Cause of increase: (Neutrophilia) Acute infection, inflammatory conditions, e.g., arthritis (rheumatoid and others), rheumatic fever. Any "itis," including gout, trauma, leukemia and stress.

Cause of decrease: (Neutropenia) Overgrowth of bacteria, anemia, viral involvements (like hepatitis or measles) radiation therapy, chemical or drug toxicity.

Lymphocytes
Cause of increase: (Lymphocytosis) Viral or bacteria involvements, multiple myeloma, lymphatic cancers, infectious hepatitis, radiation exposure.

Cause of decrease: (Lymphocytopenia) Sepsis, lupus, leukemia, drug or chemical toxicity, steroid use, and radiation exposure.

Eosinophils
Cause of increase: (Eosinophila) Parasites, allergies, skin conditions, e.g., eczema. Also, leukemia.

Cause of decrease: (Eosinopenia) Allergic reactions, stress, hyperthyroidism.

Basophils
Cause of increase: (Basophilia) Leukemia, fibrocystic conditions.

Cause of decrease: (Basopenia) Allergic reactions, stress, hyperthyroidism.

Monocytes
Cause of increase: (Monocytosis) Inflammatory processes, viral involvements, tuberculosis, parasites, ulcerative conditions.

Cause of decrease: (Monocytopenia) Drug and chemical toxicity, steroid use.

Immune cells should be working *for* us. These cells live within the ocean of the lymphatic system. When the lymphatic system becomes congested and impacted this will highly compromise the function of immune cells in many ways.

Parasites, including bacteria and protozoas, are secondary to the cause. In other words, toxicity and/or acidosis are the cause of immune system weakness. Parasites and immune response are secondary. The answer to these conditions is always detoxification. **Detoxification always cures the cause.**

RBC (RED BLOOD CELLS) — Red blood cells, or erythrocytes, carry oxygen to the cells. These are measured by the total number of RBCs in $1mm^3$ of venous blood. Within each red blood cell are numerous molecules of hemoglobin. These molecules are full of iron that binds oxygen and carries it forth. Many things affect red blood cells. They can become weakened, become out of shape, and begin sticking together, etc. However, this is mainly due to acidosis and low enzyme function within the vascular system.

Weakness and the other factors mentioned will affect the RBC's ability to carry and transport oxygen, remove carbon dioxide, and other functions. This can create a multitude of problems from low oxidation reactions to acidosis and anemia. One can experience any number of symptoms ranging from chronic fatigue, fatigue of the thyroid and adrenals, to debility. As stated, inflammatory conditions from acidosis are major factors affecting RBCs.

Dehydration will lead to increased RBCs and overhydration will lead to decreased RBCs. Diet, organ failure, cancer, anemia, hemorrhages, and drug and chemical therapy will decrease RBCs.

Again, detoxification is the only true answer to restoring red blood cells to their true, individual potentiality. Alkalization separates them while increasing hemoglobin content and capacity. Detoxification cleans the liver and spleen, and removes the chemicals and any metals that affect RBCs, or any cell for that matter.

Detoxification will restore total blood work to within normal ranges again, without compromising homeostasis.

HEMOGLOBIN — The red blood cells contain molecules called hemoglobin. Hemoglobin is a conjugated protein that consists of *hemo*, which bonds with iron, and *globin*, a simple protein (amino acid). There are hundreds of different types of hemoglobin. However, basically they bond to oxygen and glucose and transport these elements to the cells for energy and oxidation purposes. The clinical implications of this test are closely related to the RBC count.

Increased levels may suggest COPD, CHF, dehydration, or other conditions. A decrease in hemoglobin may suggest anemia, cancer, lupus, kidney disease, splenetic conditions, and nutritional deficiency. Normal hemoglobin levels are called normochromic, high levels are hyperchromic, and low levels are called hypochromic.

Old RBCs are broken down (phagocytized) by macrophages in the spleen, liver or red bone marrow. When this happens, the iron from the hemoglobin is reused immediately to produce new RBCs, or is stored in the liver. The globin portion is converted back to amino acids. The heme that is left is converted to bilirubin, which is then excreted by the bile.

HCT (HEMATOCRIT) — Hematocrit is the percentage of RBCs (erythrocytes) in any given volume of blood. Your hematocrit should closely relate to your RBC count and hemoglobin count. Increased levels may indicate dehydration, severe diarrhea, trauma or shock, burns, or other conditions. A decrease in hematocrit levels may indicate anemia, cirrhosis of the liver, cancer, hyperthyroidism, hemorrhage, bone marrow failure, rheumatoid arthritis, malnutrition, or normal pregnancy.

MCV (MEAN CORPUSCULAR VOLUME) — The MCV test is a measurement of the volume or size of a single red blood cell. This is beneficial in classifying anemias. The greater the MCV volume, the larger (or macrocytic) the cells are; and the lower the MCV volume the smaller (or microcytic) a red blood cell is. MCV volumes are calculated by dividing the hematocrit by the total RBC count. MCVs may indicate liver conditions, alcoholism, pernicious anemia, or other problems. A lower MCV finding may suggest iron deficiency anemia.

MCH (MEAN CORPUSCULAR HEMOGLOBIN) — MCH signifies the average amount (weight) of hemoglobin within an individual red blood cell.

MCHC (MEAN CORPUSCULAR HEMOGLOBIN CONCENTRATION) — The MCHC is a measurement of the average percentage or concentration of hemoglobin within an individual cell. This factor is obtained by dividing the total hemoglobin concentration by the hematocrit.

RDW (RED BLOOD CELL DISTRIBUTION WIDTH) — This is a measurement of the width of the red blood cells. This is helpful in classifying the type of anemia that one might have.

PLATELETS (THROMBOCYTES) — Platelets are essential to the ability of the blood to clot. They are the bridges and spider webs for perforations of tissue. They bind so the body can repair. Low platelet levels are indicative of bone marrow and/or spleen weakness or disease. Infections, drugs and hemorrhages are also related to low platelet counts. Below 50,000 is critical.

MPV (MEAN PLATELET VOLUME) — MVP deals with platelet size reflecting bone marrow weakness or function.

L.P.D. Profiling Panels

CHOLESTEROL (LDL AND HDL) — Cholesterol is essential for the formation of steroids (anti-inflammatory: anabolic type), bile acids and cellular wall membranes.

Cholesterol can only be used by the body in its free form. It is synthesized by the liver or metabolized from dietary cholesterol (meats mainly). This free cholesterol is then bound or connected to transporters (lipoproteins) for transport through the blood to the cells. Note: In cooked meats, lipids become bonded and are no longer free.

There are two types of lipoproteins: **LDLs** Low-density proteins, and **HDLs** High-density proteins. Seventy-five percent of the body's free cholesterol binds to the low-density proteins and 25 percent to the high-density proteins. LDLs bring the most abundant type of cholesterol. It leads some to think that the elevation of this type of bound cholesterol is an indicator of arteriosclerotic disease. This thinking is unreasonable to me. When you examine why cholesterol is produced and how it is used by the body, you realize that cholesterol production is linked to steroid use, in particular, to inflammatory responses, and to the rebuilding of cells when cell destruction has taken place.

Because the liver synthesizes and metabolizes cholesterol, low cholesterol levels can be associated with liver diseases (like inflammation, hypo-function, narcosis, and cancer), as well as malabsorption, hyperthyroidism, some anemias, sepsis and stress.

Increased levels of cholesterol may create or indicate low adrenal function, inflammatory conditions, nephrosis, biliary cirrhosis, dietary habits (over-consumption of meats), pregnancy, hypothyroidism, high blood pressure, or other conditions.

What elevated or decreased cholesterol levels indicate is quite different than what they cause. For example, low blood pressure is indicative of adrenal medulla weakness and sodium imbalances, which can reflect adrenal cortex weakness. When the cortex of the adrenal glands is weak, the body's response to inflammation from acidosis (mostly dietary and hormonal) will be low. Therefore, the production of cholesterol by the liver will increase, thus increasing blood serum levels. Cholesterol is an anti-inflammatory lipid used by the body in response to inflammation and cellular destruction.

In time, without correcting the above, blood pressure will swing from low to high (arteriosclerotic syndrome). One can also experience diabetes, hyperthyroidism, hypercholesterol-emia, hyperlipidemia, high blood pressure, heart attack, strokes, arteriosclerosis, nephrosis, and other conditions.

The answer to the above of course will always lead you back to the same thing—detoxification. Alkalize and energize, and your body will clean and rebuild itself.

TRIGLYCERIDES (TG) — Triglycerides are similar to cholesterol in that they are lipids. Triglycerides act as a source of stored energy and for healing inflammatory conditions. Triglycerides (like cholesterol) also bind with lipoproteins for transportation throughout the body. These lipoproteins include: **VLDs**—Very low-density lipoproteins and **LDLs**—Low-density lipoproteins.

Triglycerides are synthesized by the liver from glycerol and other fatty acids. Being similar to cholesterol, triglycerides have the same biological and pathogenic response. Anything that causes acidosis (from alcohol consumption to meat eating) will elevate lipids.

Thyroid Profile Panels

T3 (TRIIODOTHYRONINE) — The T3 or triiodothyronine study shows the amount of T3 in the blood. This is used to determine if there is overactive or underactive thyroid involvement.

T4 (THYROXINE) — This study shows the amount of T4 (thyroxine) present in the blood. Elevated levels have been associated with hyperthyroidism and Wilson's Syndrome—the in-

ability of the body to convert T4s into T3s. Low levels of T4 have been associated with hyperthyroidism. T4, as with most hormones, needs protein transporters. TBG or thyroid-binding globulin (a protein) is one of the transporters of T4 or thyroxine. Elevated serum proteins from acidosis or protein toxicity may increase T4 or T3 levels.

T3 uptake reflects the thyroid-binding globulin (TBG) and thyroid-binding prealbumin (TBPA) in the blood. This test is done to weed out elevated or decreased T3 or T4 levels by other factors, such as, oral contraceptives, pregnancy, or kidney disease.

TSH (THYROID-STIMULATING HORMONE) AND TRH (THYROTROPIN-RELEASING HORMONE) — TSH is a thyroid-stimulating hormone produced in the anterior portion of the pituitary gland. This hormone (TSH) activates or stimulates the thyroid gland to produce and release thyroxine (T4s). When the thyroid is weak (hypothyroidism) or the pituitary is hyperactive, TSH levels will be elevated. This is in response to the need for more thyroid hormone, thyroxine, which is vital to metabolism and heart function. Low levels of triiodothyronine (T3) and thyroxine (T4) stimulate TRH and TSH release.

TSH study is also used to determine primary hypothyroidism (from the thyroid itself), or secondary hypothyroidism (hypothalamic caused).

Remember that all things work together in creation to form one God. This is true also of your body and its glands. Specific glandular function can be a result of the gland itself being toxic and weak, or due to other related glands that are affecting it. Because all things are interwoven and interlocked, conventional "treatment" never works.

NOTE: In thirty years of clinical observation, it is my opinion that blood T3, T4 and TSH levels are the least accurate of thyroid tests. This is why the Basal Temperature Test was created. (See

Appendix A.) I have seen a tremendous number (80 percent) of hypothyroid cases missed by the medical profession because they treated the blood test, not their patient.

PART III
SHORTCOMINGS OF BLOOD ANALYSIS

Using blood analysis to determine body conditions and diagnose tissue weaknesses is one of the least accurate of the diagnostic tools available today. However, when combined with tissue analysis, Iridology, physical symptomology, reflexology, and kinesiology, it can provide as close a total picture as you can get of the internal condition of your body.

With blood analysis alone one can only hypothesize what *might* be going on in the body, and this of course *greatly* depends upon the interpreter. A blood type analysis does not accurately reflect electrolyte imbalances, hormone levels, glucose fructose utilization, and the true nature of the immune response. Each of these factors can affect, and thus skew, the results.

Electrolyte Imbalances

Your blood can show normal levels of calcium, for example, but at the cellular level you could be highly deficient. Blood level minerals do not show utilization or storage factors. Serum levels of minerals can change due to emotional issues, blood-drawing techniques, and homeostatic (balance) needs. Also, excess mineral and toxic metal accumulation is hard to detect from blood analysis because of the removal by the spleen, liver or other tissues for storage or protection. Your body must keep the blood and serum as clean and balanced as possible or death can result.

Hormone Levels

Your blood is the most inaccurate medium in showing hypoactive hormone production. Thyroid (T4 and T3) hormone activity is much better indicated by the Basal Temperature Test, which was created for this purpose. (See Appendix A.) Adrenal steroid and neurotransmitter production are also not measured properly by blood tests.

Glucose/Fructose Utilization

Your blood can show serum glucose levels, but test results can't indicate the degree of transport.

True Immune Response

Your blood can show high or low levels of immune cells (basophils, for example), but can't indicate why the immune system is responding as it is. Most immune responses are interpreted wrongly, especially without the understanding of detoxification.

Your blood carries many cellular metabolites, parasites, liver wastes and the like. These are filtered out through your spleen, kidneys, intestines and lungs. Because of this your blood's environment is always changing, giving rise to the ever-changing chemistry of the body.

Your blood analysis can be a great tool to help you to put the "pieces" of the puzzle together. It can help you determine excessive carbon buildup, excessive tissue breakdown, and electrolyte disturbances through low serum levels. It can alert you to liver, heart, kidney and muscle tissue breakdown. It can also give you clues to systemic acidosis and immune response creating inflammatory issues, and much more.

APPENDIX E

Tissue Mineral Analysis (TMA)

Your hair is little different from any other tissue in the body, requiring virtually the same elements for growth and repair. Since the hair is the second most metabolically-active tissue in your body, it can be used as a "record" of metabolic activity. The first inch or so of your hair can give you a good picture of the last two months or so of your body's metabolic activity. As it grows, it "locks in" the history of intra- and extra-cellular metabolic activity.

Hair analysis is more reliable than blood analysis in indicating tissue (cellular) level utilization, storage and excretory factors. Hair is considered excretory tissue. It can show mineral, heavy metal and toxic element levels within the body. The FBI uses hair analysis in forensic labs to determine the ingestion of toxic and deadly metals and substances like arsenic. It is so accurate that they can determine the year and almost the month of ingestion and the level changes thereof. Hair analysis can also be more definitive than blood and urine in indicating the body's storage of toxic elements. The EPA (Environmental Protection Agency) uses hair as the tissue of choice in determining toxic metal exposure.

Many factors can affect proper hair analysis by contaminating or altering the results. These include hair treatment products, such as dyes, bleaches, and shampoos.

It is important to know what goes on at the cellular level, and the hair will indicate this. The cellular level is where it is all "happening." Dr. Emanuel Cheraskin has stated in his book, *Diet and Disease,* "Minerals have interrelationships with every other nutrient. Without optimum mineral levels within the body, the other nutri-

ents are not effectively utilized." Minerals play an active role in production of hormone synthesis and activity (and vice versa). Some minerals are "electric" transporters as well as stimulators. Minerals also play a role in enzyme activity.

Tissue mineral analysis can play a vital role in understanding some of your body's symptoms. Most naturopaths and many other healthcare practitioners use hair (tissue) analysis as part of their practice. These analyses include dietary recommendations, but the diets suggested are not based upon natural health principles.

Conclusion

Blood, hair, saliva and urine analysis should be correlated with an iris analysis, and clinical (body) observation, as well as with the body's symptoms. It is easy to be misled with only a partial understanding of systemic conditions when using body fluids alone as diagnostic tools.

Detoxification can also drastically change blood, hair, saliva, and urine analysis and to the untrained physician or health care practitioner, it can fool them into thinking the body is in trouble when it is only cleaning itself. Blood cholesterol levels and cancer markers (antigens) can drastically increase in the initial stages of detoxification, but will drop into normal ranges when the body is cleaned out.

There is only one true healing modality . . . detoxification. It will bring the body's chemistry back into homeostasis (balance), and will remove the toxic metals, elements and substances that don't belong there.

Seek God, health and happiness.

Weights and Measurements

1 pound	=	453 grams
1 ounce	=	28.3 grams
128 ounces	=	1 gallon
16 ounces	=	1 pound
1 quart	=	2 pints
1 pint	=	2 cups
1 teaspoon	=	60 drops
6 teaspoons	=	1 ounce
1 tablespoon	=	3 teaspoons
1 fluid ounce	=	2 tablespoons
1 cup	=	16 tablespoons
30 milliliters	=	1 ounce
1 milliliter	=	1/30 fluid ounce
1/4 dram	=	1/500 pint
1 tablespoon	=	15 milliliters
15.4 grains	=	1 gram
1 gram	=	100 milligrams (mg.)
1 full dropper	=	approx. 60 drops
2 tablespoons of tincture	=	1/2 cup of tea

1 teaspoon = 5 milliliters = 1/6 fluid ounce = 1 dram

1 teaspoon of powder = about two "00" capsules = about 50 milligrams (mg.)

1 "00" capsule = approximately 500 mg. = 8 grains

APPENDIX G

Glossary

ABCs   a localized collection of pus and liquefied tissue in a cavity.

Abortifacients   cause induced abortion (premature expulsion of the fetus).

Absorbents   herbs used to produce absorption of exudates (accumulated fluids) or diseased tissues. (Black Elm, Mullein, Slippery Elm, etc.)

Absorption   nutritionally, the process by which nutrients are absorbed through the intestinal tract into the bloodstream to be used by the body. If nutrients are not properly absorbed, nutritional deficiencies (malabsorption) will result. This can affect the body's fuels and building materials as well, leading to enervation, starvation and deterioration.

Abstergents   detergents.

Acetylcholine   an ester of choline occurring in various organs and tissues of the body. It is thought to play an important role in transmission of nerve impulses at synapses and myoneural junctions.

Acidophilus   lactobacillus acidophilus bacteria, also called "friendly colonic flora," is used to replace destroyed bacteria. Should be used by milk drinkers only.

Acidosis   excessive acidity of body fluids, due to an accumulation of acids (as in diabetic acidosis or renal disease) or an excessive loss of bicarbonate (as in renal disease). The hydrogen ion concentration is increased, and thus the pH is decreased. Acidosis leads to an immune response called inflammation.

Acids   a class of compounds that have low pH, usually sour to the taste, and in their pure form, are often corrosive (citric acid, benzoic acid, formic acid, uric acid, phosphoric acid, carbonic acid, etc.). They can be either organic or inorganic compounds. Acids can irritate and inflame the tissues of the body. They also can become free radicals. Acids found in plant tissues (especially fruits), however, tend to prevent the secretion of fluids and shrink tissues. A buildup of acids leads to acidosis.

Acute   having a rapid onset, severe symptoms, and a short course (not chronic). Pain occurs in acute and regenerative conditions. "Acute" is actually the beginning stages of disease.

Adaptogen   a substance with qualities that increase resistance and resilience to stress. Adaptogens strengthen cells, tissues, organs and glands. Adaptogens work through support of the adrenal glands, especially. (Garlic, Echinacea, Ginkgo, Goldenseal, Pau D'Arco and Ginseng.)

Adrenal Glands   a pair of triangular-shaped glands that sit on top of each kidney. Glands of internal secretion whose effects mimic those of the sympathetic nervous system; increase carbohydrate use of energy. Also, regulate carbohydrate and fat metabolism and salt/water balance, as well as steroid hormones. They are the source of neurotransmitters like epinephrine (adrenaline) and steroids like cortisol, estrogen, and progesterone, among others.

Adrenaline   a neurotransmitter secreted by the adrenal glands that produce the "fight or flight" response. Also called Epinephrine.

Adsorb   attachment of a substance to the surface of another material.

Adulterant   an unacceptable additive or replacement of a specified herb (also: substitute).

Aerobic   1. requiring oxygen for metabolism and survival; 2. concerning organisms living in the presence of oxygen; 3. metabolizing oxygen for energy.

Alcohols found in plant volatile oils.

Aldosterone a hormone secreted by the adrenal glands that causes the retention of sodium and water.

Alimentary Canal (or GI Tract) the digestive tube from the mouth to the anus, including mouth cavity, pharynx, esophagus, stomach, small and large intestines, and rectum.

Alkaline pertaining to or having the reaction of an alkali. Neutralizes acids. In the scenario of duality, this is considered *yin* or cooling.

Alkaloids 1. a powerful and potent group (thirteen) of plant constituents. Their properties are very broad ranging from hallucinogenic alkaloids at one end, to painkillers, to deadly poisonous alkaloids at the other end. 2. Alkaloids react with acids to form salts that are used for medical purposes.

Allopathy/Allopathic 1. System of treating disease by inducing a pathologic reaction that is antagonistic to the disease being treated. 2. Conventional medicine or alternative medicine when compared to nature.

Alterative tending to restore normal health; cleanses and purifies the blood; alters existing nutritive and excretory processes gradually restoring normal body functions (Echinacea, Goldenseal, Sanicle, Yellow Dock, among other herbs).

Amenorrhea absence or suppression of menstruation.

Amino Acids a group of nitrogen-containing chemical compounds that form the basic structural units of proteins.

Anabolic 1. the building up of body tissues. The utilization or constructive phase of metabolism; 2. the conversion and utilization of nutrients to repair, rebuild or to build and maintain cells, tissues, organs and glands; 3. Energy is used and needed during this phase or process.

Anaerobic 1. requiring no oxygen to function; 2. living without oxygen.

Analeptics used for restorative purposes or for food.

Analgesic relieves pain when taken orally.

Anaphrodisiacs herbs used to lessen sexual functions and desires (Black Willow, Garden Sage, Oregon Grape, Scullcap, others).

Androgens steroid hormones, such as testosterone or androsterone, that control the development and maintenance of male characteristics. Also called *androgenic hormone*.

Anesthetics herbs to produce anesthesia, or unconsciousness.

Anhydrotic stops sweating (Agrimony, Buchu, Butcher's Broom, others).

Anionic 1. a magnetic condition created by negative ions or an acidic environment that creates coagulation. 2. to solidify, bond; similar to anabolic; 3. in reference to acidosis.

Anodyne relieves pain when applied externally.

Antacids herbs used to neutralize acid in the stomach and intestinal tract (Angelica, Fennel, Peppermint, Slippery Elm, others).

Anterior before, or in front of.

Anthelmintics helps destroy and dispel parasites (including vermicides and vermifuges) (Bistort, Wormwood, Black Walnut).

Anthraquinones purgative in action. They appear as glycosides (linked with a sugar). Their action stimulates peristalsis; said to be utilized as natural dyes, flavones, and flavonoids.

Antiabortives herbs used to counteract abortive tendencies (Cramp Bark, False Unicorn, Red Raspberry).

Antiarthritics herbs used to relieve and heal arthritic conditions and gout (Black Cohosh, Chaparral, Dandelion, Yellow Dock).

Antibacterial destroying or stopping the growth of bacteria.

Antibilious reduces biliary or jaundice condition (Blessed Thistle, Borage, Butcher's Broom).

Antibiotic inhibits the growth of or destroys bacteria.

Anticatarrhal herbs that heal and remove

catarrhal (mucous) conditions in the body (Black Haw, Burdock Root, Hyssop, Licorice, Oregon Grape, others).

Antibody protein produced by the body to fight antigens by creating an immune response.

Antidepressant relieves symptoms of depression (St. John's Wort).

Antidote a substance that neutralizes or counteracts the effects of a poison.

Antiemetic lessens nausea and prevents or relieves vomiting (Jamaican Ginger, Cayenne, Fennel).

Antifungal destroying or preventing the growth of fungi.

Antigen any foreign substance that when introduced into the body causes the formation of antibodies against it.

Antigalactagogue prevents or decreases secretion of milk.

Antihemorrhagic stops bleeding and hemorrhaging (Cayenne, Bistort Root, Witch Hazel).

Antihistamine neutralizes the effects of histamine in an allergic response.

Antihydropics herbs used to eliminate excess body fluids or dropsy (Barberry, Blessed Thistle, Celandine, Hawthorne).

Anti-inflammatory counteracting or diminishing inflammation or its effects. Having vascular constrictive properties.

Antileptics helps relieve fits.

Antilithics herbs used to prevent the formation of stones in the kidneys and bladder (Couchgrass, Elecampane, Golden Rod, Gravel Root).

Antimicrobial destroys or prevents the growth of microorganisms.

Antineoplastic preventing the development, growth or proliferation of malignant cells.

Antioxidant an agent that prevents free-radical or oxidative damage to body tissue and cells. A group of substances called proanthocyanidins (grape seed and maritime pine bark), as well as vitamins A, C, E and beta carotene, are all antioxidants.

Antiparasitical destructive to parasites (Black Walnut Hulls, Pumpkin Seeds, Usnea Lichen).

Antiperiodic relieves malarial-type fevers and chills; prevents regular recurrences (Celandine, Angelica, Goldenseal).

Antiphlogistic relieves inflammation (Chaparral, Chickweed, Comfrey).

Antipyretic reduces fever.

Antirheumatics herbs used to prevent, relieve and cure rheumatism (Angelica, Black Willow, Blue Cohosh, Butcher's Broom).

Antiscorbutic helps prevent or correct scurvy (c.a. vitamin C) (Sarsaparilla, Cleavers, Sheep Sorrel).

Antiscrofulous herbs used to heal scrofula (tubercular condition of the lymph nodes) (Agrimony, Blue Flag, Dandelion, Elder Flowers, Red Clover).

Antiseptics helps prevent the growth of microbes and cripples their activity while in contact with them. Helps oppose sepsis. (Buchu, Burdock Leaves, Chamomile, Cayenne, Echinacea).

Antispasmodic relieves spasms of voluntary and involuntary muscles and relieves nervous irritability. (Wild Lettuce, Lobelia, Scullcap.)

Antisyphilitics herbs used to relieve and cure syphilis or other venereal diseases (Goldenseal, Juniper Berry, Kava Kava, Oregon Grape).

Antithrombotic prevents blood clots.

Antitoxic neutralizes a poison from the system (Alfalfa, Chlorophyll).

Antitussive prevents or relieves coughing.

Antivenomous herbs used as antidotes to animal, vegetable and mineral poisons (Plantain, American Pennyroyal, Chaparral).

Antiviral inhibits a virus (Pau D'Arco, Echinacea, Black Walnut Hull).

Antizymotics herbs used to destroy or arrest the action of bacterial (disease-producing) organisms (Black Walnut Hulls/Leaves, Cloves, Garlic, Mullein).

Anxiolytic an anti-anxiety agent.

Aperient a mild or gentle laxative (Buckthorn,

Cascara Sagrada, Mountain Flax).

Aperitive a substance that stimulates the appetite.

Aphrodisiacs herbs used to correct conditions of impotence and strengthen sexual power and desire (Damiana, False Unicorn, Saw Palmetto, Yohimbe).

Arachidonic Acid an essential fatty acid formed from unsaturated acids of plants, and present in peanuts. It is a precursor of prostaglandins.

Aromatics strong fragrance. Helps stimulate the gastrointestinal mucous membrane aiding in digestion and the expelling of gas from the stomach and bowels. (Anise, Fennel, Peppermint).

Ascaris roundworm (also called maw-worm and eelworm) found in the small intestine causing colicky pains and diarrhea, especially in children.

Ascites excessive accumulation of serous fluid in the peritoneal cavity.

Asthenia lack or loss of strength, usually involving muscular system.

Astringent firms tissues and organs; reduces discharges and secretions. Acts upon the albumen. Affects the cleansing and detoxification of tissues. (Agrimony, Bugleweed, Horsetail, White Oak Bark, Witch Hazel).

Atonic without normal tension or tone.

Atrophy a wasting; a decrease in size of an organ or tissue; the degeneration of cells, tissues, glands, etc.

Autoimmune a process in which antibodies develop against the body's own tissues. This process is a natural response to body cells that are dying. This creates an immune response for elimination of that cell so the body can replace it.

Autonomic independent and spontaneous.

Autonomic Nervous System the part of the nervous system that controls involuntary bodily functions. It regulates the function of glands, especially the salivary, gastric, and sweat glands, and the adrenal medulla, smooth muscle tissue, and the heart. The autonomic nervous system

may act on these tissues to reduce or slow activity or to initiate their function.

Ayurvedic a traditional system of medicine in India; literally means "a science of life." Eastern Indian herbology.

Bactericide destroys bacteria.

Balsamic herbs that mitigate, soothe and heal inflamed parts (Avocado Leaves, Balm of Gilead, Spikenard).

Basal cells Original, primary cells that constitute the body.

Basophils 1. immune cells involved in inflammatory immune responses. Basophils release histamine and other chemicals (which dilate blood vessels to accomplish this). 2. also found in the anterior lobe of the pituitary gland. These cells produce corticotrophin, the substance that stimulates the adrenal cortex to secrete adrenal cortical hormone. 3. A type of white blood cell (leukocyte) characterized by possession of coarse granules that stain intensely with basic dyes.

B-cells a specialized white blood cell of the immune system that produces antibodies. These are the "Marines" of your immune cells.

Bentonite volcanic clay known for its absorptive properties. Used in nutrition for its absorption of toxic elements.

Beta cells the cells in the pancreas that manufacture insulin.

Bilirubin the breakdown product of the "heme" in the hemoglobin molecule of red blood cells.

Bile a bitter, yellow substance that is released by the liver into the intestines for the digestion of fats and the alkalization of HCL (hydrocloric acid) and other acids from the stomach.

Bioflavonoids biologically active flavonoids that are essential for the stability and absorption of vitamin C. They are well known for their strengthening effect on the blood capillaries, and although not technically vitamins, they are sometimes referred to as vitamin P.

Bitter Principles named for their bitter properties. These bitter properties stimulate digestive secretions throughout the gastrointestinal tract, while stimulating the gall bladder and liver (bile secretion). Bitters are divided into various categories with some belonging to the terpenes, cothers, and iridoids. Research has shown that some bitters have antibiotic, antifungal and anti-tumor activities.

Bitter Tonic bitter herbs which in small amounts stimulate digestion and liver function. Helps to regulate fire/inflammation in the body, as well. (Angostura, Barberry, Gentian)

Bitters herbs that have a bitter taste and have the power of stimulating the gastrointestinal mucous membrane and liver tissue, without affecting the general system (Gentian, Chaparral, Wormwood).

Blisters herbs that cause inflammatory exudation (blistering) of serum from the skin when applied locally; used as revulsants; react with acids (Black Mustard, Blue Violet Root, White Byrony, others).

Blood Pressure the force exerted by blood as it presses through and against the walls of your blood vessels. (See: Systolic and Diastolic.)

Blood Sugar sugar in the form of glucose present in the blood. (Normally 60 to 100 milligrams/100 milliliters of blood. However, blood sugar can rise after a meal to as much as 150 milligrams/100 milliliters of blood. This may vary.)

Bolus an herbal suppository injected into the rectum or vagina for healing purposes.

Bromelain the protein-digesting enzyme found in pineapple.

Bronchiole one of the smaller subdivisions of the bronchial tubes.

By-product a secondary product or result.

Calefacients used externally to cause a sense of warmth by increasing capillary circulation (Cayenne).

Calmative soothing, sedative action.

Candida yeast-like fungus that causes sugar and starch cravings. Can grow prolifically through the lymph system.

Carbohydrates 1. plant glucose, fructose, starches, cellulose, etc. Gums and mucilages are also forms of carbohydrates used for additional cellulose energy stored as ATP or glycogen. 2. carbon-based constituents used for fuels (energy) by the body.

Carbuncle painful infection of the skin and subcutaneous tissues with production and discharge of pus and dead tissue, similar to a boil (faruncle) but more severe and with a multiple sinus formation; usually caused by an accumulation of toxicity where Staphylococcus aureus is present.

Carcinogen a cancer-producing substance.

Cardiac pertains to the heart and its actions. Herbs or substances that help stimulate and tone the heart. (See: Cordial)

Cardiac Depressants herbs that lessen and are sedative to the heart's action (Blood Root, Bugleweed, Poke Root).

Cardiac Glycosides (similar to Saponins) First discovered in 1785 in the herb Foxglove. Their action on cardiac tissue has been well established. Cardiac glycosides are formed by a combination of steroidal agylcone and a sugar (sugar regulates its bioavailability). Cardiac glycosides increase the force, power and strength of the heart muscle without increased oxygen demand.

Cardiac Stimulants herbs used to increase and give greater power to the heart's action (Bugleweed, Cayenne, Pipsissewa).

Cardiovascular relating to the heart and blood vessels.

Carminative relieves intestinal gas, pain and distention; promotes peristalsis (Pennyroyal, Lovage, Myrrh).

Catabolic 1. the breaking down or destructive phase of metabolism; 2. includes digestive and all the processes used to break down complex substances into simple, usable ones; 3. Energy is generally released during this process. (For example: glucose is catabolized to water, carbon dioxide, and energy.)

Cataplasm another name for a poultice.

Catarrh a mucus discharge from the mucous

membranes as a result of inflammation, acids, or irritants (foreign proteins). This has special reference to the air passages of the head and throat. (For example: hayfever, rhinitis, influenza, bronchitis, pharyngitis, asthma). Milk and refined sugars create an over-production of mucus discharge, congesting various body tissues.

Cathartic strong laxative which causes rapid evacuation of bowels (Black Hellebore, Culvers Root, Senna Leaves).

Cationic 1. state of flux and breakdown whereby nutrients and elements are dispersed systemically; similar to catabolic; 3. in reference to alkalization.

Caustics herbs that burn or destroy living tissue (Celandine Juice, Cashew Juice, Yellow Anemone Herb).

Cell Proliferants herbs that promote rapid healing and regeneration of the body (cells). (Aloe Vera, Comfrey, Elecampane, Saw Palmetto).

Cephalics herbs that are particularly healing to cerebral conditions and diseases (Red Sage, Rosemary, Rue, Stinging Nettle, Juniper Berry).

Chlorophyll the "green" pigment in plants; used in nutrition to absorb toxins and as a vulnerary; it can be taken as a supplement, as a source of magnesium and trace elements. It has strong detoxifying properties; pulls mucus and heavy metals out of the body.

Cholagogue promotes flow and discharge of bile from liver into intestines (Beets, Fringetree, Mandrake).

Cholesterol a crystalline substance that is soluble in fats; produced by all vertebrates. It is a necessary constituent of cell membranes, and facilitates the transport and absorption of fatty acids. It can be synthesized in the liver and is a normal constituent of bile. It is important in metabolism, serving as a processor of various steroid hormones. Excess cholesterol is a potentially big threat to health. This occurs in acidosis (inflammation) where adrenal cortex weakness is observed.

Chronic 1. an advanced state of hypoactivity of tissue, organs and glands; 2. the stage before degeneration and cancer.

Chyme the mixture of partly digested food and digestive secretions found in the stomach and small intestine during digestion of a meal. It is a varicolored, thick, but nearly liquid mass.

Cimcifuga means "to drive away bugs," neutralizes rattlesnake bites, scorpion stings. (Plantain, Black Cohosh, Borage, Wood Betony.)

Cod Liver Oil natural oils from cod fish which contain essential fatty acids and vitamins A and D; also contains the Omega-3 oils.

Coenzyme a molecule that works with an enzyme to enable the enzyme to perform its function in the body. Coenzymes are necessary in the utilization of vitamins and minerals. Vitamins are considered coenzymes as they affect the ability of an enzyme to activate.

Colitis inflammation of the colon.

Coloring Agents herbs used for coloring or dyeing purposes (Bilberry—dark blue or purple; Blood Root—deep red or bronze; Turmeric—golden yellow).

Colostrum a clear fluid, rich in antibodies and nutrients, produced in the breasts as the first "milk." Colostrum stimulates and builds the immune system of the infant.

Complex Sugars where two or more simple sugars (glucose, fructose, or galactose) are combined. Starches and artificial sugars are a good example of complex sugars (dextrose, maltose, sucrose, etc.). Complex sugars lead to the overproduction of mucus and carbonic acid, which congest and acidify the body.

Compounds 1. a substance composed of two or more units or parts combined in definite proportions by weight and having specific properties of its own. Compounds are formed by all living organisms and are of two types, organic and inorganic. 2. made up of more than one part.

Compress a pad of linen applied under pressure to an area of skin and held in place.

Complete Protein a source of dietary protein that contains a full complement of the eight essential amino acids. Based upon flesh as the end result of a vegetable diet.

Complex Carbohydrate 1. a carbohydrate that contains several bonded natural sugars (glucose and fructose). These are exceedingly difficult for the body to break down. Excessive consumption leads to acidosis through the creation of excessive carbonic acid, which is a by-product of sugar breakdown. 2. The carbohydrates in starches and fiber are complex carbohydrates; also called polysaccharides. 3. requires adrenal steriods to metabolize.

Condiments herbs used to season or flavor foods (Coriander, Parsley, Sweet Basil, Sage, Rosemary).

Congestion 1. the presence of an excessive amount of blood or tissue fluid in an organ or in tissue. 2. In natural health, congestion refers to the accumulation of mucus, acids, toxins, chemicals, heavy metals, parasites, and the like. Leads to nodal swelling, masses, and tumor formation.

Connective Tissue the type of tissue that performs the function of providing support, structure, and cellular cement to the body.

Constringents astringents.

Convalescence the period of recovery (or immobility) after the termination of a disease or an operation.

Convulsants cause convulsions.

C.O.P.D. Chronic Obstructive Pulmonary Disease.

Cordials herbs that combine the properties of a warm stomach and a cardiac stimulant (Angostura, Borage, Gentian).

Correctives (corrigents) herbs used to lessen and/or alter the severity of action of other herbs, especially cathartics or purgatives. Some correctives include: American Pennyroyal, Bay Leaves, and Cascara Sagrada.

Corticosteroid Hormones a group of hormones produced by the adrenal glands that control the body's use of nutrients and the excretion of salts and water in the urine. Used for inflammatory processes by the body.

Cosmetics herbs that are skin tonics and are used to improve the complexion and beautify the skin (Agar Agar, Balm of Gilead, Comfrey).

Coumarins (aromatic constituents) anti-clotting factors in small doses and used as rat poison in large doses.

Counterirritants herbs that cause irritation by local application in one part and therapeutically relieve pain in another more deep-seated part (Prickly Ash, Rue, Lobelia).

Cultigen an organism, especially a cultivated plant, such as a Garlic, not known to have a wild or uncultivated counterpart.

Cyst an abnormal lump or swelling, filled with fluid or semi-solid "cheesy" material, in any body organ or tissue, caused from acidosis, mucus and oftentimes excessive hormones.

Craniosacral concerning the skull and sacrum.

Cruciferous means "cross-shaped." Used to refer to a group of vegetables (including broccoli, Brussels sprouts, cabbage, cauliflower, turnips, and rutabagas) that have cross-shaped blossoms, and contain substances that have been shown to prevent colon cancer.

Cystitis inflammation of the urinary bladder.

Cytotoxic a substance toxic to cells.

Cytokines chemical messengers that are involved in the regulation of almost every system in the body and are important in controlling local and systemic inflammatory response.

Debility weakness of tonicity in functions or organs of the body.

Decoction teas prepared by boiling the botanical (herbs) with water for a specified period of time, followed by straining or filtering; generally ingested as a tea.

Degeneration deterioration of a structure or function of any part of the body based in the decline of the cells or other structures that constitute that part. Opposite of regeneration.

Dehydration excessive loss of water from the body created mainly by acidosis.

Dementia senility; loss of mental function.

Demulcent soothes, protects and nurtures irritated and inflamed membranes and tissues.

Dental Anodynes herbs used locally to relieve pain from an exposed nerve filament in the tooth (toothache) (Broom, Cajuput, Ginger, Oil of Cloves).

Deobstruents help remove obstructions from the body (Barberry, Butcher's Broom, Plantain).

Deodorants herbs that eliminate foul odors (Blackberry, Chlorophyll, Echinacea).

Depressants sedatives.

Depresso-Motors herbs that diminish muscular movement by action on the spinal centers (*also see*: Nervine and Antispasmodic) (Gum Wood, Lobelia, Poke Root).

Depuratives cleanses or purifies blood by promoting eliminative functions (Blessed Thistle, Blue Flag, Dandelion).

Dermatomycoses skin infection caused by fungi.

Desiccants herbs that are able to dry surfaces by absorbing moisture (Agar Agar, Bladderwrack Powder, Corn Starch, Marshmallow, Slippery Elm Powder).

Detergent cleansing to wounds, ulcers or skin itself (Amaranth plant, Bitter Root, Poke Root).

Detoxicant removes toxins.

Detoxification the process of cleansing and alkalizing the body. The removing of obstructions (e.g., acids, mucus, parasites, chemicals, minerals, metals, thoughts and emotions) that block energy and the proper function of cells and the individual. A necessary requirement in returning to vibrant health.

Detoxify 1. to remove the toxic quality of a substance; 2. treatment of a toxic overdose of any medicine but especially of the toxic state produced by drugs of abuse or acute alcoholism.

Diaphoretic causes perspiration and increases elimination through the skin (Centaury, Coltsfoot, Sassafras).

Diastolic the second (or bottom) number in a blood pressure reading. It is the blood pressure in the heart and arteries when the heart relaxes between contractions. It is the pressure in your "pipes" (vascular system).

Digestants contains substances (i.e., ferments, acids, enzymes and bitters) which aid in digestion of food (Coriander, Sage, Cinnamon).

Digestion the process by which food is broken down mechanically and chemically in the gastrointestinal tract and converted into absorbable form, or their simplest forms.

Diluents herbs that dilute secretions and excretions (Flax Seed).

Discutients herbs that dispel or resolve (dissolve) tumors and abnormal growths (Bayberry, Chickweed, Coltsfoot, Burdock Root).

Disinfectants herbs that eliminate or destroy the noxious properties of decaying organic matter and thereby prevent the spreading or transfer of toxic matter or infection (Black Walnut Hulls/Leaves, Cajuput, Myrrh, Rue, Uva Ursi).

Diuretics promote activity of the kidney and bladder, and increase urination through the excretion of water. (Tansy, Uva Ursi, Stone Root, Dandelion).

Diverticuli pathological sac-like out-pouchings of the wall of the colon caused by impactions and weaknesses of the intestinal wall.

Doctrine of Signatures theory that the appearance of a plant indicates its inherent properties.

Dopamine A neurotransmitter produced in the medulla portion of the adrenal glands. Used to treat hypotension and Parkinson's disease.

Drastics herbs that are hyperactive cathartics producing violent peristalsis, watery stools and much griping pain (Castor Oil, Hedge Hyssop, Red and White Bryony).

Dropsy generalized edema in cellular tissue or in a body cavity.

Dyskinesia defect in voluntary movement.

Dysmenorrhea painful or difficult menstruation (False Unicorn, Cramp Bark, Wild Yam Root, Red Raspberry).

Dyspepsia imperfect or painful indigestion; not a disease in itself but symptomatic of other diseases or disorders.

Dyspnea sense of difficulty in breathing, often associated with lung or heart disease. Also a sign of congestion and acidosis.

Edema retention of fluid in tissues (swelling). A result of acidosis. The body's effort to alkalize.

Electrolytes Soluble salts dissolved in the body's fluids. Electrolytes are the form in which most minerals circulate in the body. They are capable of conducting electrical impulses (includes salts of sodium and potassium). These are considered the positively charged electrons (positive ions which have less electrons). They facilitate and carry electrical charges better than negative ions, which have more electrons dominating protons. They are called cations and create an alkaline medium.

Elimination 1. excretion of waste products by the skin, kidneys, and intestines. 2. also refers to the elimination of carbon dioxide from the lungs.

Elements in chemistry, a substance that cannot be separated into substances different from itself by ordinary chemical processes. Elements exist in free and combined states. More than 100 have been identified. Elements found in the human body include oxygen, aluminum, carbon, cobalt, hydrogen, nitrogen, calcium, phosphorus, potassium, sulfur, sodium, chlorine, magnesium, iron, fluorine, iodine, copper, manganese, and zinc.

Emetic induces vomiting (Black Mustard, Blood Root, Mistletoe).

Emmenagogue helps promote and regulate menstruation (Saw Palmetto, False Unicorn, Nettle).

Emollient soothes, softens and protects the skin, or soothes the irritated mucosa.

Emulsion a combination of two liquids that do not mix with each other, such as oil and water; one substance is broken into tiny droplets and is suspended within the other. Emulsification is the first step in the digestion of fats.

Enervate to deprive of strength, vigor, etc.; to weaken physically and mentally.

Endocrine System the system of glands that secrete hormones, steroids, and neurotransmitters directly into the bloodstream. They include the pituitary, thyroid, thymus and adrenal glands, as well as the pancreas, ovaries and testes.

Endorphin natural opiates produced in the brain that function as the body's own natural painkillers; they also have a calming effect upon the muscles and tissues of the body.

Enteritis inflammation of the small intestine.

Enterorrhagia hemorrhage from the intestine.

Enuresis involuntary urination.

Enzyme an organic catalyst produced by living cells but capable of acting independently. Enzymes are complex proteins that are capable of inducing chemical changes in other substances without being changed themselves. Enzymes are present in digestive juices, where they act upon food substances, causing them to break down into simpler compounds. They are capable of accelerating the speed of chemical reactions.

Ephidrosis abnormal amount of sweating.

Epidermis the outermost layer of the skin.

Epigastric upper middle region of abdomen.

Epinephrine Known as adrenaline, it is a neurotransmitter secreted by the adrenal medulla in response to stimulation of the sympathetic nervous system. Low levels cause some of the physiological expressions of fear and anxiety and have been found in excess in some anxiety disorders. It's also produced by tissues other than the adrenals. It is responsible for the Fight or Flight Syndrome/response.

Epithelial Cells the cells that cover the entire surface of the body and that line most of the internal organs.

Epstein-Barr Virus the virus that causes infectious mononucleosis and that is associated with Burkitt's lymphoma and nasopharyngeal cancer.

Errhines herbs that increase nasal secretions from the sinuses (Blood Root, Horseradish, Ginger).

Essential a term for nutrients needed for building and repairing that cannot be manufactured by the body, and that therefore must be supplied in the diet. At present, there are at least forty-two known essential nutrients. (There are many different opinions of what truly is "essential" and what is created by the body itself as a natural side-effect of metabolism.)

Essential Fatty Acids (EFA) unsaturated fatty acids (linoleic, linolenic, and arachidonic) which cannot be synthesized in the body and are considered essential for maintaining health.

Essential Oils also known as volatile oils, ethereal oils, or essences. They are usually complex mixtures of a wide variety of organic compounds (e.g., alcohols, ketones, phenols, acids, ethers, esters, aldehydes and oxides) that evaporate when exposed to air. They generally represent the odoriferous principles of plants and have a broad range effect upon the body, especially the nervous system.

Estrogen female hormone (steroid) responsible for stimulating the development and maintenance of female secondary sex characteristics. Aggressive and acid-forming vasodilating properties.

Evacuants remedies which evacuate; mostly applies to purgatives.

Evening Primrose Oil the seed oil of Evening Primrose, rich in gamma linolenic acid.

Excito-Motors herbs that increase motor reflex and spinal activity.

Exocrine a term applied to glands whose secretion reaches an epithelial surface, either directly or through a duct. Opposite of endocrine.

Exophthalmic protrusion of the eyeball.

Expectorant promotes discharge of phlegm and mucus from lungs and throat (Mullein, Red Root, Lungwort).

Extract a preparation in which the properties of an herb are drawn out by solvents, heat, or other processes.

Fats 1. Adipose tissue of the body, which serves as an energy reserve. 2. Grease, oil. 3. In chemistry, triglyceride ester of fatty acids; one of a group of organic compounds closely associated in nature with the phosphatides, cerebrosides, and sterols. The term lipid is applied in general to a fat or fat-like substance. Fats are insoluble in water but soluble in either chloroform, benzene, or other fat solvents. Fats are hydrolyzed by the action of acids, alkalies, lipases (fat-splitting enzymes) and superheated steam.

Fat-soluble capable of dissolving in the same organic solvents as fats and oils. Not soluble in water.

Fatty Acids any one of many organic acids from which fats and oils are made.

Febrifuge reduces fever (Fringe Tree, Feverfew, Tansy).

Fermentation the oxidative decomposition of complex substances through the action of enzymes or ferments, produced by microorganisms; bacteria, molds, and yeasts are the principal groups of organisms involved in fermentation.

Fiber the indigestible portion of plant matter. Fiber is an important component of a healthy diet because it is capable of binding to toxins and carrying them out of the body. Acts as an electrical intestinal broom.

Fistula abnormal (tube-like) passage between two internal organs, or from an organ to the surface of the body.

Flavin one of a group of natural water-soluble pigments occurring in milk, yeasts, bacteria, and some plants.

Flavonoidial and Flavone Glycosides Glycosides have a broad range effect on the body. Each glycoside has its own individual effect as well. Some are antispasmodic, diuretic, increase circulation, and act upon cardiac tissue. Flavonoid complexes known as bioflavonoids are essential to vitamin C absorption and calcium absorption (all occur in nature together). Some flavonoid glycosides (bioflavonoids) include hesperidin, rutin, and vitamin P.

Free Radicals a group of atoms that are highly chemically reactive because they have at least one unpaired electron. Because they join so readily with other compounds, free radicals can attack cells and cause a lot of damage in the body. They form in heated fats and oils, and as a result of exposure to atmospheric radiation and environmental pollutants, among other things. (A human ingests over 125 lbs. of chemicals per year. Talk about free radicals!)

Fungus   one of a class of organisms that include yeasts, mold, and mushrooms. A number of fungal species, such as Candida albicans, are capable of causing severe disease in immuno-compromised hosts.

Galactagogue   promotes secretion of milk (Anise Seed, Fennel, Vervain).

Galactophyga   herbs that diminish or arrest the secretion of milk (Bilberry, Cassia Bark, Cranes-bill).

Gastralgia   pain in the stomach.

Gastritis   inflammation of the stomach lining.

Gastroenteritis   inflammation of the mucous lining of the stomach and intestinal tract.

Gland   an organ or tissue that secretes a substance for use elsewhere in the body rather than for its own functioning.

Giardia   a genus of flagellate protozoa some of which are parasitic, found in the intestinal tract of humans and domestic animals; transmitted by ingestion of cysts in fecally- contaminated water and food; interferes with the absorption of fats; boiling water inactivates them.

Gleet   the mucous discharge in the urine from urethra, in cases of chronic gonorrhea.

Glucose   a simple sugar that is the principal source of energy for the body's cells.

Gluten   vegetable albumin, a protein that can be prepared from wheat, rye, barley, and oats.

Glycogen   a polysaccharide (complex carbohydrate) that is the main form in which glucose is stored in the body, mostly in the liver and muscles. It is converted back into glucose as needed to supply the body with energy.

Gout   inflammation of the joints. Joints affected may be at any location, but gout usually begins in the knee or foot.

Hair Analysis   a method of determining the levels of minerals, including both toxic metals and essential minerals, in the body by measur-ing the concentrations of those minerals in the hair. Unlike mineral levels in the blood, those in the hair reflect the person's status over several preceding months and their utilization at the cellular level.

Heavy Metals   metallic elements whose specific gravity (a measurement of mass as compared with the mass of water or hydrogen) is greater than 5.0. Some heavy metals, such as arsenic, cadmium, lead, and mercury, are extremely toxic.

Hemetics   herbs rich in iron and manganese and which augment and enrich the red corpus-cles of the blood (blood-builders) (Agrimony, Quassia, Yellow Dock, Dandelion).

Hemiplegia   paralysis of one half of the body.

Hemoglobin   the red (iron-containing) pig-ment in blood that carries oxygen from the lungs to the tissues of the body. Hemoglobin is a con-jugated protein consisting of heme (which is an iron carrier) and globin (which is a simple pro-tein carrier).

Hemolytic   1. a substance which destroys red blood cells; 2. related to the destruction of red blood cells.

Hemostatic   stops the flow of blood; type of as-tringent that stops internal bleeding or hemor-rhaging.

Hepatics   herbs used to strengthen, tone and stimulate the secretive functions of the liver, causing an increased flow of bile (Goldenseal, Dandelion, Milk Thistle, Oregon Grape).

Herbal Therapies   the use of herbal combina-tions for healing or cleansing purposes. Herbs can be used in tinctures, tablets, capsules or ex-tract form, as well as in baths, poultices, teas, etc.

Herpatics   herbs that are healing to skin erup-tions and scaling diseases such as ringworm. (Buckthorn Bark, Chickweed, Cleavers, Com-frey).

Histamine   a chemical released by the immune system that acts on various body tissues. It has the effect of constricting the smooth bronchial tube muscles, dilating small blood vessels, thus allowing fluid to leak from various tissues, and increasing the secretion of stomach acid.

Holistic Medicine a form of therapy aimed at treating the whole person (mind, body and spirit), not just the part or parts in which symptoms occur.

Homeostasis equilibrium of internal environment.

Hormone chemical messengers released by the glands of the endocrine system. They are released directly into the bloodstream and carried to the tissues they affect. Hormones fall into two categories: proteins and steroids. All hormones are extremely potent. They are effective in very small amounts.

Hormonal Agents herbs that contain phytosterols, or hormones used by the plant for its own growth, are compatible with female hormones and appear to work as building blocks to provide ready-made material for hormonal production. Some herbs, like Chaste Tree Berry, are thought to work on the level of the pituitary gland (the "mother of the female hormones"), and can produce either an oestrogenic or progestogenic effect, as the body turns it to its own use. Those known as oestrogenic are used to treat estrogen deficiency problems and are certainly effective (False Unicorn Root). Wild Yam provides the only known natural plant source of progesterone.

Hormonal System consists of a series of tissues, glands, and cells. The glands produce chemicals (hormones) that are secreted into the bloodstream. These chemicals are either directly released into the bloodstream (through endocrine glands) or released through tubes called ducts (exocrine glands). The hormones stimulate other cells or organs. They regulate many of the body's activities, including growth, development, and homeostasis. There may be as many as 100 hormones in the human body, but not all have been determined. The major exocrine glands are all associated with the digestive system. The major hormone-secreting endocrine

glands in the body are the thyroid, adrenal, pituitary, pineal, parathyroid, and pancreas (pancreas is both exocrine and endocrine). There are two gender-specific endocrine glands—the ovaries in females, and the testes in males.

Hydragogue promotes watery evacuation of bowels.

Hydrochloric Acid (HCL) a normal constituent of gastric juice. The amount of HCL concentration in the stomach varies, depending on several factors, including rate of secretion of gastric juice and the type of food eaten. It converts pepsinogen into pepsin and produces an acid medium favorable for the activity of pepsin; dissolves and disintegrates nucleoproteins and collagen; hydrolyzes sucrose; precipitates caseinogen; inhibits multiplication of bacteria, especially putrefactive organisms that ferment lactic acid and certain pathogenic forms; stimulates secretion by the duodenum; inhibits the action of ptyalin and thus stops salivary digestion in the stomach.

Hyperchlorhydria excess of hydrochloric acid in gastric secretion (insufficient gastric acid output).

Hyperglycemia an abnormal concentration of sugar in the blood.

Hypertension chronic high blood pressure often caused by stress.

Hypertensive used to increase blood pressure.

Hyperthyroidism (overactive thyroid) a condition caused by excessive secretion of the thyroid glands, which increases the basal metabolic rate, causing an increased demand for food to support this metabolic activity. Signs and symptoms—goiter, fine tremor of the extended fingers and tongue, increased nervousness, weight loss, altered bowel activity, heat intolerance, excessive sweating, increased heart rate. Inorganic iodine deposits, drugs, chemicals and congestion create acidosis and stimulation of this gland. Hyperthyroidism always leads to hypothyroidism or the weakening of the thyroid gland.

Hypnotics powerful nervine relaxants and

sedatives that induce sleep (Wild Lettuce, Passion Flower, Valerian).

Hypoactive   1. "Hypo" is Greek for below, beneath or under. 2. underactive gland or organ.

Hypoglycemia   abnormally low level of glucose in the blood; "low blood sugar."

Hypothalamus   the area of the brain that contains neurosecretions that are of importance in the control of certain metabolic activities, such as maintenance of water balance, sugar and fat metabolism, regulation of body temperature, secretion of releasing and inhibiting hormones, and the hunger response. It houses the pituitary gland and is considered the "master switch board."

Hypothyroidism   a condition due to deficiency of the thyroid secretion, resulting in a lowered basal metabolism. Symptoms may include obesity or difficulty losing weight, dry skin and hair, low blood pressure, slow pulse, sluggishness of all functions, depressed muscular activity, and depression.

Hypertension   high blood pressure. Usually defined as a regular resting pressure of 140/90.

Hypotensives   used to reduce blood pressure.

Iatrogenic literally, "physician induced." This term can be applied to any medical condition, disease, or other adverse occurrence that results from medical treatment.

Immunostimulant   an agent that stimulates the immune system in a non-specific manner.

Infection   invasion of body tissues by disease-causing organisms such as viruses, protozoa, fungi or bacteria.

Inflammation   1. tissue reaction to injury; 2. Inflammation is not infection. It is a reaction of your immune system in your body to an acidic compound or injury to tissue. The succession of changes that occur in living tissue when it is injured in any way. The inflamed area undergoes continuous change as the body repair processes start to heal and replace injured tissue. 3. Inflammation is a conservative process modified by whatever produces the reaction, but it should not be confused with infection; the two are relatively different conditions, although one may arise from the other. Acidosis is one of the greatest causes of inflammation. Inflammation is counter-balanced by the body with steroids, cholesterol, electrolytes and antioxidants.

Infusion   an herbal tea.

Insulin   a hormone produced by the pancreas that regulates the metabolism of glucose (sugar) in the body. Acts as a carrier through cell membrane walls.

Interferon   1. a protein produced by the cells in response to viral infection that prevents viral reproduction and is capable of protecting uninfected cells from viral infection. Includes alpha, beta, and gamma; 2. a group of proteins released by white blood cells that combat a virus; 3. a potent immune-enhancing substance that is produced by the body's cells to fight off viral infection and cancer.

Intestinal Flora   the "friendly" bacteria and other microorganisms normally present in the intestines that are essential for the digestion and metabolism of different nutrients and foodstuffs.

In Vitro   outside a living body and in an artificial environment, like a laboratory (e.g., in test tubes).

In Vivo   in a living body of an animal, plant or human, outside of a controlled environment or laboratory.

Incontinence   the inability to control urination or defecation.

Indolent   sluggish; causing little or no pain, slow to heal.

Inferior   below.

Insecticides   herbs that are used to destroy or repel insects (Black Walnut Hulls/Leaves, Black Cohosh, Rue, Quassia).

Intercostal   between the ribs.

Interstitial   placed or lying between (spaces within an organ or tissue); around the outside of cells.

Interleukin a type of cytokine that enables communication among leukocytes and other cells active in inflammation or the cell-mediated immune response. The result is a maximized response to a microorganism or other foreign antigen.

Intracellular within cells.

Irritants herbs that produce a greater or lesser degree of vascular excitement when applied to the epidermis or skin surface (Cascara Sagrada, Kava Kava resin, Stinging Nettle, Stone Root).

Jaundice a condition caused by elevation of bilirubin in the body and characterized by a yellowing of the skin.

Jejunum the second portion of the small intestines (from duodenum to the ileum). It's about eight feet long and comprises two-fifths of the small intestine.

Laxatives mild purgatives. Promote bowel movements.

Lesions a circumscribed area of pathologically altered tissue; an injury or wound; a single infected patch in a skin disease.

Lipid any one of a group of fats or fat-like substances characterized by their insolubility in water and sollubility in fat solvents such as alcohol, ether, and chloroform. The term is descriptive rather than a chemical name such as protein or carbohydrate. Includes true fats (esters of fatty acids and glycerol); lipoids (phospholipids, cerebrosides, waxes); and sterols (cholesterol, ergosterol).

Lipotropic promoting the flow of lipids to and from the liver.

Lithotriptics dissolves or discharges urinary and biliary concretion (like kidney stones). Helps dissolve calculi within the body. (Bitter Root, Butcher's Broom, Cleavers).

Local Anesthetics herbs that produce loss of sensation (anesthesia) when applied locally to a surface (Caraway Oil, Coca, Kava Kava).

Lymph fluid contained in lymphatic vessels, that flows through the lymphatic system to be returned to the blood. The lymph is to the immune cells what blood serum is to red blood cells. Lymph cleans itself through the kidneys, colon and skin.

Lymphatic System that system including all structures involved in the conveyance of lymph from the tissues to the bloodstream. It includes the lymph capillaries, lacteals, lymph nodes, lymph vessels, and main lymph ducts (thoracic and right lymphatic duct).

Lymph Nodes organs located in the lymphatic vessels that act as filters, trapping and removing foreign materials. They also form lymphocytes, which are immune cells that develop the capacity to seek out and destroy specific foreign agents. Lymph nodes are like septic tanks that hold and neutralize toxins and foreign proteins by immune cells and/or enzymes.

Lymphocyte a type of white blood cell found in lymph, blood, and other specialized tissues, such as the bone marrow and tonsils. There are several different categories of lymphocytes, designated B-lymphocytes, T-lymphocytes, and null (or non-B, non-T) lymphocytes. These cells are crucial components of the immune system. B-lymphocytes are primarily responsible for antibody production, whereas the T-lymphocytes are involved in the direct attack against invading organisms. It is the T-helper cell, a subtype of T-lymphocyte, that is the primary cell infected and destroyed by human immuno-deficiency virus (HIV), the virus that causes AIDS (man made).

Kidneys a pair of organs sitting at the back of the abdominal cavity that form urine from blood plasma. Each kidney's more than one million small filtering units (called glomeruli) process chemical wastes and excess water in the body, which produces urine. They are the major regulators of the water and electrolytes, and maintain the acid-base content of the blood and body fluids. The kidneys are one of the body's four eliminative organs. Lack of proper elimination means a stagnant lymphatic system.

Kupffer's Cells About 50 percent of all macrophages are found in the liver as Kupffer cells.

Macrophages 1. a monocyte that has left the circulation and settled and matured in a tissue; 2. Along with neutrophils, macrophages are the major phagocytic cells of the immune system. They have the ability to recognize and ingest all foreign antigens through receptors on the surface of their cell membranes; these antigens are then destroyed by lysosomes. Their placement in the peripheral lymphoid tissues enables macrophages to serve as the major scavengers of the blood, clearing it of abnormal or old cells and cellular debris as well as pathogenic organisms. 3. They also serve a vital role by processing antigens and presenting them to T cells, activating the specific immune response. They also release many chemical mediators that are involved in the body's defenses, including interleukin-1 and complement.

Malabsorption nutritionally, an inability to absorb nutrients from the intestinal tract into the bloodstream. Primarily due to impactions, inflammation and poor pancreatic digestion.

Maturating herbs that promote the maturation or ripening (bringing to a head) of tumors, boils, ulcers, carbuncles, etc. (Bayberry Bark, Burdock Root, Plantain, Yellow Dock).

Menorrhagia excessive bleeding during menstruation.

Meridians in Chinese medicine, the specific pathways of energy flow in the body. The fourteen channels in the body through which *qi* (universal energy or God force) runs.

Metabolism the physical and chemical processes necessary to sustain life, including the production of cellular energy, the synthesis of important biological substances, and degradation of various compounds.

Minerals 1. an inorganic element or compound (especially one that is solid) occurring in nature. (Inorganic, not of animal or plant origin.); 2. an inorganic substance required by the body in small quantities.

Molecule 1. the smallest quantity into which a substance may be divided without loss of its characteristics; 2. a chemical combination of two or more atoms that form a specific chemical compound.

Monocytes white blood cells that are one of the first lines of defense in the inflammatory process.

Monoplegia paralysis of a single limb.

Montmorillonite lake clays used in nutrition as a source of trace minerals.

Mucus a viscid fluid secreted by mucous membranes and glands, consisting of mucin, leukocytes, inorganic salts, water, and epithelial cells. This mucus acts as a protectant and detoxificant.

Mucilages herbs having mucilaginous (soothing) properties on inflamed mucous membranes and tissues (Bladderwrack, Comfrey, Evening Primrose, Marshmallow).

Mydriatic dilates (enlarges) the pupil (Belladonna, Coca, Scopola).

Myotics herbs that cause contraction of the ciliary muscles of the eye (makes the pupil smaller) (Arena Nut, Jaborandi).

Narcotics depresses central nervous system, thus relieving pain and promoting sleep (Belladonna, Coca, Grindelia).

Nauseants herbs that produce nausea or an urge to vomit when taken in large doses (similar to emetics) (Lobelia, Quassia, Vervain).

Nephritis inflammation of the kidney (Bugleweed, Culver's Root, Horse Chestnut).

Nervine a tonic for the nerves. Helps to relieve pain and regulate the nervous system. Also strengthens functional activity of nervous system. May be stimulant or sedative. (Skullcap, Lobelia, Valerian).

Neurasthenia severe nerve weakness; nervous exhaustion.

Neuromuscular concerning both the nerves and muscles.

Neuropathy a complex of symptoms caused by abnormalities in motor or sensory nerves. Symptoms may include tingling or numbness, especially in the hands or feet, followed by gradual, progressive muscular weakness.

Neurotransmitter 1. a chemical substance that transmits nerve impulses from one nerve cell to another (includes acetylcholine, dopamine, gamma-aminobutyric acid, epinephrine, nor-epinephrine, and serotonin); 2. substances that transmit nerve impulses to the brain.

Neurotics acts upon the nervous system.

Neutrophils are responsible for much of the body's protection against infection. They play a primary roll in inflammation, are readily attracted to foreign antigens (chemotaxis), and destroy them by phagocytosis.

NK Cells natural killer cells.

Norepinephrine a neurotransmitter produced by the adrenal medulla, similar in chemical and pharmacological properties to epinephrine, but it is chiefly a vasoconstrictor and has little effect on cardiac output.

Nutraceutical 1. a food- or nutrient-based product or supplement designed or used for a specific clinical or therapeutic purpose; 2. using the active principle from an herb; increasing its potency; then adding it back to form a high potency formula.

Nutrients substances needed by the body to maintain life and health.

Nutritives increases weight and density; nourishes the body. Helps supply material for tissue rebuilding.

Oestrogenic a substance affecting female sexual functions.

Opthalmic healing to disorders and diseases of the eyes (Bilberry, Eyebright, Marshmallow).

Osteomyelitis inflammation of the bone, especially the marrow.

Osteoporosis a disorder in which minerals leach out of the bones, making them progressively more porous and fragile. A result of acidosis and hypothyroidism.

Ovaries 1. located in the pelvic cavity of women; responsible for development of sex characteristics; some effects on growth; 2. produces the ovum (egg) and secretes the female hormones estrogen and progesterone.

Oxidation a chemical reaction in which oxygen reacts with another substance, resulting in a chemical transformation. Many oxidation reactions result in some type of deterioration or spoilage.

Oxytocin pituitary hormone that stimulates uterine contractions (to induce and assist labor in childbirth) and the production of milk.

Oxyuris genus of nematode intestinal worms which includes pinworms (also called threadworm and seatworm).

Pancreas Both an exocrine and endocrine organ, it secretes enzymes (amylase, lipase) that aid in the digestion of food in the small intestine; it also produces hormones (glucagon, insulin) which, when taken up by the bloodstream, help regulate carbohydrate metabolism by controlling blood sugar levels.

Parasite an organism that lives and feeds upon the weaknesses and toxicity of another organism, known as the host, without contributing to survival of the host. Within the human body parasites can invade weakened cells or live in a toxic lymph system.

Parasiticides herbs that kill or destroy animal and vegetable parasites within the body.

Parasympathetic Nervous System part of the autonomic nervous system that normally acts as a balance for the sympathetic system once a crisis has passed or in non-stressful situations. It brings about constriction of the pupils, slowing of the heart rate, and constriction of the bronchial tubes. It also stimulates the formation and release of urine and activity of the digestive tract. For example, saliva flows more easily and its quantity and fluidity increase.

Parathyroid gland located on the back side of the thyroid gland, it secretes a hormone, parathormone, that regulates calcium and phosphorus metabolism. Indirectly affects muscular irritability. Weaknesses include hypoparathyroidism or hyperparathyroidism.

Pathogen a microorganism or substance (foreign protein) capable of producing an immune response; creating pathological changes.

Paturient stimulates uterine contractions that induce and assist labor (Birthwort, Black and Blue Cohosh, Rue).

Pectoral healing to problems in the broncho-pulmonary area.

Pepsin the chief enzyme of gastric (stomach) juice, which converts proteins into proteoses and peptones. It is formed by the cells of gastric glands and produces its maximum activity at a pH of 1.25 to 2.25.

Peristalsis a progressive wavelike contraction of the smooth muscles of the digestive tract or the colon muscles that move food byproducts along and expel waste matter.

Peristaltics herbs that stimulate and increase peristalsis, or muscular contractions (as in the bowels) (Aloe, Cascara Sagrada, olive oil, Turkey Rhubarb powder).

Petechiae bruising.

pH (potential of hydrogen) a scale used to measure the relative acidity or alkalinity of substances. The scale goes from 0 to 14, with 7 being considered neutral. Below 7 indicates more acidic, above 7 indicates more alkaline.

Phagocytosis the destruction of bacteria (microorganisms) and/or particles through ingestion and digestion by a phagocyte (an immune cell).

Phenolic Compounds phenol or phenolic compounds make up many important constituents of botanicals. These phenolic compounds are antiseptic, anti-inflammatory, anti- spasmodic, and pain-killing in their actions. Phenolic compounds combined with a sugar can form glycosides.

Phytochemical any one of many substances present in fruits and vegetables that have various health-promoting properties. Phytochemicals appear to protect against certain types of cancer. Most plant constituents could be called phytochemicals.

Pineal Gland an endocrine gland in the brain, shaped like a pinecone. The pineal gland synthesizes melatonin. Melatonin is inhibited when light strikes the retina. This small gland is considered by many to be the spiritual gland. One of the seats or doorways for Spirit in the physical world.

Pituitary Gland a small, gray, rounded body attached to the base of the brain secreting hormones that regulate the thyroid, adrenals, and other endocrine organs. It is often referred to as the "Master Gland" of the body and secretes a number of hormones that regulate many bodily processes including growth, reproduction and various metabolic activities.

Plaque a fatty, fibrous, cholesterol-containing mass in the lining of the arteries and other tissues. The buildup of plaque in the arteries is a leading cause of cardiovascular occlusions, causing strokes and heart attacks. Plaque deposits on the teeth can lead to gum disease. Alzheimer's disease is associated with the accumulation of plaque in the brain tissue causing a lack of nutrition to cells.

Platelets round, oval disks found in the blood of vertebrates. They are fragments of megakaryocytes, large cells found in the bone marrow. Platelets play in important role in blood coagulation, hemostasis, and blood thrombus formation.

Poultice an external (topical) herbal concoction applied to an injury, burn, tumor, boil, etc.

Portal concerning entrance to an organ, especially that through which blood is carried to liver.

Posterior towards the rear or caudal end; opposed to anterior. In humans, toward the back; dorsal. Situated behind, coming after.

Progesterone 1. an anti-inflammatory steroid; 2. aids in the growth and development of female reproductive organs and secondary sexual characteristics; 3. causes growth and maturation of the endometrium of the uterus during the menstrual cycle. Sometimes used to treat menstrual disorders and menopause issues.

Prophylactic agents that ward off disease.

Prostaglandin any number of hormone-like

chemicals that are made in the body from essential fatty acids and that have important effects on many organs. They influence the secretion of hormones and enzymes, and are important in regulating the inflammatory response, blood pressure, and blood clotting time.

Protectives herbs that serve as protective coverings to abraded, inflamed or injured parts when applied locally to a surface (Acadia, Castor Oil, Flaxseed, Marshmallow).

Proteins complex nitrogen-based organic compounds made up of different combinations of amino acids. Proteins are basic elements of all animal and vegetable tissues. Biological substances such as hormones and enzymes are also composed of protein. The body makes the specific proteins it needs for growth, repair, and other functions from amino acids that are either extracted from dietary protein or manufactured from other amino acids. Proteins also serve as carriers (e.g., hemoglobin, insulin, etc.).

Pruritis severe itching.

Pungents herbs that cause a sharply pricking, acrid and penetrating sensation to the sensory organs (Black Pepper, Cardamom, Cayenne, Mustard).

Purgative a substance that promotes the vigorous evacuation of the bowels; usually used to relieve severe constipation.

Putrefaction 1. decay and rot; 2. decomposition of animal matter, especially protein associated with malodorous and poisonous products such as the ptomaines, mercaptans, and hydrogen sulfide, caused by certain kinds of bacteria and fungi; also, the process of breaking down protein compounds by rotting.

Pyelitis inflammation of the pelvis, of the kidney and its calices.

Qi or ch'i in Chinese, the concept of life force; vital energy.

Red Blood Cells blood cells that contain the red pigment hemoglobin and transport oxygen and carbon dioxide in the bloodstream.

Regeneration rebuilding and strengthening the body. Requires an alkaline medium with electrically "alive" nutrients.

Refrigerant reduces body temperature and relieves thirst (Barberry, Borage, Couch Grass, Chickweed).

Relaxant tends to relax and relieve tension, especially muscular tension.

Resolvents help promote resolution, or dissipation, of pathological growths (Chickweed, Elder, Milk Thistle, St. John's Wort).

Restorative an agent that is effective in the regaining of health and strength; restores normal physiological activity (Astragalus Root, all Ginsengs, and Goldenseal).

Rhinitis inflammation of nasal mucosa.

Rhizome an underground stem, often creeping.

Rouleau adhesion or sticking together of red blood cells. Caused by acidosis, which creates an anionic atmosphere in which lipids, amino acids, minerals, etc., adhere to cell walls and each other.

Rubefacient with local application stimulates capillary dilation and action (drawing blood from deeper tissues and organs and thereby relieving congestion and inflammation), causing skin redness (Black Bryony, Cayenne, Cloves, Stinging Nettle, Horseradish, Sassafras, Jamaican Ginger).

Saponins compounds in plants important for their anti-inflammatory and expectorant properties. Saponins have been used in the synthesis of cortisone and in some cases, the sex hormones.

Saturated Fat 1. a fat that is solid at room temperature. Most saturated fats are of animal origin, except for a few, such as coconut oil and palm oil, that come from plants. 2. fully bonded fatty acids.

Scorbutic concerning or affected with scurvy.

Scrofula variety of tuberculous adenitis.

Sedative calms or tranquilizes by lowering functional activity.

Septicemia presence of pathogenic bacteria in the blood; blood poisoning.

Serotonin a neurotransmitter found primarily

in the brain; considered essential for relaxation, sleep, and concentration.

Serum   the fluid portion of the blood.

Sialogogue   promotes secretion and flow of saliva (Blue Flag, Elder Bark, Turkey Rhubarb).

Simple Carbohydrate   a type of carbohydrate that, owing to its basic chemical structure, is rapidly digested and absorbed into the bloodstream. For example: glucose, galactose, and fructose.

Smooth Muscle Tissue (*Muscularis Mucesae*) also known as the Involuntary (visceral, smooth) Muscle System. These are the muscles in the stomach and intestines, the walls of arteries and veins, and several other places in the body. They respond automatically, without conscious control (although a person does have partial control over some of these muscles). They are usually unstriated and smooth, especially those muscles in the gut.

Solution   a liquid or gas, which consists of one or more substances (solutes). The liquid in which the substances are dissolved is called the solvent and the substance dissolved, the solute.

Somatic   related to non-reproductive cells or tissues.

Somnifacient   soporifics.

Soporifics   herbs that induce a relaxing sleep (Catnip, Hops, Passion Flower, Valerian).

Sorbefacients   cause absorption.

Spasmolytic   tending to check spasms. (See: Antispasmodic.)

Specifics   herbs which have a direct curative influence upon certain individual tissue weaknesses.

Spermatorrhea   abnormally frequent involuntary loss of semen without orgasm.

Spondylosis   abnormal immobility and fixation of vertebral joints.

Squamous Cells   a flat, scaly, epithelial cell.

Steroids   hormones derived from lipids and produced by the adrenal cortex and the sex glands. They have a wide range of effects. Steroids can act as anti-inflammatories, and affect metabolism, and reproduction, as well as systemic anabolism and catabolism. Systemic steroids are produced in the adrenal glands. Reproductive steroids are produced in the gonads.

Sternutatories   herbs that are irritating to the mucous membranes in nasal passages, which cause sneezing (Wood Betony, Bayberry, Cayenne, Sneezewort).

Stimulants   herbs that increase functional activity and energy in the body (strengthens metabolism and circulation) (Boneset, Brigham Tea [Ephedra], Feverfew, Ginseng, Prickly Ash, Red Clover, Rosemary, Wormwood, Yarrow).

Stimulation   irritating action on muscles, nerves, or sensory end organs by which activity in a part is evoked.

Stomachics   help strengthen the functions of the stomach. Help promote digestion, appetite, and relieve indigestion.

Styptics   help arrest bleeding through a strongly astringent action. Also contracts blood vessels (Black Walnut, Comfrey, Plantain, Stinging Nettle).

Subcostal   beneath the ribs.

Substitute   a plant that is an acceptable replacement for another herb (See: Adulterant.)

Sudorifics   help cause active or droplet perspiration. Stimulate production and secretion of perspiration.

Sugars (simple)   sugar in its simplest form biologically.

Sugars (complex)   two or more simple sugar molecules bonded together (e.g., maltose, dextrose, sucrose, etc.).

Superior   above.

Sympathetic Nervous System   part of the autonomic nervous system that tends to act as an accelerator for those organs needed to meet a stressful situation. The sympathetic division dominates during stressful situations, such as anger or fright, and the body responses contribute to fight or flight, with unimportant activities such as digestion markedly slowed. Most sympathetic neurons release the neurotransmitter norepinephrine.

Syndrome   a group of signs and symptoms that occur together in a pattern characteristic of a particular "disease" or abnormal condition related to a specific effect.

Synergistic   the simultaneous action of two or more substances whose combined effect is greater than the sum of each working alone.

Systems of the Human Body   fourteen in all; nine major systems. They are: Circulatory, Digestive, Eliminative (Intestinal, Lymphatic, Urinary, Integumentary, and Immune), Glandular, Muscular, Nervous, Reproductive, Respiratory, and Skeletal.

Systemic   relating to or affecting the entire body.

Systolic   the period of greatest pressure in the arterial vascular system affected directly by the adrenal medula and neuro-transmitter release.

Taeniafuges and Taeniacides   herbs that expel (taeniafuges) or kill (taeniacides) tapeworms in the intestinal tract (Castor Oil, Cucumber Seeds, Male Fern, Pumpkin Seeds).

Tannins   substances in plants that possess astringent properties. Tannins bind and act upon various chemicals and proteins to form protection to the skin and mucus membranes. Tannins are known to help reduce diarrhea, internal bleeding, reduce inflammation, burns, and stimulate the healing of wounds. Tannins act with infectious conditions.

Tapeworm   any of several ribbon-like worms that infest the intestines of invertebrates, including humans. They can grow to 20-30 feet long.

T-Cells   white blood cells that facilitate the immune system. They start out as B-cells, travel to the thymus gland and mature into T-cells. T-cells reflect conditional immune response.

Testes   located in the male scrotum. A gender-specific endocrine gland for development of sex characteristics; some effects on growth.

Testosterone   an androgen found in the testes. Testosterone is an aggressive, steroid-type hormone produced in the adrenal cortex of both men and women; responsible for sperm production and secondary sex characteristics in males.

Tetters   skin disease with pimples or blisters such as herpes, ringworm, or eczema.

Thyroid Gland   largest of the endocrine glands; located in the neck. This gland produces hormones, principally thyroxin. A hormone called calcitonin is also produced in the thyroid and is vital in calcium utilization. The main function of the thyroid hormones is to regulate metabolism for the production of heat and energy in the body tissues. When enlarged, the thyroid gland is called a goiter. The thyroid increases metabolic rate and indirectly influences growth and nutrition.

Thymus   organ located above the heart, mid sternum; important in the development of the immune response. It is essential to the maturation of T-cells.

Tincture   a preparation made by soaking (macerating) an herb in a specified amount of grain alcohol to extract its properties.

Tinea capitis   fungal skin disease of the scalp.

Tinnitus   ringing or tinkling sound in the ear.

Tonics   stimulate nutrition and increase systemal tone, energy and vigor. Enhances the entire system (Angelica, Centaury, Boneset, German Chamomile, Red Clover, Sanicle, Self-Heal, Stinging Nettle, Yarrow).

Toxemia   1. a toxic condition of the body arising from the consumption of meats, dairy products, refined sugars, candies, soda pops, grains, chemical medications, vaccinations, drugs, etc. Smoking tobacco and/or marijuana also add to systemic toxicity; 2. a condition of acidosis.

Toxicity   the quality of being poisonous. Toxicity reactions in the body impair bodily functions and/or damage cells, thereby impairing health. (*Also see:* Toxemia.)

Toxin   a poisonous substance of an animal or plant origin.

Trace Elements   minerals required by the body in very small amounts.

Triglyceride   a compound consisting of three fatty acids plus glycerol. They are the form in which fat is stored in the body, and are the primary type of lipid in the diet. These stored fats are used for additional energy if needed by the body. They act like batteries, storing energy until needed.

Unsaturated Fat any dietary fat that is liquid at room temperature. Unsaturated fats come from vegetable sources and are good sources of essential fatty acids. (Flaxseed oil, sunflower oil, safflower oil, and evening primrose oil.)

Uric Acid a waste product of the metabolism of proteins. The kidneys eliminate uric acid from the body. High protein consumption and obstructed kidneys lead to conditions such as gout (acidosis), etc.

Uremia 1. toxic condition associated with renal insufficiency produced by the retention in the blood of nitrogenous substances normally excreted by the kidneys. 2. reflections of high protein consumption or the breakdown of tissue.

Utilization the ability of the body to use a nutrient or fuel. Most utilization depends on hormones, steroids, or neurotransmitters. Consumption and absorption is not utilization.

Vasoconstrictor an agent that narrows blood-vessel openings, restricting the flow of blood through them.

Vasodepressant/Vasodilator lowers blood pressure by dilation (widening) of blood vessels.

Vermicides herbs that kill intestinal worms.

Vermifuge herbs which cause the expulsion of or repels intestinal worms and tapeworms.

Vesicants agents that causes blistering, such as poison ivy, oak or sumac.

Villi the short filamentous process found on certain membranous surfaces that act as filtering mechanisms (found in the lungs, intestines, etc.).

Vitality 1. that which distinguishes living things from the nonliving. 2. animation, action.

3. state of being alive. 4. a state of dynamic health.

Vitamin any of a group of organic substances other than proteins, carbohydrates, fats, minerals, and organic salts which are essential for normal metabolism, growth, and development of the body.

Volatile Oils aromatic oils used as essential oils therapeutically or in perfumes. Volatile oils have been used for centuries. Antiseptics; help stimulate the production of white blood cells. Causes digestive juice increase; said to relax overactive peristalsis. They are also known to have an affect on the central nervous system (sedate or stimulate). Volatile oil compounds are made from simple to complex molecules including isoprene, isopentane and terpenes.

Voluntary (skeletal) Muscle System muscles in the body that respond to conscious control from the brain, i.e., the muscles contract or lengthen, depending on the chemical messages they receive from the brain. These muscles usually look striated or striped when viewed under a microscope. They are attached to the bones by tendons.

Vulnerary assists in healing of wounds by protecting against infection and stimulating cell growth (Agrimony, Balm of Gilead, Bladderwrack, Cleavers, Comfrey, Elder, Rue).

White Blood Cell a blood cell that functions in fighting infection and in wound repair. Better known as immune cells, of which there are many types.

Yeast a type of single-celled fungus. Certain types of yeast can cause infection, most commonly in the mouth, vagina, or gastrointestinal tract. Common yeast infections include vaginitis and thrush. Candidiasis is a condition related to a yeast overgrowth of Candida albicans.

Prefixes and Suffixes

a-	Without, lack of	-cilia-	Hair-like projection
ab-	Away from, not	circum-	Around, about
-able	Capable	-clast-	Smash, break
acou-	Hearing	co-	With, together
ac-	Pertaining to, having	com-, con-	With, together
acro-	Extremities, all parts	contra-	Against, opposite
ad-	To, toward, near to	-crine	To secrete
aden-	Gland	crypto-	Hidden
-al	Expressing relationship	cysto-	Bladder or sac
-algia	Pain	-cyte-, cyto-	Cell
ambi, ambo	Around, on both sides	de-	Away from
an-	Without, not, lack of	derm-	Skin
ana-	Up, back, again	di-	Two, twice, double
angio-	Vessel	dia-	Through, apart, across
ante-	Before, forward	dis-	Apart from, opposite of
anti-	Against, counteracting	-duct-	Draw, tube, canal
arthr-	Joint	dura-	Hard
-ary	Associated with	-dynia	Pain
-asis	Condition, state of	dys-	Difficult, out of order
auto-	Self, self caused	e-, ec-	Out, away from
bi-	Two, double	ecto-	On outer side
bio-	Life	-ectomy	Cut out
-blast-	Bud, germ	-edem-	Swell
brachy-	Short	em-	In or blood
brady-	Slow	-emia	Blood
burso-	Sac	ent-	Inside, within, inner
carcin-	Cancer	endo-	Within
cardio-	Heart	entero-	Intestine
cata-	Down, lower, under	epi-	Upon, in addition to
-cele	Hollow, hernia, tumor	erythro-	Red
cephal-	Head	eu-	Well, good, normal
cerebro-	Brain	ex-	Out, away from
chol-	Bile	exo-	Outside, on outer side
cholecyst-	Gallbladder	extra-	Outside
chondr-	Cartilage	-ferent	Carry
-cide	Kill	-fistul-	A narrow passage, pipe

flex, flect	Bend, turn	megal	Enlarged
-form	Shaped like, resembling	melan-	Black
gastro-	Stomach	meso-	Middle, mid
-genesis	Produce, origin	meta-	Beyond, after, change
gloss-	Tongue	micro-	Small
glyco-	Sugar, sweet	mito-	Thread, filament
-gram	A drawing, record, write	mono-	One, single, alone
-graph	Instrument that records	-morph-	Form, shape
hem(at)-	Blood	multi-	Many, much
hemi-	Half, part of	myelo-	Marrow, spinal cord
hepato-	Liver	myo-	Muscle
hetero-	Different, opposite	narco-	Numbness
hist-	Tissue	neo-	New
homeo-	The same as, like	nephro-	Kidney
hydro-	Wet, water	neuro-	Nerve
hyper-	Over, more than normal, excessive	oculo-	Eye
hypo-	Under, below, deficient, beneath	odonto-	Tooth or teeth
		-oid	Expressing resemblance
-ia	Expressing condition	oligo-	Few, scanty, little
-iatr-	Treat, cure, heal	-ology	Study of
-id	Expressing condition	-oma	Tumor
im-	Not	-op-	See
in-	In, into	ophthalm-	Eye
infero-	On the outside, below	onco-	Mass, tumor, or swelling
infra-	Below, beneath	ortho-	Straight, normal
inter-	Between, among	-ory	Referring to
intra-	Within	-ose	Full of
-ism	Condition, state of	-osis	A condition of
iso-	Equal	osteo-	Bone
-itis	Inflammation	oto-	Ear
-ity	Expressing condition	-ous	Full of, abounding in,
kerato-	Cornea of the eye	para-	Beside, beyond, near to
kin-, cin-	To move	-pathy	Disease
leuko-	White	-pect-	Chest, breast, thorax
-liga-	Bind	-penia	Deficiency, decrease
lip-	Fat	per-	Throughout, excessive
-logy	Study of	peri-	Around, surrounding
-lysis	Breaking up, loosening, dissolving	-phag-	Eat
		-phas-	Speak, utter
macro-	Large	-phil-	Like, love
mal-	Bad	phleb-	Vein
malaco-	Soft, a soft condition	-phobia	Fear
mast-	Breast	-plas/plasia	Form, grow
		-platy	Flat, broad

-plegia	Paralyze, loss of power	squam-	Scale
-plexus	Interweaving, network	-stasis	Stop, stand still
-pne,-pnea	Breathe	steno-	Narrow
pneumo-	Air, gas, or lungs	steth-	Chest
pod-	Foot	-stomy	To make an artificial opening
-poie-	Make	sub-	Under, below, less
poly-	Many, much	super-	Above, upper, excessive
post-	After, behind	supra-	Above, upon, over
pre-, pro-	Before, in front of	sym-, syn-	Together, with
procto-	Anus, rectum	tachy-	Fast, swift
pseudo-	False	-tein	To stretch
psycho-	Mind, soul	tele-	Distant, far away
-ptosis	Falling, drooping	therm-	Heat
pulmon-	Lung	thorac-	Chest
pyo-	Pus	thromb-	Lump, clot
re-	Back, again, contrary	-tomy	Cut, incise
ren-	Kidney	tox-	Poison
retro-	Backward, contrary to the usual course	-tract	Draw
		trans-	Across, through, beyond
-rrhagia	Burst forth, pour	tri-	Three, third
-rrhea	Flow, discharge	tres-	Hole, opening
-rupt	Break	-troph-	Nourishment
sarco-	Flesh or fleshy	-trophy	Development, growth
sclero-	Hard	-tropic	Changing, influencing
scol-, scoli	Curved, twisted	-tum	Swell
-scope	Examine	ul, ule	Small, little
-sect	to cut or divide	-uria	Urine
semi-	Half, partially	utero-	Uterus
sept-	dividing wall or membrane	vaso-	Vessel
-sin	curve, fold, bend	vene-, vena-	Vein
somato-	Body	-vesic-	Bladder
somni-	Sleep	viscer-	Internal organ
splen-	Spleen	-vulse	Twitch or pull

Bibliography

Aihara, Herman. *Acid & Alkaline.* CA: George Ohsawa, Macrobiotic Foundation, 1986.

Alexander, Joe. *Blatant Raw Foodist Propaganda!* CA: Blue Dolphin Publishing, 1990.

Amber, Reuben. *Color Therapy.* NM: Aurora Press, 1983.

Anderson, Mary. *Colour Healing.* NY: Harper & Row Publishers, 1975.

Andrews, Ted. *How to Heal with Color.* MN: Llewellyn Publications, 1992.

Arlin, Dini, Wolf. *Nature's First Law: The Raw Food Diet.* CA: Maul Brothers Publishing, 2nd edition, 1997.

Arlin, Stephen. *Raw Power! Building Strength and Muscle Naturally.* CA: Maul Brothers Publishing; 2nd edition, 2000.

Balz, Rodolphe. *The Healing Power of Essential Oils.* WI: Lotus Light Press, 1st edition, 1996.

Bensky, Dan & Barolet, Randall. *Chinese Herbal Medicine: Formulas and Strategies.* WA: Eastland Press, Inc., 1990.

Bethel, May. *Healing Power of Herbs.* CA: Melvin Powers, Wilshire Book Co., 1968.

Blunt, Wilfrid and Sandra Raphae. *The Illustrated Herbal.* NY: W.W. Norton & Company, 1979.

Boxer, Arabella and Philippa Back. *The Herb Book. A Complete Guide to Culinary Herbs.* NJ: Thunder Bay Press, 1994.

Bragg, Paul and Patricia. *The Miracle of Fasting.* Health Science, 3rd edition, 1999.

Brennan, Barbara Ann. *Hands of Light.* NY: Bantam Books, 1987.

Brown, Deni. *New Encyclopedia of Herbs and Their Uses.* NY: Dorling Kindersley Publishing, 1995.

Brown, Donald. *Herbal Prescriptions for Better Health.* CA: Prima Publishing, 1996.

Carrington, Hereward. *The Natural Food of Man.* CA: Health Research, 1963.

Christopher, John. *School of Natural Healing.* UT: Christopher Publications, 1996.

Cohn, Robert. *Milk—The Deadly Poison.* NJ: Argus Publishing, Inc., 1998.

Copen, Bruce. *A Rainbow of Health.* England: Academic Publications, 1974.

Culpepper, Nicholas. *Culpepper's Color Herbal.* MA: Storey Books, 1997.

Culpepper, Nicholas. *Culpepper's Complete Herbal and English Physician.* UK: FoulSham & Co., Ltd., 1995.

Deoul, Kathleen. *Cancer Cover-Up (Genocide).* MD: Cassandra Books, 2001.

Dodt, Colleen. *The Essential Oils Book: Creating Personal Blends for Mind and Body.* VT: Storey Communications, Inc., 1996.

Douglass, William Campbell. *Milk of Human Kindness Is Not Pasteurized.* GA: Last Laugh Publishers, 1985.

Dubelle, Lee. *Proper Food Combining Works—Living Testimony.* CO: Nutri Books, Corp., 1987.

Dubin, Dale. *Rapid Interpretation of EKG's.* FL: Cover Publishing Co., 6th edition, 2000.

Dykeman, Thomas, Elias, and Peter. *Edible Wild Plants.* Benedict Lust Publications, Inc., 1990.

Ehret, Arnold. *Mucusless Diet Healing System.* Benedict Lust Publications, Inc., 2001.

Ehret, Arnold. *Rational Fasting*. Benedict Lust Publications, Inc., 2001.

Ehret, Arnold. *The Definite Cure of Chronic Constipation*. Benedict Lust Publications, Inc., 2002.

Fathman, George and Doris. *Live Foods: Nature's Perfect System of Human Nutrition*. NY: Cancer Care Inc., 1986.

Feeney, Mary. *The Cardiac Rhythms: A Systematic Approach to Interpretation*. PA: W.B. Saunders Co., 3rd edition, 1997.

Foster, Steven. *Herbal Renaissance*. UT: Gibb Smith Publisher, Revised edition, 1993.

Foster, Steven, and Yue Chongxi. *Herbal Emissaries: Bringing Chinese Herbs to the West*. VT: Healing Art Press, 1992.

Fratkin, Jake. *Chinese Herbal Patent Formulas —A Practical Guide*. CO: Shya Publications, 1985.

Gaeddert, Andrew. *Chinese Herbs in the Western Clinic*. CA: Get Well Foundation, 1998.

Gladstar, Rosemary. *Herbal Healing for Women*. NY: Fireside Simon and Schuster Inc., 1993.

Glasby, John. *Dictionary of Plants Containing Secondary Metabolites*. PA: Taylor and Francis Inc., 1991.

Grauer, Ken. *A Practical Guide to ECG Interpretation*. Year Book Medical Pub., 2nd edition, 1998.

Griffin, LaDean. *Please Doctor, I'd Rather Do It Myself . . . With Herbs!* UT: Hawkes Publishing, Inc., 1979.

Gurudas. *Flower Essences and Vibrational Healing*. CA: Cassandra Press, 2nd edition, 1989.

Harborn, Jeffrey, and Herbert Baxter, editors. *Phytochemical Dictionary: A Handbook of Bioactive Compounds from Plants*. PA: Taylor and Francis, 2nd edition, 1999.

Heinerman, John. *Medical Doctor's Guide to Herbs*. UT: Woodland Publishing, 1987.

Hey, Barbara. *The Illustrated Guide to Herbs*. NJ: New Horizon Press.

Hobbs, Christopher. *Ginkgo: Elixir of Youth*. CA: Botanica Press, 1990.

Hobbs, Christopher. *Handbook for Herbal Healing*. Culinary Arts Ltd., 1994.

Hobbs, Christopher. *Milk Thistle—The Liver Herb*. CA: Botanica Press, 2nd edition, 1993.

Hoffmann, David. *The New Holistic Herbal*. MA: Element Book Ltd., 3rd edition, 1991.

Holmes, Peter. *Jade Remedies: A Chinese Herbal Reference for the West (Volume 1)*. CO: Snow Lotus Press, Inc., 1997.

Horowitz, Leonard G. *Emerging Viruses, AIDS & Ebola, Nature, Accident or Intentional?* MA: Tetrahedron, Inc., 1998.

Hotema, Hilton. *Long Life in Florida*. Health Research, Reprint edition, 1962.

Hunt, Ronald. *The Seven Keys to Color Healing*. NY: HarperCollins, 1989.

Jensen, Bernard. *Beyond Basic Health*. CA: Bernard Jensen, 1988.

Jensen, Bernard. *Developing a New Heart Through Nutrition and a New Lifestyle*. CA: Bernard Jensen, 1995.

Jensen, Bernard. *Doctor-Patient Handbook*. CA: Bernard Jensen Enterprises, 1978.

Jensen, Bernard. *Goat Milk Magic*. CA: Bernard Jensen, 1994.

Jensen, Bernard. *Herbs: Wonder Healers*. CA: Bernard Jensen, 1992.

Jensen, Bernard. *Iridology: The Science and Practice in the Healing Arts (Volume II)*. CA: Bernard Jensen Enterprises, 1982.

Jensen, Bernard. *Iridology Simplified*. CA: Bernard Jensen, 1980.

Jensen, Bernard. *What is Iridology?* Illustrated. CA: Bernard Jensen, 1984.

Katz, Michael and Ginny. *Gifts of the Gemstone Masters*. OR: Gemisphere, 1989.

Keville, Kathi. *Herbs for Health and Healing*. PA: Rodale Press, Inc., 1996.

Kloss, Jethro. *Back to Eden*. Benedict Lust Publications, Inc., 1981.

Kroeger, Hanna. *Parasites—The Enemy Within*. CO: Hanna Kroger, 1991.

Kulvinskas, Viktoras. *Life in the 21st Century*. IA: 21st Century Publications, 1981.

Kulvinskas, Viktoras. *Love Your Body or How To Be A Live Food Love*. IA: 21st Century Publications, 1972.

Kulvinskas, Victoras. *Survival Into the 21st Century*. IA: 21st Century Publications, 1975.

L'Orange, Darlena. *Herbal Healing Secrets of the Orient*. NJ: Prentice Hall, 1998.

Liberman, Jacob. *Light—Medicine of the Future*. NM: Bear and Company, 1992.

Lopez, D.A., R.M. Williams and M. Miehike. *Enzymes—The Fountain of Life*. Germany: The Neville Press, Inc., 1994.

Lu, Henry. *Chinese System of Food Cures—Prevention and Remedies*. NY: Sterling Publishing Co., Inc., 1986.

Mauseth, James. *Botany: An Introduction to Plant Biology*. MA: Jones & Barlett Pub., 3rd edition, 2003.

McBean, Eleanor. *The Poisoned Needle*. Health Research, Reprint edition, 1993.

McDaniel, T.C. *Disease Reprieve*. PA: Xlibris Corporation, 1st edition, 1999.

Meyer, Clarence. *The Herbalist*. IL: Meyer-books, 1986.

Miller, Neil Z. *Vaccines: Are They Really Safe and Effective? (A Parents Guide to Childhood Shots)*. NM: New Atlantean Press, Revised and updated edition, 2002.

Monte, Tom. *World Medicine—The East /West Guide to Healing Your Body*. NY: G.P. Putnam's Sons, 1993.

Murray, Michael. *Natural Alternatives for Weight Loss*. NY: William Morrow and Company, Inc., 1996.

Meyer, Joseph. *The Old Herb Doctor*. IL: Meyerbooks, 2nd edition, 1984.

Naturopathic Handbook of Herbal Formulas: A Practical and Concise Herb User's Guide. CO: Kivaki Press, 3rd edition, 1994.

Olsen, Cynthia. *Australian Tea Tree Oil Guide*. WI: Lotus Press, 3rd edition, 1998.

Parachin, Victor. *365 Good Reasons To Be A Vegetarian*. NY: Avery Penguin Putnam, 1997.

PDR for Herbal Medicines. NJ: Medical Economics Co., 2nd edition, 2000.

Pedersen, Mark. *Nutritional Herbology: A Reference Guide to Herbs*. IN: Wendell W. Whitman Co., 3rd edition, 1998.

Pizzorno, Joseph. *Total Wellness*. CA: Prima Publishing, 1996.

Rector, Linda. *Renewing Female Balance*. CA: Healthy Healing Publications, Inc., 4th edition. 1997.

Rector, Linda. *Renewing Male Health and Energy*. CA: Healthy Healing Publications, Inc., 2nd edition, 1997.

Royal, Penny. *Herbally Yours*. UT: Sound Nutrition, 3rd edition, 1982.

Sandman, Amanda. *A-Z of Natural Remedies*. NY: Longmeadow Press, 1995.

Sanecki, Kay. *The Book of Herbs*. NJ: Quantum Books Ltd., 1996.

Santillo, Humbart. *Food Enzymes: The Missing Link to Radiant Health*. AZ: Hohm Press; 2nd edition, 1993.

Santillo, Humbart. *Natural Healing with Herbs*. AZ: Hohm Press, 1991.

Scalzo, Richard. *Naturpathic Handbook of Herbal Formulas—A Practical and Concise Herb User's Guide*. CO: Kivaki Press, 3rd edition, 1994.

Schauenberg, Paul. and Paris, Ferdinand. *Guide to Medicinal Plants*. CT: Keats Publishing, Inc., Reprint edition, 1990.

Shelton, Herbert. *Food Combining Made Easy*. Ontario: Willow Publishing, 1982.

Swahn, J.O. *The Lore of Spices*. MN: Stoeger Publishing Company, 2002.

Tenny, Louise. *Today's Herbal Health*. UT: Woodland Publishing, 5th edition, 2000.

Thie, John. *Touch for Health*. CA: Devorss and Co., Publishers, 1979.

Thomas, Lalitha. *10 Essential Herbs*. AZ: Hohm Press, 2nd edition, 1995.

Tierra, Michael. *Planetary Herbology*. WI: Lotus Press, 1987.

Tierra, Michael. *The Way of Herbs*. NY: Pocket Books; Revised edition, 1998.

Tilden, John. *Toxemia: The Basic Cause of Disease*. FL: Nat'l Health Assoc, 1974.

Tompkins, Peter and Christopher Bird. *The Secret Life of Plants*. NY: HarperCollins, 1989.

Twitchell, Paul. *Herbs the Magic Healer.* CA: Eckankar, 1971.

Walker, Norman. *Colon Health: The Key to a Vibrant Life*. TN: Associated Publishers Group, 2nd edition, 1997.

Walker, Norman. *Water Can Undermine Your Health*. AZ: Norwalk Press, 1996.

Walker, N.W. *Become Younger.* AZ: Norwalk Press, 2nd edition, 1995.

Walker, N.W. *The Vegetarian Guide to Diet and Salad*. Longman Trade/Caroline House, Revised edition, 1995.

Walker, N.W. *Fresh Vegetable and Fruit Juices: What's Missing in Your Body?* Longman Trade/Caroline House, 1995.

Walker, N.W. *Pure and Simple: Natural Weight Control*. AZ: Norwalk Press, 1981.

Walker, N.W. *The Natural Way to Vibrant Health*. Longman Trade/Caroline House, 1995.

Weiss, Rudolf Fritz. *Herbal Medicine*. NY: Thieme Medical Pub., 2nd edition, 2001.

Werbach, Melvyn and Michael Murray. *Botanical Influences on Illness—A Sourcebook of Clinical Research*. CA: Third Line Press, 2nd edition, 2000.

Wigmore, Ann. *The Hippocrates Diet and Health Program*. NJ: Avery Penguin Putnam, 1984.

Wigmore, Ann. *The Wheatgrass Book*. NJ: Avery Penguin Putnam, 1984.

Wolfe, David. *The Sunfood Diet Success System*. CA: Maul Brother's Publishing, 3rd edition, 2000.

Books about raw food eating are available at:
Nature's First Law
1475 North Cuyamaca Street
El Cajon, CA 92020
www.naturesfirstlaw.com
1-800-205-2350

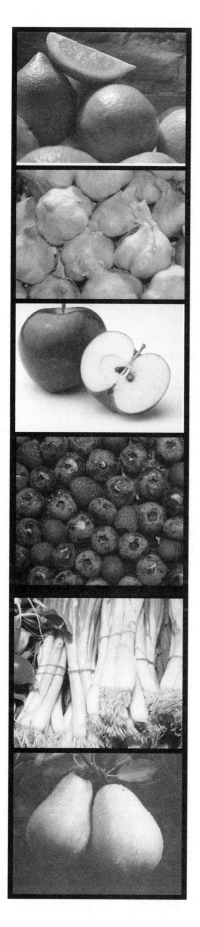

Index

B

B-cell response, 35–36
B-cells, 38
bacilli, 147
bacteria, 146, 149
 types of, 146–47
Banana Ice Cream, 230
bananas, 105
Basal Temperature Study, 6, 292
Basal Temperature Test, 44
basil oil, 295
basophils, 38, 326
baths, steam, 278–79
beans, 226–27
bearberry, 253
benzene, 131
benzyl/benzoic, 128
bergamot oil, 295
berries, 214. *See also* fruit
beryllium (B), 85
beta cells, 47
BHA/BHT (butylated hydroxyani-
 sole), 128
bilberry, 237
bile, 28
bile salts, 70
bilirubin, 325
bioelectromagnetics, 293–94
bioflavonoids, 77
biological transmutation, 105
biotin, 77
birch oil, 295
bitter principles, 97
black cohosh, 237–38
black current seed oil, 70
black walnut hull, 238, 274
bladder, 41–42, 172, 179
 herbal formula for, 260–61
blood, 177
 herbal formula for, 257
blood analysis, 321–22
 shortcomings, 330
blood pressure, 6–7, 45, 151, 198,
 201
 herbal formula for, 258
blood serum composition, 23
blood test(s)
 how to interpret, 322, 324–29
 sample, 323
blood typing, 322
body care products, natural, 312
body fuels, 161
body language, 169–73

body systems, structures and functions of, 15–17
bone cells, 58
bone marrow, 59
bone structures, 59
bones
 growth and repair, 59–60
 terminology, 59
 types of, 58–59
books, in Resouce Guide, 306
borage oil, 70
boron (B), 85–86
bovine growth hormone (rBGH),
 112
bowel formulas, herbal, 209–10,
 262–63
bowel management, healthy,
 208–9
bowels, 208
 ways to cleanse, 209–11
brain, herbal formula for, 257
brain tissue, regeneration of, 104
breatharianism, 3–4, 12
breathing, deep, 277–78
bronchi, 57
bronchioles, 57
bronchitis, 185
bugleweed, 238
BUN (blood urea nitrogen), 324
burdock, 238
butcher's broom, 238–39

C

cadmium (Cd), 86
caffeine, 119, 129
calcium (Ca), 79–80, 111, 324
 ionized, 324
 utilization, 103, 111
cancellous bone, 59
cancer, 111, 153–55, 188
 causes, 123, 153–55
 detox for prevention and
  cure, 155–57, 200–201,
  205, 207
 pancreatic, 200–201, 205
 tumor markers, 321
cancer patients, 103, 104, 106
 family support, 156
Candida, 145
capillaries, 22
caramel, 129
carbohydrates, 13. *See also* starches; sugar(s)

digestive and metabolic
  by-products, 66
 metabolism, 65
carbon (C), 80
carbon dioxide, 63, 324
carbonic acid, 63
carbonic anhydrase, 23
cardiac muscles, 53
cardiovascular system, 21–24, 178.
 See also circulatory system; heart
 herbal rejuvenation for, 264–65
carnivores, 9
carrageenan, 129
Carrot/Squash Soup, 231
cascara sagrada, 239
castor oil packs, 282–83
catabolic breakdown, 46, 72, 102
catalysts, 100–102
cationic reaction, 99
cations, 102
Cauliflower Soup, 230
cayenne pepper (capsicum), 119,
 239
cell division, types of, 20
cell salts, 93
 basic, 93–95
cell wall membrane, 18
cells, 18–20, 139
 how nutrients enter, 19–20
cellulose, 66, 73, 129
central nervous system (CNS), 55
cervix, 56
chamomile oil, 295
chaparral, 239–40
chemical medicines, 1, 6. *See also*
 medications
chemical toxicity, 125–32. *See also*
 toxicity
chemicals, toxic, 125–26, 131–32
 everyday, 126
 protecting yourself from, 133–34
 sources of information
  about, 128
 top 20 hazardous
  substances, 126
 types of, 125–32
children's products, 306
Chinese herbs, 310
chiropractic, 297
chlorine/chloride (Cl), 80, 129, 324
 of potash, 93
 of soda, 93
chocolate, 119
cholecystokinin, 25, 26, 28

enteritis, 192
enzymes, 19, 25, 67, 70, 72–74, 159
  exogenous, 73–74
  inactive, 73
  systemic, 72
eosinophils, 23, 38, 326
epidermis, 42
epithelial tissue, 21
erythrocytes, 22–23
essential oils, 97, 294–97
estrogen, 48, 152
eucalyptus oil, 295
evening primrose oil, 70
excessive thinness, 163–65A
excretion. See elimination
exercise, 277
expectoration, 195

F

fallopian tubes, 56
false unicorn (helonias), 242
family support, 156
fasts/fasting, 204
  how to "break," 206
  preparation before, 205
  types of
    all fruit, 204
    all raw-food, 204
    juice, 205, 207
    water, 188, 205
  when to "break," 205–6
fatigue, 196–97
fats (lipids), 13, 14, 68, 150, 151
  composition, 68
  digestive and metabolic by-products, 71
  metabolism, 69–71
  sources, 69–70
  types of, 68–69
fatty acids, 68
  essential, 69, 70
fennel oil, 295
fenugreek, 242
fevers, 166, 194, 202
fiber, 224
Fisher, Barbara Loe, 122
flavones, 97
flax seed oil, 70
flora, intestinal, 112
flower essences, 301, 306
flu vaccine, 121
fluorine/fluoride (F), 87, 131
  of lime, 93

folic acid, 76
food additives, 127. See also specific additives
food combining, 217–19
food contaminants, 127
food processing, commercial, 79
food(s)
  alkaline and acid forming, 215–16. See also pH factors, of foods
  colors of, 300
  consciousness and, 103–5
  electromagnetic energy of various, 104, 158
  energy of, 103–5
  how much and how often, 221
  which to eat, 214
  whole, living, 106–8
formed elements, 22, 23
fragrances, artificial, 131
frankincense oil, 295
Frozen Bananas, 230
frozen foods, 105
fructose, 64–66, 330
frugivores, 8, 10
fruit, 104, 187–88
  alkaline and acid forming, 216
  food combining and, 218, 219
  washing, 133
  which to eat, 214
fruit diet, 157–58, 188, 200
fruit juices, 222–25
fruit salad, 229
fruitarianism, 4
fundus, 56
fungus, 145, 149

G

galactose, 66
galbaunum oil, 295
gallbladder, 28, 171, 177
gallbladder flush, 280–81
gamma globulins, 37
garlic, 242–43
gastric juices, 70
gastritis, 192
gastrointestinal (GI) disorders, 192
gastrointestinal (GI) tract, 171, 177, 208, 212
  and diabetes, 162
gem stone therapy, 301–2
gentian, 243
geranium oil, 295
ginger, 243

ginger oil, 295
ginkgo biloba, 243–44
glands, 50–52. See also specific glands
  emotions and, 168–69
  endocrine and exocrine, 43
  language of the, 170–73
glandular system, 17, 49, 164–65A
  herbal rejuvenation for, 265–66
glandular weaknesses, 6
glandulars, 313
Glisson's capsule, 27
glucose, 27, 63, 64, 66, 322
glucose/fructose utilization, 330
glycerol, 70
glycogen, 27
glycoproteins, 36
glycosides, 97
"God eaters," 4
goldenseal, 244
Golgi apparatus, 18
gotu kola, 244–45
grains, 164, 226
grape juice, 225
grape juice fast, 207
grapefruit oil, 295
"green foods." See super-foods
green products, 308
growth hormone, bovine, 112
guacamole, 229
Gulf War Syndrome, 122, 146
gums, 129

H

hair analysis, 331
hawthorn berry, 245
HCT (hematocrit), 327
healing, 20
"healing crisis," 7, 185, 191, 192, 197–99
  cases of cleansing, 200–201
  cleansing effects
    mild, 199
    moderate, 199–200
    strong, 199–200
  end results of cleansing process, 201–2
  smart cleansing, 202–3
  what to avoid during, 202
Health Questionnaire, 174–81
healthy habits, 276–79
heart, 21–22, 172–73, 178. See also cardiovascular system
  herbal formula for, 260
heart center, open vs. closed, 168

oxidation, 101–2
oxygen (O), 81

P

PABA (para-amino benzoic acid), 78
pancreas, 25–26, 47, 165A, 171, 176
role of, 159–61
pancreatic enzymes, 67
pancreatic juice, 26
pancreozymin. *See* cholecystokinin
pangamic acid, 76
paralysis. *See* spinal cord injuries
parasite elimination, 6, 233, 262, 271
parasites, 111, 142, 144–45. *See also specific types of microorganisms*
most common, 149
parasympathetic nervous system, 55, 56
parathyroid gland, 44–45, 111, 161, 165A, 170, 174–75
parsley, 249
patchouly oil, 296
pau d'arco, 249
PEG (polyethylene glycol), 130
peppermint oil, 296
pepsin, 73
pepsinogen, 73
peptidase, 25, 73
peptide, 25
peptones, 24
pesticides, 127, 128, 202. *See also* organic food
petrochemicals, 127
pH, 101, 102, 184, 294. *See also* acidosis; alkaline/acid balance
and cancer, 155
cooking and, 110
digestion and, 13
hormones and, 47
and nerve damage and regeneration, 158
protein consumption and, 114, 116
testing, 150
and utilization, 14
pH factors, 141
of foods, 99–100, 106, 141, 150, 187–91, 215–16
phagocytosis, 33
pharynx, 58
phenols, 97

phosphate
of iron, 93–94
of lime, 94
of magnesia, 94
of potash, 94
of soda, 94
phosphorus (P), 81–82
phytochemicals, 95–98
pineal gland, 44
pipsissewa, 249
pituitary gland, 43–44, 161, 165A
plantain, 249–50
plants, 133
plasma, 22, 23
plasma membrane, 18
plastics, 132
platelets, 328
Poison Control Centers, 134–37
poison ivy, 197
poke root (pokeweed), 250
polarity therapy, 303–4
polio vaccine, 121, 154
pollution, 84
polysaccharides, 65–66
potash
chloride of, 93
phosphate of, 94
sulphate of, 94
potassium (K), 82, 322, 324
potential energy, 61
pro-enzymes, 73
progesterone, 48, 152
propylene glycol, 130
propylgallate, 130
prostaglandins, 34
prostate gland, 56
protease, 67, 73. *See also* proteus
proteids and non-proteids, 113
protein(s), 13, 67, 113. *See also* high protein diets
complete, 118
digestion, 67, 114. *See also* protease; proteus
digestive and metabolic by-products, 67
food combining and, 219
total, 325
usability, 114–16, 163–64
proteus, 147
protozoa, 149
PSA (prostate-specific antigen), 321
ptyalin, 73

R

radiation, 1–2, 131, 294
Rainbow Fruit Salad, 229
Raw Dressing, 229
raw food diet, 5, 106, 157–58
raw food resource centers, 316–17
raw food resources, 313–16
raw foods, 62
RDW (red blood cell distribution width), 328
recipes, 228–31
red blood cells (RBCs), 22–23, 327
red clover, 250
red dye #40 (Allura Red AC), 130
red pepper. *See* cayenne pepper
red raspberry, 250–51
reflexology, 279, 303
regeneration, 182
components of, 183
reishi mushroom, 251
Relish, 228
reproductive system, 17, 56–57, 151–52
herbal formulas for, 258–60
herbal rejuvenation for, 269
respiratory system, 17, 57–58, 173, 179–80. *See also* lungs
herbal rejuvenation for, 269–70
ribosomes, 18
rice, brown, 231
RNA (ribose), 66
rose oil, 296
rosemary oil, 296
rosewood oil, 296

S

saccharin, 131
sage oil, 296
salad, 228
salivary glands, 24
salts, 98
sandalwood oil, 296
sandwich, veggie, 229
saponins, 98
saturated fats, 68
saunas, 278–79
saw palmetto, 251
Schroeder, Henry, 84
secretin, 25, 26
secretory vesicles, 18–19
seeds, 104, 214
selenium (Se), 91
self-antigens, 35

senna, 252

shavegrass, 245–46

shiitake mushroom, 252

Short-Grain Whole Brown Rice, 231

Siberian ginseng, 252

silica/silicon (Si), 91–92

silicic acid, 94

simian virus number 40 (Sim-40/ SV 40 virus), 123, 154

skeletal system, 17, 58–60
   herbal rejuvenation for, 270

skin, 166, 173, 178. *See also* integumentary system
   disorders, 166–67, 173, 178
   elimination and detoxification, 166, 167
   moisturizers, 166–67

skin brushing, dry, 278

skullcap, 251–52

slant boarding, 279

slippery elm, 252

Smoothies, 230

soaps, natural, 312

soda, 119
   chloride of, 93
   phosphate of, 94
   sulphate of, 95

sodium (Na), 82–83, 322

sodium bicarbonate, 26, 73

sodium erythorbate, 131

sodium fluoride, 131

sodium laureth/lauryl sulfate (SLES/SLS), 131

solvents, 125

soups, 230, 231

soy beans
   cooked and processed, 227
   properties of raw, 227

soy myth, the, 227–28

soy protein and soy bean oil, processes used in obtaining, 227–28

spearmint oil, 296–97

spinal cord injuries, regeneration in, 2, 106, 143, 157, 201. *See also* nerve tissue

spirilla, 147

spiritual perspective, 146

spirituality, health and, 285–89. *See also* energy

spirochetes, 147

spleen, 31

sprouts and sprouting, 226, 317

spruce oil, 297

squash soup, 231

St. John's wort, 251

staphylococci, 146–47

starches, 66, 164
   food combining and, 219
   modified food starch, 130

steam baths, 278–79

Steamed Veggies, 231

stem cells, 23

steroids, 150

stimulants, 119–20

stinging nettles, 248

Stir-Fried Veggies, 231

stomach, 24–25
   herbal formula for, 262–63
   streptobacilli, 147
   stress, 84

sucrase, 25

sucrose, 66

sugar(s), 63–65, 161
   complex, 65–66, 164
   refined, 31, 120
   simple, 63, 164

sulfur (S), 83, 272

sulphate
   of lime, 94
   of potash, 94
   of soda, 95

sunlight, 279

super-foods, 143

surgery, 2

sweeteners, artificial, 64

swelling, 197

sympathetic nervous system, 55–56

T

T-cells, 38

talc, 131

tannins (tannic acid), 98, 131

tarragon oil, 297

tea tree oil (melalenca), 297

TEA (triethanolamine), 129

teas, 119
   herbal, 319
     making, 235

tendons, 53

terpenoids, 98

testes/testicles (gonads), 48–49

testosterone, 48–49

thermotherapy. *See* fevers

thoracic duct, 30

thrombocytes, 328

thyme oil, 297

thymus gland, 32, 45

thyroid, 44–45, 111, 161
   functioning, 6, 44, 111, 164–65A, 170, 174–75, 197, 226
   herbal formula for, 263–64

thyroid profile panels, 329–30

tin (Sn), 92

tissue mineral analysis (TMA), 331

tissue salts. *See* cell salts

tissues, types of, 21

titration, 215

toluene, 131

tongue examination, 206

tonics, herbal, 271

toxicity, 140, 162. *See also* chemical toxicity

toxins, physical, 126. *See also* chemicals, toxic

trachea (windpipe), 58

TRH (thyrotropin-releasing hormone), 329

triglycerides (TG), 329

trypsin, 73

trypsinogen, 26

TSH (thyroid-stimulating hormone), 329

tumor markers, 321

turmeric, 253

U

underweight persons, 165

unsaturated fats, 68

ureters, 41

urethra, 42

uric acid, 114

urinary (tract) system, 16, 41–42, 172
   herbal rejuvenation for, 270

urine, 41

uterus, 56–57

utilization, 14

uva ursi, 253

V

vaccination facts, 154

vaccinations, harmful effects of, 121–24, 146, 154

valerian, 253

vanadium (V), 92

vascular system, 22

vegetable juice combinations, 225

vegetable juices, 222–25

Vegetable Soup, 230
vegetables, 104, 157–58, 231
    alkaline and acid forming, 216
    food combining and, 219
    washing, 133
    which to eat, 214
Veggie Sandwich, 229
veins, 22
ventricles, 21
venules, 22
vessels, 22
vibrational therapies, 304
vibrios, 147
video sources, 306
villi, 25
vinyls, 132
viruses, 145–46, 196, 272
    in catalyst for immune response,
    145

vitamins, 74–77
vomiting, 193
    what to do for, 193–94

W

Walker, Norman W., 206
water
    contaminants, 127
    purified, 132, 134, 281–82
water systems, 319–20
water therapy, 302–3, 320
weight gain. *See also* obesity
    emotional components, 165-65A
weight loss. *See* excessive thinness
white blood cells (WBCs), 23,
    38–39, 326–27
white lotus oil, 297
white oak bark, 254

white pond lily, 253–54
wild tansy oil, 297
wood betony, 254
worms, 147–49
wormwood, 254–55

Y

yeast, 145
yellow dock, 255
yucca, 255

Z

zinc (Zn), 92–93

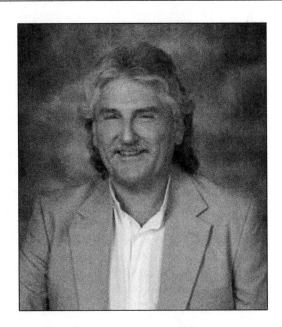

About the Author

Robert S. Morse, N.D., D.Sc., I.D., M.H., is a board certified and accredited Naturopathic physician, a biochemist, iridologist, and a master herbalist. In his forty years of practice, his groundbreaking work has helped thousands overcome cancer, diabetes, M.S., Crohn's Disease, Scleroderma, and other serious illnesses. Dr. Morse was a personal friend of the late Dr. Bernard Jensen, the "Father of the science of Iridology" in the United States, and a great advocate of living foods. Dr. Jensen referred to Dr. Morse as "one of the world's greatest healers."

Robert Morse is a member of The International Association of Naprapathic Physicians and the American Naturopathic Medical Association. He is an Honorary Member of (ASPEMT) Associacao Profissional dos Especialistas da Medicina Tradicional (Portugal). In 1998 he was given an Honorary Degree from the Medical Association of Portugal for his professional work in Tissue Regeneration.

Since 1974, he has owned and operated a Natural Health Clinic, God's Herbs, and Nature's Botanical Pharmacy located in Port Charlotte, Florida. Dr. Morse teaches physicians, healthcare practitioners and other healers the Art of Detoxification and Cellular Regeneration through his International School of Detoxification. Over 500 people have graduated from his International School. He has a passion for education and teaches the general public weekly through his YouTube video channel, 'robertmorsend'. He started the channel in 2011 to help the world get well and has already had over 1,300,000 views of his videos.

Thirty-five years ago, Dr. Morse created extra strong, tissue specific, botanical formulas for his rejuvenation clinic. These formulas have received worldwide acclaim and are used by physicians, clinics, and individuals throughout the world. He lives in Port Charlotte, Florida.

His website is www.drmorsesherbalhealthclub.com.